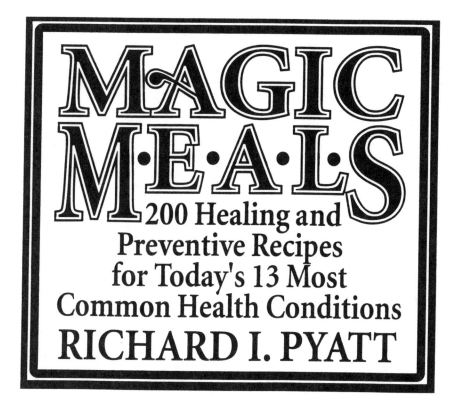

MAGIC MEALS

200 Healing and Preventive Recipes for Today's 13 Most Common Health Conditions

RICHARD I. PYATT

PARKER PUBLISHING COMPANY
West Nyack, New York 10995

10 9 8 7 6 5 4 3 2

Library of Congress Cataloging-in-Publication Data

Pyatt, Richard I.,
    Magic meals : 200 healing and preventive recipes for today's 13
most common health conditions / Richard Pyatt.
        p.   cm.
    Includes bibliographical references and index.
    ISBN 0-13-554676-1 (paper). — ISBN 0-13-554684-2 (case)
    1. Diet therapy. 2. Nutrition. 3. Medicine, Preventive.
I. Title.
RM219.P93 1993
    615.8′54—dc20
                                                            92-21198
                                                            CIP

ISBN 0-13-554684-2 (case)
ISBN 0-13-554676-1 (pbk.)

Parker Publishing Company
Career & Personal Development
West Nyack, NY 10995
Simon & Schuster, A Paramount Communications Company

Printed in the United States of America

ABOUT THE AUTHOR

Richard I. Pyatt began his media writing career when he became a radio writer-announcer and a writer-director-producer in the field of radio and television in New York.

While working in media in New York, Pyatt initiated radio and television courses at Pace University in New York City where he taught speech communication. He subsequently taught radio and television writing courses at various colleges and is currently associate professor in radio/television at Iona College in Yonkers, New York.

Pyatt spent more than 15 years at WNYC-AM, FM, and TV in New York City as staff announcer, writer, producer, assistant program manager, and director of programming. An accomplished writer and investigative broadcast journalist, he is a recipient of the Associated Press Award for writing and producing the most outstanding investigative radio series on drug addiction. His radio program "Healthline" has been recognized by the Public Health Association, which honored him with its Merit Award for the best series on health.

Well known in broadcast and print media, Pyatt has been heard on WOR, WFAS, and WNBC radio, and his writing appears in *USA Today*, the *Daily News*, the Gannett Westchester chain, and numerous magazines.

Pyatt has received grants from the Corporation of Public Broadcasting, National Public Radio, the British Information Service, and Oxford University Publishing to write, produce, and host radio documentaries and drama.

Pyatt earned a B.A. degree from New York University of New York City and an M.S. degree in communication from New York University and has done graduate work in literature at Pace University. He has published three books on health and related subjects. He is a member of the Authors Guild and the Authors League of America, the American Medical Writer's Association, the New York Press Club, and the Broadcast Education Association.

He is currently the host of "Meet Your Health Professional," a cable television program distributed throughout New York City, Westchester County, and the cable network of New Jersey with an audience of over one and a half million viewers.

OTHER BOOKS BY THE AUTHOR

Medical Breakthroughs from the NIH

The People's Medical Answer Book: Plain Answers to One Thousand One Hundred Common Questions from Thirty-Six Leading Specialists

CONTENTS

Introduction   **xxiii**

   200 Recipes   xxiii
   Easy-To-Read Nutritional Charts   xxiii
   Instant USRDA Percentages Column   xxiv
   Quick and Easy Cookbook   xxiv
   U.S. Recommended Dietary Allowance Charts   xxiv
   Food Chart Ranking Highest Amount of Vitamins   xxv
   Tips and Myths   xxv
   Primer on Fats, USRDAs, Meat, Amino Acids   xxvi
   How to Read the Nutritional Chart   xxvi

Chapter One   Healing and Preventive Recipes for Cancer   **1**

   Simple Cabbage Soup   4
   Nutrients Contained in: Simple Cabbage Soup   5

   Dynamic Cabbage and Potatoes   6
   Nutrients Contained in: Dynamic Cabbage and Potatoes   7

   Red Peppers with Pasta Sauce   8
   Nutrients Contained in: Red Peppers with Pasta Sauce   9

   Be All That You Can Beet Soup   10
   Nutrients Contained in: Be All That You Can Beet Soup   11

   Magical Broccoli with Pepper and Onion   12
   Nutrients Contained in: Magical Broccoli with Pepper and Onion   13

   Double Orange Sweet Potato   14
   Nutrients Contained in: Double Orange Sweet Potato   15

   Kale Delight   16
   Nutrients Contained in: Kale Delight   17

   Asparagus with Sweet Red Peppers   18
   Nutrients Contained in: Asparagus with Sweet Red Peppers   19

   Asparagus, Carrots, and Celery   20
   Nutrients Contained in: Asparagus, Carrots, and Celery   21

   Steamed Green Cabbage   22
   Nutrients Contained in: Steamed Green Cabbage   23

Cauliflower with Curry and Spices   24

Nutrients Contained in: Cauliflower with Curry and Spices   25

Brussels Sprouts with Onions and Spices   26

Nutrients Contained in: Brussels Sprouts with Onions and Spices   27

Chapter Two   Healing and Preventive Recipes for Stroke   29

Spaghetti, Potato, and Onion Round   32

Nutrients Contained in: Spaghetti, Potato, and Onion Round   33

A Different Cabbage and Pork   34

Nutrients Contained in: A Different Cabbage and Pork   35

Pork and Prunes   36

Nutrients Contained in: Pork and Prunes   37

Turkey Breast, Wheat Germ, and Shiitake   38

Nutrients Contained in: Turkey Breast, Wheat Germ, and Shiitake   39

Black Fungus Lima Bean Soup   40

Nutrients Contained in: Black Fungus Lima Bean Soup   41

Spear and Oval Salad   42

Nutrients Contained in: Spear and Oval Salad   43

Open Sesame Turkey   44

Nutrients Contained in: Open Sesame Turkey   45

A Bean Bake   46

Nutrients Contained in: A Bean Bake   47

Kidney Beans, Barley, and Wheat   48

Nutrients Contained in: Kidney, Barley, and Wheat   49

Celery, Pepper, and Lentil Refreshment   50

Nutrients Contained in: Celery, Pepper, and Lentil Refreshment   51

On Guard with Swordfish   52

Nutrients Contained in: On Guard with Swordfish   53

Spaghetti, Asparagus, and Beetgreens with Almonds   54

Nutrients Contained in: Spaghetti, Asparagus, and Beetgreens with Almonds   55

Peas, Potatoes, and Tomatoes   56

Nutrients Contained in: Peas, Potatoes, and Tomatoes   57

Stir-Fry Tofu and Beans   58

Nutrients Contained in: Stir-Fry Tofu and Beans   59

Double-Flavor Onion and Garlic   60

Nutrients Contained in: Double-Flavor Onion and Garlic   61

Chapter Three Healing and Preventive Recipes for High Blood Pressure   63

Blackeyes   66
Nutrients Contained in: Blackeyes   67

Reliable Broccoli   68
Nutrients Contained in: Reliable Broccoli   69

Favorite Fava Beans   70
Nutrients Contained in: Favorite Fava Beans   71

Garlic and Pork Combine   72
Nutrients Contained in: Garlic and Pork Combine   73

Rice, Garlic, Carrots, and Curry   74
Nutrients Contained in: Rice, Garlic, Carrots, and Curry   75

Asparagus with Shiitake Mushrooms   76
Nutrients Contained in: Asparagus with Shiitake Mushrooms   77

Spicy Curried Rice   78
Nutrients Contained in: Spicy Curried Rice   79

Quick Beans and Spinach   80
Nutrients Contained in: Quick Beans and Spinach   81

Lentil Mushroom Powerhouse   82
Nutrients Contained in: Lentil Mushroom Powerhouse   83

Barley and Mushroom Casserole   84
Nutrients Contained in: Barley and Mushroom Casserole   85

Simple Lentils with Garlic   86
Nutrients Contained in: Simple Lentils with Garlic   87

Garlic Straight   88
Nutrients Contained in: Garlic Straight   89

Rice and Greenery   90
Nutrients Contained in: Rice and Greenery   91

Garlic and Trout   92
Nutrients Contained in: Garlic and Trout   93

Miracle Chicken Livers   94
Nutrients Contained in: Miracle Chicken Livers   95

Chapter Four Healing and Preventive Recipes for Heart Disease   97

Minced and Mashed Chicken with Bean Curd   100
Nutrients Contained in: Minced and Mashed Chicken with Bean Curd   101

Broiled Mackerel   102

Nutrients Contained in: Broiled Mackerel   103

Potato, Pepper, and Onion Gathering   104

Nutrients Contained in: Potato, Pepper, and Onion Gathering   105

Kerstin's Tomato Spinach   106

Nutrients Contained in: Kerstin's Tomato Spinach   107

Sweet Potato Smoothie   108

Nutrients Contained in: Sweet Potato Smoothie   109

Steamy Greens   110

Nutrients Contained in: Steamy Greens   111

Lemon, Lettuce, and Chicken Breasts   ·   112

Nutrients Contained in: Lemon, Lettuce, and Chicken Breasts   113

Tore's Turnips   114

Nutrients Contained in: Tore's Turnips   115

Stir-Fry Tofu with Asparagus   116

Nutrients Contained in: Stir-Fry Tofu with Asparagus   117

Pearly Barley with Okra, Zucchini, and Tomatoes   118

Nutrients Contained in: Pearly Barley with Okra, Zucchini, and Tomatoes   119

Tuna Stuffed Tomatoes   120

Nutrients Contained in: Tuna Stuffed Tomatoes   121

Stir-Fry Variation with Zucchini, Carrots, and Leeks   122

Nutrients Contained in: Stir-Fry Variation with Zucchini, Carrots, and Leeks   123

Heart-Rending Potatoes, Tomatoes, and Peas   124

Nutrients Contained in: Heart-Rending Potatoes, Tomatoes, and Peas   125

Turnip, Carrot, and Squash Free-for-All   126

Nutrients Contained in: Turnip, Carrot, and Squash Free-for-All   127

Salmon Steaks   128

Nutrients Contained in: Salmon Steaks   129

Bean Insurance   130

Nutrients Contained in: Bean Insurance   131

Sweet Sweet Potatoes   132

Nutrients Contained in: Sweet Sweet Potatoes   133

Chapter Five   Healing and Preventive Recipes for Diabetes   135

Barley, Okra, and Mushroom Salad   138

Nutrients Contained in: Barley, Okra, and Mushroom Salad   139

Tofu and Friends   140

Nutrients Contained in: Tofu and Friends   141

Kidney Beans with a Flair   142

Nutrients Contained in: Kidney Beans with a Flair   143

Six Who Passed While the Lentils Boiled   144

Nutrients Contained in: Six Who Passed While the Lentils Boiled   145

Soybean Strength   146

Nutrients Contained in: Soybean Strength   147

Oysters Non-Rockefeller   148

Nutrients Contained in: Oysters Non-Rockefeller   149

Okra and Cauliflower with Your Macaroni   150

Nutrients Contained in: Okra and Cauliflower with Your Macaroni   151

Happy Greens   152

Nutrients Contained in: Happy Greens   153

Sweet Potatoes and Onions   154

Nutrients Contained in: Sweet Potatoes and Onions   155

Linking with Kale   156

Nutrients Contained in: Linking with Kale   157

Apple of Your Eye   158

Nutrients Contained in: Apple of Your Eye   159

A Stirring Dish   160

Nutrients Contained in: A Stirring Dish   161

Orient Bean Express   162

Nutrients Contained in: Orient Bean Express   163

Lemon Flounder   164

Nutrients Contained in: Lemon Flounder   165

Green and Orange Special   166

Nutrients Contained in: Green and Orange Special   167

Chapter Six Healing and Preventive Recipes for Osteoporosis   169

Shrimp and Bok Choy   172

Nutrients Contained in: Shrimp and Bok Choy   173

Salmon with Broccoli, Wheat Germ, and Cheese   174

Nutrients Contained in: Salmon with Broccoli, Wheat Germ, and Cheese   175

Halibut Swimming in Chard   176

Nutrients Contained in: Halibut Swimming in Chard   177

Lovely Avocado Sprouts   178

Nutrients Contained in: Lovely Avocado Sprouts   179

Tuna, Cheese, and Pepper Powerhouse   180

Nutrient Contained in: Tuna, Cheese, and Pepper Powerhouse   181

Kasha and Pea Pods   182

Nutrients Contained in: Kasha and Pea Pods   183

Cauliflower Mushroom Marriage   184

Nutrients Contained In: Cauliflower Mushroom Marriage   185

Brussels Sprouts and Jack   186

Nutrients Contained in: Brussels Sprouts and Jack   187

Nutty Bok Choy   188

Nutrients Contained in: Nutty Bok Choy   189

Mellow Melon Salad   190

Nutrients Contained in: Mellow Melon Salad   191

Fish and Rice Sitdown   192

Nutrients Contained in: Fish and Rice Sitdown   193

Rice Under Almonds   194

Nutrients Contained in: Rice Under Almonds   195

Brussels Sprouts Parmesan   196

Nutrients Contained in: Brussel Sprouts Parmesan   197

Vegetable Haymaker   198

Nutrients Contained in: Vegetable Haymaker   199

Mustards and Collards   200

Nutrients Contained in: Mustards and Collards   201

Garlic Tofu Soup   202

Nutrients Contained in: Garlic Tofu Soup   203

Chapter Seven   Healing and Preventive Recipes for Rheumatoid Arthritis   205

Fish and Chicks   208

Nutrients Contained in: Fish and Chicks   209

Spicy Onion Salmon   210

Nutrients Contained in: Spicy Onion Salmon   211

Nuts to Apples   212

Nutrients Contained in: Nuts to Apples   213

Green and Yellow Vibrancy   214

Nutrients Contained in: Green and Yellow Vibrancy   215

Corn the Great   216
Nutrients Contained in: Corn the Great   217

Baked Winter Comfort   218
Nutrients Contained in: Baked Winter Comfort   219

Peachy Sweet Potatoes   220
Nutrients Contained in: Peachy Sweet Potatoes   221

Little Sprouts   222
Nutrients Contained in: Little Sprouts   223

Bow Ties and Black Hats   224
Nutrients Contained in: Bow Ties and Black Hats   225

A Touch of Walnuts   226
Nutrients Contained in: A Touch of Walnuts   227

Cabbage and Wild Friends   228
Nutrients Contained in: Cabbage and Wild Friends   229

Salmon Potassium King   230
Nutrients Contained in: Salmon Potassium King   231

Easy Sardines   232
Nutrients Contained in: Easy Sardines   233

Blues Are Not Bad   234
Nutrients Contained in: Blues Are Not Bad   235

Mackerel and Mushrooms   236
Nutrients Contained in: Mackerel and Mushrooms   237

Chapter Eight Healing and Preventive Recipes for Gallbladder   238

Red Baked Acorn Squash   240
Nutrients Contained in: Red Baked Acorn Squash   241

Yellow Jewels   242
Nutrients Contained in: Yellow Jewels   243

No Small Matter Shrimp   244
Nutrients Contained in: No Small Matter Shrimp   245

On the Half Shell   246
Nutrients Contained in: On the Half Shell   247

Back to Your Roots   248
Nutrients Contained in: Back to Your Roots   249

Savory Beef Fillet   250
Nutrients Contained in: Savory Beef Fillet   251

Pleasant Crabs   252
Nutrients Contained in: Pleasant Crabs   253

Greens L'Italia   254
Nutrients Contained in: Greens L'Italia   255

Green and Brown Beans   256
Nutrients Contained in: Green and Brown Beans   257

Breast Over Broccoli   258
Nutrients Contained in: Breast Over Broccoli   259

OK Lima Beans   260
Nutrients Contained in: OK Lima Beans   261

Carrots' Cousin   262
Nutrients Contained in: Carrots' Cousin   263

Ole for Sole   264
Nutrients Contained in: Ole for Sole   265

Soup of Beans   266
Nutrients Contained in: Soup of Beans   267

Simple Zucchini and Carrots   268
Nutrients Contained in: Simple Zucchini and Carrots   269

Lobster for a Change   270
Nutrients Contained in: Lobster for a Change   271

Chapter Nine   Healing and Preventive Recipes for Constipation   274

Carrot Cabbage   276
Nutrients Contained in: Carrot Cabbage   277

The Big Herb with Beans   278
Nutrients Contained in: The Big Herb with Beans   279

Arabian Pockets   280
Nutrients Contained in: Arabian Pockets   281

Semolina with Color   282
Nutrients Contained in: Semolina with Color   283

Grandma's Oats   284
Nutrients Contained in: Grandma's Oats   285

Bulgur Variations   286
Nutrients Contained in: Bulgur Variations   287

Bran Oat Wheatloaf   288
Nutrients Contained in: Bran Oat Wheatloaf   289

Chicken Con Carne   290
Nutrients Contained in: Chicken Con Carne   291

Really Stuffed Green and Red Pepper   292
Nutrients Contained in: Really Stuffed Green and Red Pepper   293

Pork Apple Love Affair   294
Nutrients Contained in: Pork Apple Love Affair   295

Pork and Prunes   296
Nutrients Contained in: Pork and Prunes   297

Scotch Pearl Soup   298
Nutrients Contained in: Scotch Pearl Soup   299

North African Stew   300
Nutrients Contained in: North African Stew   301

Peppers and Prunes   302
Nutrients Contained in: Peppers and Prunes   303

Double Rice   304
Nutrients Contained in: Double Rice   305

Chapter Ten Healing and Preventive Recipes for Cataracts   307

Dandy Halibut   310
Nutrients Contained in: Dandy Halibut   311

Munchy Mollusks   312
Nutrients Contained in: Munchy Mollusks   313

Savory Baked Chicken   314
Nutrients Contained in: Savory Baked Chicken   315

Untamed Wild Rice   316
Nutrients Contained in: Untamed Wild Rice   317

Poor Man's Octopus   318
Nutrients Contained in: Poor Man's Octopus   319

Clam Special   320
Nutrients Contained in: Clam Special   321

Perch Fry   322
Nutrients Contained in: Perch Fry   323

Elegant Asparagus   324
Nutrients Contained in: Elegant Asparagus   325

Yam What I Yam   326
Nutrients Contained in: Yam What I Yam   327

Roots of Another Kind   328

Nutrients Contained in: Roots of Another Kind   329

Red Miners and Mangoes   330

Nutrients Contained in: Red Miners and Mangoes   331

Handsome Beets   332

Nutrients Contained in: Handsome Beets   333

Kale and Gobble   334

Nutrients Contained in: Kale and Gobble   335

Grainy Turnips   336

Nutrients Contained in: Grainy Turnips   337

Hammy Spinach   338

Nutrients Contained in: Hammy Spinach   339

Chapter Eleven   Recipes to Enhance Fertility   341

Vegetable and Grain Medley   344

Nutrients Contained in: Vegetable and Grain Medley   345

Deep Baked Greenery   346

Nutrients Contained in: Deep Baked Greenery   347

Whole Steamed Flounder   348

Nutrients Contained in: Whole Steamed Flounder   349

Oyster Salsa   350

Nutrients Contained in: Oyster Salsa   351

Chicken Breast Deluxe with Bean Sprouts   352

Nutrients Contained in: Chicken Breast Deluxe with Bean Sprouts   353

Turkey Lentil Bake   354

Nutrients Contained in: Turkey Lentil Bake   355

Roots and Fruits   356

Nutrients Contained in: Roots and Fruits   357

Barley, Tofu, and Shiitake Mushroom Soup   358

Nutrients Contained in: Barley, Tofu, and Shiitake Mushroom Soup   359

Shrimp Vegetable Stew   360

Nutrients Contained in: Shrimp Vegetable Stew   361

Seedy Cabbage   362

Nutrients Contained in: Seedy Cabbage   363

Sprouting Peppers   364

Nutrients Contained in: Sprouting Peppers   365

Baked Potatoes with Skin and Wheat Germ   366
Nutrients Contained in: Baked Potatoes with Skin and Wheat Germ   367

Spirit of Corn with Broccoli and Almonds   368
Nutrients Contained in: Spirit of Corn with Broccoli and Almonds   369

Tuna Under Onion, Garlic, and Mushrooms   370
Nutrients Contained in: Tuna Under Onion, Garlic, and Mushrooms   371

Stuffed Red Dynamos   372
Nutrients Contained in: Stuffed Red Dynamos   373

Chicken Livers with Peppers and Mushrooms   374
Nutrients Contained in: Chicken Livers with Peppers and Mushrooms   375

Chapter Twelve   Healing and Preventive Recipes for Anemia   377

Chicken and Beef Meet   380
Nutrients Contained in: Chicken and Beef Meet   381

Steak and Vegetable Gravy   382
Nutrients Contained in: Steak and Vegetable Gravy   383

Fruited Chicken   384
Nutrients Contained in: Fruited Chicken   385

Plain and Simple Sole   386
Nutrients Contained in: Plain and Simple Sole   387

Turkey's Dark Side   388
Nutrients Contained in: Turkey's Dark Side   389

Little Liver   390
Nutrients Contained in: Little Liver   391

Big Liver   392
Nutrients Contained in: Big Liver   393

American Swedish Meatballs   394
Nutrients Contained in: American Swedish Meatballs   395

Chili Turkey   396
Nutrients Contained in: Chili Turkey   397

Cruciferous Cabbage Roll   398
Nutrients Contained in: Cruciferous Cabbage Roll   399

Fava Chicken   400
Nutrients Contained in: Fava Chicken   401

Stuffed Reds   402
Nutrients Contained in: Stuffed Reds   403

Onion Lover's Chicken   404

Nutrients Contained in: Onion Lover's Chicken   405

Lean and Mean Haddock   406

Nutrients Contained in: Lean and Mean Haddock   407

Fish and Peas   408

Nutrients Contained in: Fish and Peas   409

Chapter Thirteen   Healing and Preventive Recipes for the Immune System   410

Halibut and Mustard Greens   412

Nutrients Contained in: Halibut and Mustard Greens   413

Sweet Potato Brew   414

Nutrients Contained in: Sweet Potato Brew   415

Citrus Baked Bluefish   416

Nutrients Contained in: Citrus Baked Bluefish   417

Orange Spinach   418

Nutrients Contained in: Orange Spinach   419

Onion Garlic Potatoes with Corn   420

Nutrients Contained in: Onion Garlic Potatoes with Corn   421

Universal Potatoes Baked with Cabbage   422

Nutrients Contained in: Universal Potatoes Baked with Cabbage   423

Southern Oysters   424

Nutrients Contained in: Southern Oysters   425

Three Green Chicken with Walnuts and Oranges   426

Nutrients Contained in: Three Green Chicken with Walnuts and Oranges   427

Halloween Chicken   428

Nutrients Contained in: Halloween Chicken   429

Turkey and Oyster on Whole Wheat Toast   430

Nutrients Contained in: Turkey and Oyster on Whole Wheat Toast   431

Citrus Fruit Gathering   432

Nutrients Contained in: Cirtus Fruit Gathering   433

Magic Mushroom Bake   434

Nutrients Contained in: Magic Mushroom Bake   435

Pungent Onion Stuffed with Carrots   436

Nutrients Contained in: Pungent Onion Stuffed with Carrots   437

Lean Cod Potato Stew   438

Nutrients Contained in: Lean Cod Potato Stew   439

Trout Fruit Melange   440

Nutrients Contained in: Trout Fruit Melange   441

Sweet on Apricots   442

Nutrients Contained in: Sweet on Apricots   443

Tuna Cabbage Jackets   444

Nutrients Contained in: Tuna Cabbage Jackets   445

References   **447**

Appendix A   **453**

Appendix B   **455**

Appendix C   **457**

Index   **459**

RESOURCES AND REFERENCES

Resources

Nutrition is an active field of research spanning many disciplines. Many of the scientists, physicians, and specialists interviewed who have made key discoveries related to the effects of food nutrients as a factor in disease prevention and healing constitute prime resources for *Magic Meals*.

Bernard Brachfeld, Ph.D.: Regional director of nutrition and technical services with the Food and Nutrition Service, U.S. Department of Agriculture, Mid-Atlantic Region.

Roscoe Brady, M.D.: Research scientist and study leader of a recent enzyme and genetic study at the National Institutes of Health (NIH) in Bethesda, Maryland.

Vincent T. DeVita, Jr.: Former director of the National Cancer Institute of the NIH in Bethesda, Maryland.

K. Buol Heslin, M.D.: An opthamologist in private practice in cataract surgery in New York City; inventor of Heslin/Mackool Ocusystem. Affiliated with the New York Eye and Ear Infirmary.

Ruth L. Kirschstein, M.D.: Director of the National Institute of General Medical Sciences (NIGMS).

Richard A. Kunin, M.D.: Physician practicing in San Francisco, California, and author of *Mega-Nutrition* published by McGraw-Hill.

Niels Laurersen, M.D.: Gynecologist affiliated with the Mount Sinai Medical Center in New York and author of *Listen to Your Body*, published by Simon & Schuster.

Claude Lenfant, M.D.: Director of the National Heart, Lung, and Blood Institute of the NIH.

Franklin Williams, M.D.: Former director of the National Institute on Aging (NIA).

References

The key references materials and organizations here exclude those just mentioned.

American Journal of Clinical Nutrition, January 1991.
American Journal of Epidemiology, November 1990.

Arteriosclerosis Council Abstracts, November 1990.

British Medical Journal, September 15, 1990.

Committee on Dietary Allowances, *Recommended Dietary Allowances,* National Academy of Sciences, Washington, D.C.

George Washington University Medical Center, Washington, D.C.

Harvard Medical School, Boston, MA.

International Journal of Cancer, Vol. 43, pp. 1050–1054.

Journal of the American Dietetic Association, Supplement, September 1990.

Tufts University School of Nutrition, Boston, MA.

USDA Human Nutrition Research Center at Tufts University.

University of California at Berkeley School of Public Health.

ACKNOWLEDGMENTS

Many studies and research groups contributed to the production and publication of this book. To my former editor, Deborah Kurtz, I'm indebted for imaginative and cheerful assistance in the initial stages of this project. Doug Corcoran, my new editor at Prentice Hall, has been extremely supportive in the later stages of the work.

I also want to acknowledge my friends as well as my colleagues at Iona College who have cheerfully and willingly tested many of the recipes. My wife and daughters have been particularly generous in letting me dominate the kitchen with my creations.

FOREWORD

All of the recipes in *Magic Meals* urge the reader to become more aware of the fact that foods contain many known nutrients and many that are still unknown to scientists. It should also become apparent that taste does not have to be sacrificed for nutrition.

The RDA for any given vitamin or mineral should simply be recognized as the government estimate of the amount of essential nutrients each person in a population might be required to consume on a daily basis in order to stay optimally healthy. The RDA is only a guideline for public health and not an absolute as there are few, if any, absolutes that can be generally applied and adopted by an entire population in the area of nutrition.

The variables in the life of each individual may dictate nutrient intakes far in excess of the RDAs used in the recipe charts. The government has not even made a recommended daily allowance for several minerals and vitamins as yet. For example, no recommended daily allowance has been established for potassium. Yet the National Academy of Sciences estimates the safe, adequate daily intake to be 1,875–5,625 milligrams for adults. You will notice that this amount is easily provided by a variety of the recipes.

A more detailed explanation of how RDA came about is in the Appendix.

The reader should be mindful that eating 5 servings of fruits and vegetables a day will cover the established nutritional needs. Your charts will tell you what amounts of vitamins and minerals are contained in your choices.

Magic Meals provides a means to rapidly evaluate foods and combinations of foods and compare them to our needs as established by the USRDA figures given for the general population and by recognized health experts. The RDA chart shows the figures based upon groups classified by age range and sex.

Because there are so many variables involved in the analysis of nutrients, absolute accuracy is not possible and the nutritional charts accompanying each recipe are a very close approximation of the milligrams, micrograms, and international units found in each food. This simply means that some figures may not add up to one-hundred percent; you may see, for example, the USRDA for vitamin A reads 5,000 IU and a serving of a particular meal provides 11,402 IUs of vitamin A indicating an intake of 221 percent of the USRDA. Obviously, the precise arithmetic would read 228 percent. This difference, however, is negligible in evaluating your minimum required intake of vitamins and minerals to maintain good health.

The figures are based on the needs of a statistically average adult and include a safety factor. Individuals differ in lifestyle, in the environment they live in and in their genetic endowment. And it is important to recognize that no one meal is the answer to health. It is the collective eating pattern that will have a positive effect on our well-being.

What you have is a guide that will rapidly inform you of the approximate intake of nutrients recommended by health professionals. You will be able to immediately determine the amount of fat in a meal; how close each meal provides the USRDA of minerals and vitamins, and with this information, you are able to make intelligent plans for eating with a minimum of time and involvement.

PREFACE

Magic Meals is a book of "keys" enabling the reader to eat scientifically, without being a scientist; to eat nutritionally, without being a nutritionist; and to eat deliciously, without being a gourmet chef.

More than anything else, this is a practical, no-special-skills-needed, easy- and quick-to-make-meals cookbook containing appetizing recipes that have the power to protect and heal.

For over four years, I interviewed thousands of physicians, scientists, and researchers on my radio and television programs. For over two years, I met and had discussions with scientists at the largest biomedical research center in the world, the National Institutes of Health, in Bethesda, Maryland. The breakthroughs in nutrition and findings in many other areas of medicine making the headlines today are in my book, *Medical Breakthroughs,* from the National Institutes in Health.

The notion that foods available to you from your markets such as broccoli, carrots, and cabbage all have properties that help protect against various cancers, that fish oil can help ease arthritic stiffness, that vegetables of all kinds have a protective effect on gallbladder, that peas and beans can relieve constipation, that vitamins from fish and low-fat cheese can slow the onset of cataracts—all these findings have been researched for years. What is important now is that these developments are no longer associated only with alternative medicine groups, quackery, or "health nuts." Indeed, these findings are fast becoming an important aspect behind the strategies of mainstream medical practices.

Magic Meals shows you how to combine food to maximize the astonishing power found in the substances of many foods that have the ability to strengthen health and prevent bodily deterioration. Its 13 chapters offer 200 recipes that fight cancers, high blood pressure, stroke, diabetes, constipation, anemia, cataracts, infertility, heart disease, gallbladder problems, osteoporosis, arthritis, and impaired immunity. Each chapter offers 15 imaginative and potent recipes that, if eaten, will put you on the track to good health and keep you that way. Scientists are saying these days that food is the best medicine for longevity and health.

Among the many benefits you will get from reading *Magic Meals* is that when you are able to compute your exact nutritional needs from its easy-to-read charts, you will find that you don't have to eat large quantities of food. This, of course, not only keeps you healthy, but it saves you money.

When the word "compute" comes up in any discussion related to food, I hear people saying, "this may be worthwhile, but I don't understand grams from crackers or IUs from IOUs and I'm certainly not going to pull out a calculator every time I eat." The good news is you don't need to—I have calculated all that for you!

The best news is that hundreds of foods have been investigated by thousands of scientists and physicians; they have not, even yet, tapped all the unknown nutrients that these foods offer. Working, however, from existing information based on a wealth of scientific evidence, we can begin to streamline our eating patterns to receive the greatest benefits.

While much remains to be discovered and documented by research to reach absolutes, informed policy makers and scientists agree that, even now, there is a large body of evidence showing a link between nutrition and chronic disease. There is no question that dietary factors stand between a long life relatively disease free and a short one with attendant health problems.

The discovery that the foods we normally eat, when properly prepared and combined, can prevent and heal numerous diseases is the foundation upon which the recipes have been written and the justification for a title such as *Magic Meals*.

INTRODUCTION

This book was written so that you can reap immediate advantages from the research heralding the incredible power of food to prevent and treat numerous diseases. Researchers throughout the world are unearthing the magical healing properties buried within common foods such as carrots, broccoli, cabbage, corn, beans, spinach, and many more.

200 Recipes

Magic Meals contains 200 recipes filled with foods that scientific studies have shown to be effective against such problems as heart disease, arthritis, osteoporosis, cancers, anemia, and other common diseases. The ingredients of each meal have been carefully selected from all the healing foods now making the headlines every day. The ingredients have also been skillfully combined to heighten further their disease prevention and healing powers.

You will find in the chapter on cancers, for example, a combination of cabbage, potatoes, and onions that gives you 200 percent of the U.S. Recommended Daily Allowance (USRDA) for vitamin C, which is known to defend the body against cancerous cells. How do you know it has 200 percent of the USRDA? Simply scan the nutritional chart—another innovative feature developed for *Magic Meals*.

Easy-To-Read Nutritional Charts

Each recipe is accompanied by a comprehensive, immediate, easy-to-read nutritional chart that displays the percentages of milligrams (and micrograms) of all the vitamins and minerals contained in the dish. Just below that you will see the number of calories of fat, protein, and carbohydrates contained in the meal, and below that, an instant picture of the amount of cholesterol, amino acids, and fiber you have received from that one serving.

Instant USRDA Percentages Column

But that's not all. An adjacent column shows you what *percentages* of the USRDAs for vitamins and minerals are contained in that meal. This knowledge gives you the expertise needed to pinpoint how much or how little of each vitamin and mineral your meal produces and what adjustments, if any, you should consider. This exclusive feature of *Magic Meals* affords you the certainty of knowing how to maintain your daily nutritional requirements. (A sample chart follows the introduction.)

For example, government studies over a 12-year period indicate that fulfilling the USRDAs for potassium seems to protect against stroke. As you cook from the chapter on preventing strokes, you will find that each meal has been designed to provide ample potassium. To determine what percentage of potassium you will receive in a recipe called, "A Different Cabbage and Pork," you simply scan the USRDA column, and you will see that this meal gives you 95 percent of your daily allowance for potassium. Eating this way not only protects you against major diseases, but it is also fun.

Quick and Easy Cookbook

Magic Meals enables you to prepare delicious and powerful meals for your family's or your guest's health and satisfaction without spending all day doing it. Most of the recipes contained in the 13 chapters are either easy to cook or are made in less than an hour. I have avoided complicated preparations, sticking to those that require the least amount of time. They all, however, offer the maximum action in preventing or reversing ill health.

In addition to the effective substances found in the foods, I used the following guidelines for final selection:

1. Must be easy to cook (usually no more than 1 hour or even less).
2. Must use ingredients that are easily found in most kitchens or stores.
3. Must be cooked and eaten with pleasurable results.

U.S. Recommended Dietary Allowance Charts

Magic Meals adds yet another feature. You will find, preceding each group of recipes, in each chapter a chart showing the RDAs listed for each mineral and vitamin by group and age and the milligrams each group should have for a particular vitamin and mineral. These handy charts tell you what the RDAs are for each age group beginning with infants as well as for males and females.

Food Chart Ranking
Highest Amount of Vitamins

And at the end of each chapter, you are provided with a list of the foods ranked in the highest order for the particular vitamin featured in the recipe. For example, at the end of Chapter 3, on blood pressure, you will find all the foods listed from the highest to the lowest in sodium content. This helps you not only to avoid overeating harmful amounts of certain nutrients, but it allows you to create your own favorite healthy recipes.

The chart also gives you information that allows you to keep control over the amount of fat, cholesterol, fiber, and calories you should or should not ingest for your best nutritional well-being.

Tips and Myths

Another exciting bonus emphasized in *Magic Meals* are the tips and myths given on each recipe page. For example, from a recipe in Chapter 1, on cancer, you see this tip,

TIP: Many varieties of greens—especially kale, collards, and others in the cabbage family—are rich in beta-carotene, which the body converts to vitamin A, vitamin C, and other substances that may protect against various cancers.

Immediately below that you always get the latest news behind myths about food and health we all seem to hold. For example, do you believe the following:

MYTH: The vitamin content of fruits and vegetables is determined by the soil they grow in.

You might be surprised at the answer. These Tips and Myths actually represent a book within a book as you will find loads of valuable information concerning research on health and nutrition. These mini reports, which are easy to read and understand, are equal in importance to news you will read in many journals and reports.

Primer on Fats, USRDAs, Meat, Amino Acids

For the benefit of readers who want to examine in more detail the research findings on fat, on meat, on the importance of amino acids, as well as a little historical background on the RDAs and the USRDAs, I have simplified this information in the appendixes of the book.

All that remains now is for you to choose this evening's delicious and nourishing dinner.

How To Read the Nutritional Chart

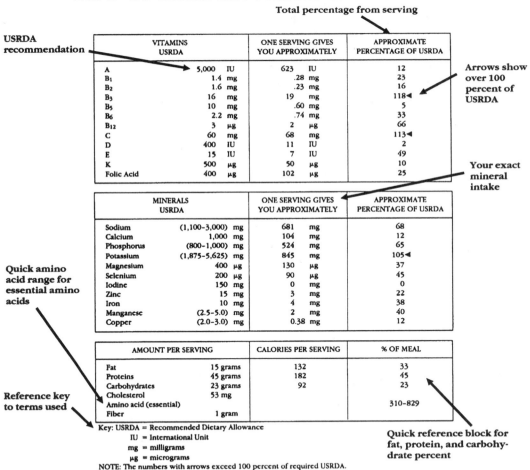

Total percentage from serving

USRDA recommendation

VITAMINS USRDA			ONE SERVING GIVES YOU APPROXIMATELY		APPROXIMATE PERCENTAGE OF USRDA
A	5,000	IU	623	IU	12
B₁	1.4	mg	.28	mg	23
B₂	1.6	mg	.23	mg	16
B₃	16	mg	19	mg	118◄
B₅	10	mg	.60	mg	5
B₆	2.2	mg	.74	mg	33
B₁₂	3	µg	2	µg	66
C	60	mg	68	mg	113◄
D	400	IU	11	IU	2
E	15	IU	7	IU	49
K	500	µg	50	µg	10
Folic Acid	400	µg	102	µg	25

Arrows show over 100 percent of USRDA

Your exact mineral intake

MINERALS USRDA			ONE SERVING GIVES YOU APPROXIMATELY		APPROXIMATE PERCENTAGE OF USRDA
Sodium	(1,100–3,000)	mg	681	mg	68
Calcium	1,000	mg	104	mg	12
Phosphorus	(800–1,000)	mg	524	mg	65
Potassium	(1,875–5,625)	mg	845	mg	105◄
Magnesium	400	µg	130	µg	37
Selenium	200	µg	90	µg	45
Iodine	150	mg	0	mg	0
Zinc	15	mg	3	mg	22
Iron	10	mg	4	mg	38
Manganese	(2.5–5.0)	mg	2	mg	40
Copper	(2.0–3.0)	mg	0.38	mg	12

Quick amino acid range for essential amino acids

AMOUNT PER SERVING		CALORIES PER SERVING	% OF MEAL
Fat	15 grams	132	33
Proteins	45 grams	182	45
Carbohydrates	23 grams	92	23
Cholesterol	53 mg		
Amino acid (essential)			310–829
Fiber	1 gram		

Reference key to terms used

Key: USRDA = Recommended Dietary Allowance
　　　IU = International Unit
　　　mg = milligrams
　　　µg = micrograms
NOTE: The numbers with arrows exceed 100 percent of required USRDA.

Quick reference block for fat, protein, and carbohydrate percent

CHAPTER ONE

Healing and Preventive Recipes for Cancer

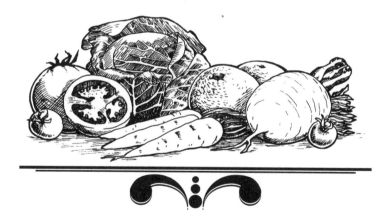

The first muse is health.
—Ralph Waldo Emerson

After decades of searching, scientists and physicians at the National Cancer Institute and research centers around the world have concluded that it is possible to begin protecting ourselves from various cancers by choosing the foods we eat.

The evidence is that a diet of fruits, vegetables, fiber, and low fat can give you the advantage in keeping cancers at bay. The strategy suggested is to select foods rich in vitamins C and E and omega-3 fatty acids and to limit your intake of calories from fat to no more than 30 percent daily. You will find, however, that many nutritional authorities asked that we aim for even lower figures.

Evidence shows that vitamin C is especially protective of cancers of the mouth, larynx, esophagus, stomach, pancreas, rectum, and uterine cervix. Studies also indicate that vitamin C is a protective factor in breast cancer. The findings showed that women who had the most vitamin C in their diets had the lowest risk of breast cancer. Women who had the least C had the greatest incidence of breast cancer risk.

Consequently, I have created recipes that feature foods with the highest amounts of vitamin C. Your chart will show the percentages for each meal of not only vitamin C but other nutrients connected with cancer protection as well, such as beta-carotene (a form of vitamin A) and vitamin E.

You will find a list of foods at the end of the chapter ranked in order of the highest amounts of vitamin C for you to create your own recipes.

RECOMMENDED DIETARY ALLOWANCES FOR VITAMIN C

GROUP/AGE	VITAMIN C (MILLIGRAMS)
Children 1–10 years	35
Males 11–14 years	45
Males 15+ years	50
Females 11–14 years	50
Females 15+ years	60
Pregnant women	80

Simple Cabbage Soup

Ingredients:

- 1 head cabbage
- 1 quart stock, beef or vegetable
- 1 onion, chopped fine
- 2 carrots, peeled and diced
- 2 turnips, peeled and diced
- 1 8-ounce can of tomatoes
- chopped parsley
- chili powder or cayenne pepper

Preparation: Boil and simmer

Time: 45 minutes

Calories: 119 per serving

Serves: 4

Directions

Bring the stock to a boil. Add the onion, carrots, turnips, cabbage, and can of tomatoes, including liquid. Lower heat to simmer, cover, and cook 30 minutes until vegetables are tender. Season with pepper to taste. Sprinkle with chopped parsley. Use chilipowder or cayenne for a livelier taste.

TIP: The *International Journal of Cancer* has concluded that eating foods rich in vitamins E and C and beta-carotene may lower risk of cervical cancer after researchers found that cervical cancer risk was about one-half lower for those on a high-vitamin-E diet, one-half lower for those on a high-vitamin-C diet, and nearly one-half lower for those on a high-beta-carotene diet.

MYTH: Vitamins supply quick energy.

FACT: Vitamins do not contain calories and thus do not supply energy quickly or otherwise, report scientists. Only carbohydrates, fat, and protein provide energy. The notion that vitamins supply energy continues to be spread by some vitamin manufacturers as well as some popular literature. Vitamins are essential for the body's energy-producing processes and work with other nutrients in foods and certain proteins produced by the body.

Nutrients Contained in: Simple Cabbage Soup

VITAMINS USRDA			ONE SERVING GIVES YOU APPROXIMATELY		APPROXIMATE PERCENTAGE OF USRDA
A	5,000	IU	12,233	IU	244◀
B₁	1.4	mg	2	mg	114◀
B₂	1.6	mg	1	mg	98
B₃	16	mg	5	mg	29
B₅	10	mg	2	mg	19
B₆	2.2	mg	2	mg	74
B₁₂	3	μg	13	μg	416◀
C	60	mg	162	mg	269◀
D	400	IU	0	IU	
E	15	IU	18	IU	119◀
Folic Acid	400	μg	165	μg	41

MINERALS USRDA			ONE SERVING GIVES YOU APPROXIMATELY		APPROXIMATE PERCENTAGE OF USRDA
Sodium	(1,100–3,000)	mg	82	mg	8
Calcium	1,000	mg	155	mg	19
Phosphorus	(800–1,000)	mg	116	mg	14
Potassium	(1,875–5,625)	mg	926	mg	115◀ˑ
Magnesium	400	μg	54	μg	15
Selenium	200	μg	5	μg	2
Iodine	150	mg	0	mg	0
Zinc	15	mg	0.62	mg	4
Iron	10	mg	4	mg	42
Manganese	(2.5–5.0)	mg	0.54	mg	10
Copper	(2.0–3.0)	mg	13	mg	4

AMOUNT PER SERVING		CALORIES PER SERVING	% OF MEAL
Fat	1 gram	7	6
Proteins	4 grams	18	15
Carbohydrates	23 grams	94	79
Cholesterol	0 mg		
Amino acid (essential)			33–55
Fiber	8 grams		

Key: USRDA = Recommended Dietary Allowance

IU = International Unit

mg = milligrams

μg = micrograms

NOTE: The numbers with arrows exceed 100 percent of required USRDA.

ˑBased on minimum of 800 mg

Dynamic Cabbage and Potatoes

Ingredients:

4–5	medium boiling potatoes, peeled and quartered
1	large head green cabbage, quartered
1	large onion
1	tsp olive oil
	black pepper
	cayenne pepper

Preparation: Boil and saute

Time: 40 minutes

Calories: 227 per serving

Serves: 4

Directions

Place potatoes in a pot and cover with water. Put the cabbage quarters on top. Bring to a boil, cover, and cook for 15 to 20 minutes, until the potatoes are just tender. Remove the cabbage and chop coarsely. Set aside. Remove potatoes and mash. Set aside. Drain the pot. To dry pot, add the oil and heat. When oil is hot, add the onion and saute until soft. Add the mashed potatoes and cabbage and blend thoroughly. Season with black pepper and a touch of cayenne. Especially tasty on winter nights.

TIP: Many varieties of greens—especially kale, collards, and others in the cabbage family—are rich in beta-carotene, which the body converts to vitamin A, vitamin C, and other substances that may protect against various cancers.

MYTH: The vitamin content of fruits and vegetables is determined by the soil they grow in.

FACT: Researchers say if the growing soil is good enough to produce a healthy plant, the vitamins and other nutrients found in that plant will be present and available. All the vitamins in plants are manufactured by the plants themselves, according to their own genetic program. An important cause of vitamin loss in plant foods is improper storage and handling after harvest.

Nutrients Contained in:
Dynamic Cabbage and Potatoes

VITAMINS USRDA			ONE SERVING GIVES YOU APPROXIMATELY		APPROXIMATE PERCENTAGE OF USRDA
A	5,000	IU	286	IU	5
B_1	1.4	mg	0.27	mg	22
B_2	1.6	mg	0.10	mg	7
B_3	16	mg	2	mg	15
B_5	10	mg	1	mg	10
B_6	2.2	mg	0.64	mg	29
B_{12}	3	μg	0	μg	0
C	60	mg	121	mg	201◄
D	400	IU	0	IU	0
E	15	IU	31	IU	18
K	500	μg	100	μg	20
Folic Acid	400	μg	149	μg	37

MINERALS USRDA			ONE SERVING GIVES YOU APPROXIMATELY		APPROXIMATE PERCENTAGE OF USRDA
Sodium	(1,100–3,000)	mg	49	mg	4
Calcium	1,000	mg	126	mg	15
Phosphorus	(800–1,000)	mg	118	mg	14
Potassium	(1,875–5,625)	mg	1,063	mg	132◄
Magnesium	400	μg	64	μg	18
Selenium	200	μg	3	μg	1
Iodine	150	mg	0	mg	0
Zinc	15	mg	0.86	mg	5
Iron	10	mg	2	mg	28
Manganese	(2.5–5.0)	mg	0.60	mg	12
Copper	(2.0–3.0)	mg	0.29	mg	9

AMOUNT PER SERVING		CALORIES PER SERVING	% OF MEAL
Fat	4 grams	36	16
Proteins	6 grams	22	10
Carbohydrates	42 grams	169	74
Cholesterol	0 mg		
Amino acid (essential)			49–74
Fiber	3 grams		

Key: USRDA = Recommended Dietary Allowance
   IU = International Unit
   mg = milligrams
   μg = micrograms
NOTE: The numbers with arrows exceed 100 percent of required USRDA.

Red Peppers with Pasta Sauce

Ingredients:

3 large red peppers, cored and cut into medium pieces
1 large onion, coarsely chopped
3 cloves garlic, chopped fine
12 ounces tomato paste
1 Tbs red wine vinegar
¼ cup of olive oil
⅓ cup of water

Preparation: Saute

Time: 1 hour, 10 minutes

Calories: 483 per serving

Serves: 4

Directions

Heat oil over moderate heat. Add onion. Cook until soft, about 15 minutes, stirring now and then. Add peppers. Cover pan, reduce heat to low, cook 15 minutes stirring occasionally until peppers are soft. Add remaining ingredients and stir until blended. Cover. Cook, for 10 to 15 minutes on low heat, stirring frequently. Remove from heat and let cool a little bit. Pulse in food processor in small amounts until sauce is coarse. Serve over pasta.

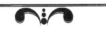

TIP: Ounce for ounce, raw green peppers have two and a half times as much vitamin C as oranges and red peppers nearly four times as much.

MYTH: It's better to let hot foods cool at room temperature rather than in a refrigerator.

FACT: Researchers at University of California say it's never a good idea to let cooked foods cool at room temperature. Improper cooling is the most common cause of outbreaks of foodborne illness. Put food in refrigerator as soon as you can, and in any case don't let food sit out more than two hours.

Nutrients Contained in: Red Peppers with Pasta Sauce

VITAMINS USRDA			ONE SERVING GIVES YOU APPROXIMATELY		APPROXIMATE PERCENTAGE OF USRDA
A	5,000	IU	3456	IU	69
B$_1$	1.4	mg	0.26	mg	21
B$_2$	1.6	mg	0.14	mg	9
B$_3$	16	mg	3	mg	20
B$_5$	10	mg	0.07	mg	0
B$_6$	2.2	mg	0.12	mg	5
B$_{12}$	3	μg	0	μg	0
C	60	mg	112	mg	186◄
D	400	IU	0	IU	
E	15	IU	6	IU	39
Folic Acid	400	μg	13	μg	3

MINERALS USRDA			ONE SERVING GIVES YOU APPROXIMATELY		APPROXIMATE PERCENTAGE OF USRDA
Sodium	(1,100–3,000)	mg	41	mg	4
Calcium	1,000	mg	40	mg	4
Phosphorus	(800–1,000)	mg	93	mg	11
Potassium	(1,875–5,625)	mg	983	mg	122◄
Magnesium	400	μg	10	μg	2
Selenium	200	μg	1	μg	0
Iodine	150	mg	0	mg	0
Zinc	15	mg	0.17	mg	1
Iron	10	mg	4	mg	40
Manganese	(2.5–5.0)	mg	0.11	mg	2
Copper	(2.0–3.0)	mg	0.06	mg	2

AMOUNT PER SERVING		CALORIES PER SERVING	% OF MEAL
Fat	41 grams	371	76
Proteins	4 grams	17	4
Carbohydrates	24 grams	95	20
Cholesterol	0 mg		
Amino acid (essential)			18–36
Fiber	1 gram		

Key: USRDA = Recommended Dietary Allowance
     IU = International Unit
     mg = milligrams
     μg = micrograms
NOTE: The numbers with arrows exceed 100 percent of required USRDA.

Be All That You Can Beet Soup

Ingredients:

- 3 cups beets, cooked fresh or canned
- 1 cup cabbage, shredded
- 1 onion
- 2 carrots
- 3 cups low-sodium chicken or vegetable broth
- 1 Tbs lemon juice
- $\frac{1}{2}$ tsp salt (optional)
- black pepper
- cayenne pepper

Preparation: Steam or cook under pressure

Time: 15 minutes

Calories: 81 per serving

Serves: 4

Directions

Chop vegetables coarsely and put them and other ingredients in pressure cooker or steamer. Cook 3 minutes in pressure cooker, 10 minutes in steamer. Put half the carrots and beets in a blender with a cup of the stock in which they were cooked. Blend for 30 seconds. Return to steamer or pressure cooker and keep on low heat. If desired, season with black pepper or cayenne pepper. This is really delicious as well as colorful. Remember, cayenne is a healthy spice.

TIP: Steam cooking is fast, fuel efficient, and healthful. You need not add oil to your foods. Because food is cooked rapidly over a small amount of water, vitamin retention is high.

MYTH: Fasting can "cleanse your system" and lead to permanent weight loss.

FACT: Researchers at the University of California say that as part of a fad diet, fasting is usually of no value. There's no evidence that a fast can "cleanse" your body in any way, although for a person in good health, there is no danger in fasting for 24 hours. Few people who actually lose weight by this means maintain their loss, and some may sustain permanent injury, say the scientists.

Nutrients Contained in: Be All That
You Can Beet Soup

VITAMINS USRDA			ONE SERVING GIVES YOU APPROXIMATELY		APPROXIMATE PERCENTAGE OF USRDA
A	5,000	IU	11,402	IU	228◄
B_1	1.4	mg	2	mg	167◄
B_2	1.6	mg	1	mg	94
B_3	16	mg	4	mg	24
B_5	10	mg	2	mg	15
B_6	2.2	mg	1	mg	68
B_{12}	3	μg	13	μg	416◄
C	60	mg	100	mg	167◄
D	400	IU	50	IU	12
E	15	IU	17	IU	112◄
K	500	μg	100	μg	20
Folic Acid	400	μg	111	μg	27

MINERALS USRDA			ONE SERVING GIVES YOU APPROXIMATELY		APPROXIMATE PERCENTAGE OF USRDA
Sodium	(1,100–3,000)	mg	303	mg	30
Calcium	1,000	mg	96	mg	12
Phosphorus	(800–1,000)	mg	80	mg	10
Potassium	(1,875–5,625)	mg	595	mg	74
Magnesium	400	μg	47	μg	13
Selenium	200	μg	6	μg	3
Iodine	150	mg	50	mg	33
Zinc	15	mg	0.45	mg	3
Iron	10	mg	4	mg	35
Manganese	(2.5–5.0)	mg	0.37	mg	7
Copper	(2.0–3.0)	mg	0.09	mg	2

AMOUNT PER SERVING		CALORIES PER SERVING	% OF MEAL
Fat	4 grams	4	5
Proteins	39 grams	11	14
Carbohydrates	17 grams	66	81
Cholesterol	0 mg		
Amino acid (essential)			20–31
Fiber	2 grams		

Key: USRDA = Recommended Dietary Allowance

IU = International Unit

mg = milligrams

μg = micrograms

NOTE: The numbers with arrows exceed 100 percent of required USRDA.

Magical Broccoli with Pepper and Onion

Ingredients:

1 head of broccoli
  (about 1 ½ lb)
1 red bell pepper,
  seeded and diced
3 green onions, sliced
  thin
2 Tbs water
1 tsp olive oil or rice oil
  parsley
  black pepper
  cayenne pepper

Preparation: Microwave

Time: 25 minutes

Calories: 61 per serving

Serves: 4

Directions

Wash and trim broccoli. Use the florets and about 1 inch of the peeled stems. Cut the florets into 1-inch pieces and the stems into thin slices. Place florets in the middle of a microwavable baking dish, keeping stems on the outside. Sprinkle a little water on top. Cover tightly with plastic wrap and microwave on high about 5 minutes. Pierce the plastic with a fork to make air holes. Let stand covered for a few minutes. Then remove cover and sprinkle the pepper and onion over the top. Cover again and microwave for 1 minute. Let stand for a few minutes. Remove cover and sprinkle with cayenne pepper, black pepper, and parsley.

TIP: Broccoli is said to be even better than cabbage as a cancer fighter. It helps protect against colon and lung cancer among others. Rich in carotenoid and other cancer-fighting agents, it is noteworthy that frozen broccoli may contain about one-third more beta-carotene than fresh broccoli.

MYTH: Automatic misting of produce in supermarkets causes the nutrients to lose vitamins.

FACT: Researchers at the University of California say that misting actually helps preserve the nutrients. Moisture keeps vegetables fresh longer. A study showed that misting broccoli increased its retention of vitamin C. Refrigeration also leads to dehydration—that's why it is suggested that you keep produce covered or in the hydrator drawer of your refrigerator.

Nutrients Contained in: Magical Broccoli with Pepper and Onion

VITAMINS USRDA			ONE SERVING GIVES YOU APPROXIMATELY		APPROXIMATE PERCENTAGE OF USRDA
A	5,000	IU	1400	IU	28
B_1	1.4	mg	0.06	mg	4
B_2	1.6	mg	0.09	mg	6
B_3	16	mg	0.50	mg	3
B_5	10	mg	0.37	mg	3
B_6	2.2	mg	0.12	mg	5
B_{12}	3	μg	0	μg	0
C	60	mg	85	mg	140◄
D	400	IU	0	IU	0
E	15	IU	1	IU	8
K	500	μg	225	μg	45
Folic Acid	400	μg	49	μg	12

MINERALS USRDA			ONE SERVING GIVES YOU APPROXIMATELY		APPROXIMATE PERCENTAGE OF USRDA
Sodium	(1,100–3,000)	mg	19	mg	1
Calcium	1,000	mg	36	mg	4
Phosphorus	(800–1,000)	mg	48	mg	6
Potassium	(1,875–5,625)	mg	254	mg	31
Magnesium	400	μg	20	μg	5
Selenium	200	μg	0.18	μg	0
Iodine	150	mg	0	mg	0
Zinc	15	mg	0.32	mg	2
Iron	10	mg	0.86	mg	8
Manganese	(2.5–5.0)	mg	0.17	mg	3
Copper	(2.0–3.0)	mg	0.05	mg	1

AMOUNT PER SERVING		CALORIES PER SERVING	% OF MEAL
Fat	4 grams	33	54
Proteins	2 grams	8	13
Carbohydrates	5 grams	20	33
Cholesterol	0 mg		
Amino acid (essential)			17–23
Fiber	1 gram		

Key: USRDA = Recommended Dietary Allowance
    IU = International Unit
    mg = milligrams
    μg = micrograms
NOTE: The numbers with arrows exceed 100 percent of required USRDA.

Double Orange Sweet Potato

Ingredients:
4 small to medium-sized sweet potatoes
½ cup orange juice
pineapple sections
curry powder
nutmeg

Preparation: Bake

Time: 1 hour

Calories: 386 per serving

Serves: 4

Directions

Preheat oven to 375°F. Cut a lengthwise groove into each potato. Drip the orange juice into the grooves and fill each groove with pineapple sections. Wrap with aluminum foil and bake until tender, about 1 hour. Sprinkle with curry or nutmeg if desired.

TIP: Research by the National Cancer Institute gives the sweet potato very high marks as a weapon against lung cancer. According to the NCI, men who ate a half cup of this tuber every day were only half as likely to develop lung cancer as were men who ate almost none.

MYTH: Preference for salt is inborn.

FACT: Salt is an acquired taste that is influenced by habitual behavior. Researchers report that many people who have eaten salty foods from a young age develop a tolerance and then a craving for the salt taste. People who are put on low-sodium diets for medical reasons find that after about six to eight weeks, they adjust to a less salty diet. In effect, they have unlearned what they learned.

Nutrients Contained in: Double Orange Sweet Potato

VITAMINS USRDA			ONE SERVING GIVES YOU APPROXIMATELY		APPROXIMATE PERCENTAGE OF USRDA
A	5,000	IU	56,071	IU	1121◄
B$_1$	1.4	mg	0.24	mg	19
B$_2$	1.6	mg	0.48	mg	34
B$_3$	16	mg	2	mg	14
B$_5$	10	mg	2	mg	18
B$_6$	2.2	mg	0.85	mg	38
B$_{12}$	3	μg	0	μg	0
C	60	mg	78	mg	129◄
D	400	IU	0	IU	0
E	15	IU	6	IU	40
Folic Acid	400	μg	57	μg	14

MINERALS USRDA			ONE SERVING GIVES YOU APPROXIMATELY		APPROXIMATE PERCENTAGE OF USRDA
Sodium	(1,100–3,000)	mg	43	mg	4
Calcium	1,000	mg	76	mg	8
Phosphorus	(800–1,000)	mg	96	mg	12
Potassium	(1,875–5,625)	mg	708	mg	88
Magnesium	400	μg	41	μg	11
Selenium	200	μg	0.70	μg	35
Iodine	150	mg	0	mg	0
Zinc	15	mg	0.92	mg	6
Iron	10	mg	2	mg	20
Manganese	(2.5–5.0)	mg	2	mg	34
Copper	(2.0–3.0)	mg	0.59	mg	19

AMOUNT PER SERVING		CALORIES PER SERVING	% OF MEAL
Fat	19 grams	11	3
Proteins	6 grams	23	6
Carbohydrates	88 grams	352	91
Cholesterol	2 mg		
Amino acid (essential)			63–91
Fiber	3 grams		

Key: USRDA = Recommended Dietary Allowance
    IU = International Unit
    mg = milligrams
    μg = micrograms
NOTE: The numbers with arrows exceed 100 percent of required USRDA.

Kale Delight

Ingredients:

3 cups kale, coarsely chopped
1 cup onion, coarsely chopped
1 tsp safflower or olive oil
juice of one lemon
chili pepper
salt
black pepper

Preparation: Saute
Time: 25 minutes
Calories: 142 per serving
Serves: 4

Directions

Heat the oil in a large skillet and when hot, cook the onions until they are lightly browned. Wash the kale and add it to the skillet with the other ingredients. Lower the heat and allow the kale to cook in the oil, stirring often for about 5 minutes until it is bright green. Add water as needed. Cover and cook until kale is tender, about 10 minutes. Pour the lemon juice over the kale and mix well. Add chili pepper, salt, and black pepper to taste. Delightful.

TIP: Vitamin C needs to be treated with care. Heat and air can take away its effectiveness very easily. When food is kept around for long periods of time, vitamin C loses its original vitamin content. Buy fresh vegetables and use them as soon as possible.

MYTH: Your taste and cravings can be depended upon to tell what nutritional food to eat.

FACT: There is no evidence that we choose foods according to our nutritional needs. It's more likely that your mouth is watering for some roast chicken because you are passing a delicatessen that offers the scent of roasts than because your body needs protein or some other nutrient.

Nutrients Contained in: Kale Delight

VITAMINS USRDA			ONE SERVING GIVES YOU APPROXIMATELY		APPROXIMATE PERCENTAGE OF USRDA
A	5,000	IU	4429	IU	88
B₁	1.4	mg	0.08	mg	7
B₂	1.6	mg	0.07	mg	5
B₃	16	mg	0.56	mg	3
B₅	10	mg	0.13	mg	1
B₆	2.2	mg	0.21	mg	9
B₁₂	3	µg	0	µg	0
C	60	mg	71	mg	118◄
D	400	IU	0	IU	0
E	15	IU	10	IU	68
K	500	µg	0	µg	0
Folic Acid	400	µg	24	µg	6

MINERALS USRDA			ONE SERVING GIVES YOU APPROXIMATELY		APPROXIMATE PERCENTAGE OF USRDA
Sodium	(1,100–3,000)	mg	23	mg	2
Calcium	1,000	mg	81	mg	10
Phosphorus	(800–1,000)	mg	42	mg	5
Potassium	1,875–5,625	mg	307	mg	38
Magnesium	400	µg	28	µg	8
Selenium	200	µg	4	µg	1
Iodine	150	mg	0	mg	0
Zinc	15	mg	0.30	mg	1
Iron	10	mg	1	mg	10
Manganese	(2.5–5.0)	mg	0.44	mg	8
Copper	(2.0–3.0)	mg	0.17	mg	5

AMOUNT PER SERVING		CALORIES PER SERVING	% OF MEAL
Fat	11 grams	96	67
Proteins	29 grams	9	7
Carbohydrates	9 grams	37	26
Cholesterol	0 mg		
Amino acid (essential)			22–32
Fiber	1 gram		

Key: USRDA = Recommended Dietary Allowance
    IU = International Unit
    mg = milligrams
    µg = micrograms
NOTE: The numbers with arrows exceed 100 percent of required USRDA.

Asparagus with Sweet Red Peppers

Ingredients:

32 asparagus spears, stems peeled and cut diagonally in 2-inch pieces

2 sweet red peppers, seeded and sliced crosswise

1 tsp safflower or olive oil

black pepper

chervil

mint

Preparation: Steam and saute

Time: 15 minutes

Calories: 51 per serving

Serves: 4

Directions

Place asparagus stems and tips in steamer and steam 5 to 7 minutes. Heat oil in skillet and saute peppers until soft. Drain the asparagus and arrange on large plates; top with the peppers. Season with pepper and chervil and mint for extra taste.

TIP: Nutritionists report that women may benefit from vitamin C more than men. They say females who consume the same amount of vitamin C as males retain higher level of the vitamins in their blood. The National Institute on Aging studied members of both sexes with high levels of vitamin C in their blood, and both had high amounts of "good" High Density Lipoproteins (HDL) cholesterol, but women's HDL levels were higher.

MYTH: Sea salt contains extra minerals.

FACT: Researchers at the University of California say no. They say that the composition of sea salt is about the same as that of table salt. It has no nutritional advantages and does not have less or more of a salt taste. Whatever small amounts of magnesium, sulphur, and potassium are present have been processed out by the time it gets to the table.

Nutrients Contained in: Asparagus
with Sweet Red Peppers

VITAMINS USRDA			ONE SERVING GIVES YOU APPROXIMATELY		APPROXIMATE PERCENTAGE OF USRDA
A	5,000	IU	1,142	IU	22
B_1	1.4	mg	0.14	mg	12
B_2	1.6	mg	0.16	mg	11
B_3	16	mg	1	mg	8
B_5	10	mg	0.23	mg	2
B_6	2.2	mg	0.22	mg	9
B_{12}	3	μg	0	μg	0
C	60	mg	80	mg	132◄
D	400	IU	0	IU	0
E	15	IU	7	IU	45
K	500	μg	80	μg	16
Folic Acid	400	μg	123	μg	30

MINERALS USRDA			ONE SERVING GIVES YOU APPROXIMATELY		APPROXIMATE PERCENTAGE OF USRDA
Sodium	(1,100–3,000)	mg	7	mg	0
Calcium	1,000	mg	35	mg	4
Phosphorus	(800–1,000)	mg	80	mg	9
Potassium	1,875–5,625	mg	439	mg	54
Magnesium	400	μg	33	μg	9
Selenium	200	μg	3	μg	1
Iodine	150	mg	0	mg	0
Zinc	15	mg	0.63	mg	4
Iron	10	mg	1	mg	12
Manganese	(2.5–5.0)	mg	0.28	mg	5
Copper	(2.0–3.0)	mg	0.15	mg	5

AMOUNT PER SERVING		CALORIES PER SERVING	% OF MEAL
Fat	1 gram	5	10
Proteins	3 grams	14	27
Carbohydrates	8 grams	32	63
Cholesterol	0 mg		
Amino acid (essential)			21–35
Fiber	1 gram		

Key: USRDA = Recommended Dietary Allowance

IU = International Unit

mg = milligrams

μg = micrograms

NOTE: The numbers with arrows exceed 100 percent of required USRDA.

Asparagus, Carrots, and Celery

Ingredients:

32 asparagus spears, cut
    in half on the diagonal
3 large carrots, sliced
2 stalks of celery
1 tsp chervil (dried)
2 Tbs fresh chopped
    parsley
juice of one lemon
black pepper

Preparation: Steam

Time: 15 minutes

Calories: 66 per serving

Serves: 4

Directions

Give the carrots and the celery a minute or two head start in the steamer. Then place the asparagus in the steamer, cover, and let steam until the vegetables are tender. Be careful not to overcook the asparagus. Remove from steamer and add the chervil and parsley; for flavor, add juice of one lemon and sprinkle with pepper. Notice the high amount of vitamin A, potassium, and folic acid in this meal.

TIP: Asparagus is considered one of the healthy foods we should include in our diet. Cancer researcher Dr. Bruce N. Ames says that its food-based nutrients such as beta-carotene and vitamin C are a good barrier to cancer. Notice the low calorie count for this recipe.

MYTH: As we grow older, we naturally start losing intelligence and memory.

FACT: Not according to researchers who say after age 30, we lose 18 million brain cells per year. We also grow billions of new dendrite connections as we age. Scientists matched healthy 70-year-olds and 20-year-olds and the older group outperformed the younger one in long-term memory tests.

Nutrients Contained in: Asparagus, Carrots, and Celery

VITAMINS USRDA			ONE SERVING GIVES YOU APPROXIMATELY		APPROXIMATE PERCENTAGE OF USRDA
A	5,000	IU	16,022	IU	320◀
B$_1$	1.4	mg	0.18	mg	14
B$_2$	1.6	mg	0.18	mg	12
B$_3$	16	mg	2	mg	11
B$_5$	10	mg	0.33	mg	3
B$_6$	2.2	mg	0.25	mg	11
B$_{12}$	3	μg	0	μg	0
C	60	mg	38	mg	62
D	400	IU	0	IU	0
E	15	IU	7	IU	44
K	500	μg	155	μg	31
Folic Acid	400	μg	127	μg	31

MINERALS USRDA			ONE SERVING GIVES YOU APPROXIMATELY		APPROXIMATE PERCENTAGE OF USRDA
Sodium	(1,100–3,000)	mg	42	mg	4
Calcium	1,000	mg	51	mg	6
Phosphorus	(800–1,000)	mg	101	mg	12
Potassium	(1,875–5,625)	mg	604	mg	75
Magnesium	400	μg	33	μg	9
Selenium	200	μg	2	μg	1
Iodine	150	mg	0	mg	0
Zinc	15	mg	0.72	mg	4
Iron	10	mg	1	mg	11
Manganese	(2.5–5.0)	mg	0.35	mg	7
Copper	(2.0–3.0)	mg	0.15	mg	5

AMOUNT PER SERVING		CALORIES PER SERVING	% OF MEAL
Fat	19 grams	5	7
Proteins	4 grams	15	23
Carbohydrates	11 grams	46	70
Cholesterol	0 mg		
Amino acid (essential)			25–38
Fiber	2 grams		

Key: USRDA = Recommended Dietary Allowance
   IU = International Unit
   mg = milligrams
   μg = micrograms
NOTE: The numbers with arrows exceed 100 percent of required USRDA.

Steamed Green Cabbage

Ingredients: 1 head cabbage
juice of one lemon
cayenne pepper

Preparation: Steam

Time: 15 minutes

Calories: 70 per serving

Serves: 4

Directions

Cut cabbage into wedges. Steam over simmering water 5 to 8 minutes, until slightly firm but tender. Drain and sprinkle with pepper and the juice of one lemon. Add a little cayenne pepper to liven things up. Cayenne pepper is recommended as a spice in many of these recipes because it has health benefits as well as being spicy. Notice the high amount of vitamin C on the chart.

TIP: Cast iron pots and skillets are good sources of iron, especially when cooking acidic foods. The iron content of a half cup of spaghetti sauce increases from 3 to 50 milligrams or more when simmered in an iron pot for a few hours.

MYTH: Speaking of iron takes us to lead and the idea that there is harmful lead ink residues in bread wrappers.

FACT: This is a problem of the past. Bakers and printing ink groups now report that they have taken the lead out of inks used on bread wrappers. You can now use the wrappers to turn inside out and use safely as storage bags.

Nutrients Contained in: Steamed Green Cabbage

VITAMINS USRDA			ONE SERVING GIVES YOU APPROXIMATELY		APPROXIMATE PERCENTAGE OF USRDA
A	5,000	IU	290	IU	5
B$_1$	1.4	mg	0.12	mg	9
B$_2$	1.6	mg	0.07	mg	4
B$_3$	16	mg	0.70	mg	4
B$_5$	10	mg	0.35	mg	3
B$_6$	2.2	mg	0.23	mg	10
B$_{12}$	3	μg	0	μg	0
C	60	mg	115	mg	192◄
D	400	IU	0	IU	0
E	15	IU	3	IU	16
K	500	μg	100	μg	20
Folic Acid	400	μg	130	μg	32

MINERALS USRDA			ONE SERVING GIVES YOU APPROXIMATELY		APPROXIMATE PERCENTAGE OF USRDA
Sodium	(1,100–3,000)	mg	41	mg	4
Calcium	1,000	mg	110	mg	13
Phosphorus	(800–1,000)	mg	55	mg	6
Potassium	(1,875–5,625)	mg	578	mg	72
Magnesium	400	μg	41	μg	11
Selenium	200	μg	5	μg	2
Iodine	150	mg	0	mg	0
Zinc	15	mg	0.43	mg	2
Iron	10	mg	1	mg	13
Manganese	(2.5–5.0)	mg	0.36	mg	7
Copper	(2.0–3.0)	mg	0.06	mg	1

AMOUNT PER SERVING		CALORIES PER SERVING	% OF MEAL
Fat	0 grams	4	6
Proteins	3 grams	12	17
Carbohydrates	14 grams	54	77
Cholesterol	0 mg		
Amino acid (essential)			22–38
Fiber	2 grams		

Key: USRDA = Recommended Dietary Allowance
    IU = International Unit
    mg = milligrams
    μg = micrograms
NOTE: The numbers with arrows exceed 100 percent of required USRDA.

Cauliflower with Curry and Spices

Ingredients: 6 cups cauliflower
                           florets
                 ¼ cup water
                 2 tsp curry
                 1 tsp ground ginger

Preparation: Steam
Time: 15 minutes
Calories: 49 per serving
Serves: 4

Directions

Steam florets over simmering water 5 to 8 minutes, or until tender. Heat curry and ginger in a ¼ cup of water, stirring for about 1 minute. Pour over cooked cauliflower. Note high amount of vitamin C and vitamin K on the chart. Vitamin K is required for blood coagulation and body growth.

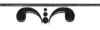

TIP: A half cup of cooked florets has only 15 calories and contains rich amounts of potassium and just a little sodium—good for blood pressure and stroke control. You can see from the chart that a half cup contains about 50 percent of your daily quota of vitamin C, which fights cancer and fatigue and helps iron fight anemia.

MYTH: Heat rubs for muscle soreness or arthritis penetrate the skin.

FACT: The Mayo Clinic reports that there's no evidence that over-the-counter heat rubs, linaments, or other such products penetrate your skin to any extent great enough to fight muscle soreness or arthritic pain. They say the tingling sensation some ointments cause may seem to help by distracting your attention from the underlying aching.

Nutrients Contained in: Cauliflower
with Curry and Spices

VITAMINS USRDA		ONE SERVING GIVES YOU APPROXIMATELY		APPROXIMATE PERCENTAGE OF USRDA
A	5,000 IU	24	IU	
B_1	1.4 mg	0.11	mg	9
B_2	1.6 mg	0.09	mg	6
B_3	16 mg	1	mg	6
B_5	10 mg	0.23	mg	2
B_6	2.2 mg	0.36	mg	16
B_{12}	3 μg	0	μg	0
C	60 mg	107	mg	178◄
D	400 IU	0	IU	0
E	15 IU	0.07	IU	15
K	500 μg	5,400	μg	1,080◄
Folic Acid	400 μg	99	μg	24

MINERALS USRDA		ONE SERVING GIVES YOU APPROXIMATELY		APPROXIMATE PERCENTAGE OF USRDA
Sodium	(1,100–3,000) mg	279	mg	27
Calcium	1,000 mg	43	mg	5
Phosphorus	(800–1,000) mg	79	mg	9
Potassium	(1,875–5,625) mg	550	mg	68
Magnesium	400 μg	23	μg	6
Selenium	200 μg	0.90	μg	0
Iodine	150 mg	0	mg	0
Zinc	15 mg	0.31	mg	2
Iron	10 mg	1	mg	10
Manganese	(2.5–5.0) mg	0.30	mg	6
Copper	(2.0–3.0) mg	0.5	mg	1

AMOUNT PER SERVING		CALORIES PER SERVING	% OF MEAL
Fat	0 grams	3	6
Proteins	3 grams	14	29
Carbohydrates	10 grams	32	65
Cholesterol	0 mg		
Amino acid (essential)			29–41
Fiber	1 gram		

Key: USRDA = Recommended Dietary Allowance

IU = International Unit

mg = milligrams

μg = micrograms

NOTE: The numbers with arrows exceed 100 percent of required USRDA.

Brussels Sprouts with Onions and Spices

Ingredients:

20 Brussels sprouts
    (5 for each serving)
1 cup of onions
    chopped roughly
1 tsp margarine or
    safflower oil
$\frac{1}{2}$ cup water
$\frac{1}{2}$ tsp marjoram
$\frac{1}{2}$ tsp cumin
    salt to taste

Preparation: Saute

Time: 20 minutes

Calories: 90 per serving

Serves: 4

Directions

Saute onions in margarine in a large skillet pan. Add the water, a little salt if you like, and the spices. Rinse the brussels sprouts and add to the pan. Cook on very low flame until the brussels sprouts are tender, about 7 to 10 minutes.

TIP: The vitamin C in foods on your plate will help block the formation of nitrosamine; researchers report that vitamins A and C will knock out free radicals* before they damage DNA (Deoxyribonucleic Acid) carrier of genetic information. The National Cancer Institute suggests at least three servings of vegetables a day, half a cup each.

MYTH: "Breast disease" is a disease.

FACT: Fibrocystic disease or benign breast disease is a misnomer. Doctors say it describes chronically lumpy breasts that may be painful and tender before menstruation. Dr. Susan Love of Harvard Medical School says these changes are normal and predictable and are "no more a disease than gray hair or age lines." The Cancer Committee of the College of American Pathologists say these conditions aren't disease but refer to a variety of changes and symptoms that occur in many women.

*Free radicals are substances in the body believed to contribute to cancer and other diseases.

Nutrients Contained in: Brussels Sprouts with Onions and Spices

VITAMINS USRDA			ONE SERVING GIVES YOU APPROXIMATELY		APPROXIMATE PERCENTAGE OF USRDA
A	5,000	IU	956	IU	19
B$_1$	1.4	mg	0.15	mg	12
B$_2$	1.6	mg	0.09	mg	6
B$_3$	16	mg	0.75	mg	4
B$_5$	10	mg	0.35	mg	3
B$_6$	2.2	mg	0.27	mg	12
B$_{12}$	3	μg	0	μg	0
C	60	mg	84	mg	140◄
D	400	IU	0	IU	0
E	15	IU	1	IU	7
K	500	μg	750	μg	150◄
Folic Acid	400	μg	66	μg	16

MINERALS USRDA			ONE SERVING GIVES YOU APPROXIMATELY		APPROXIMATE PERCENTAGE OF USRDA
Sodium	(1,100–3,000)	mg	59	mg	5
Calcium	1,000	mg	51	mg	6
Phosphorus	(800–1,000)	mg	77	mg	9
Potassium	(1,875–5,625)	mg	433	mg	54
Magnesium	400	μg	24	μg	6
Selenium	200	μg	46	μg	22
Iodine	150	mg	0	mg	0
Zinc	15	mg	0.47	mg	3
Iron	10	mg	1	mg	14
Manganese	(2.5–5.0)	mg	0.37	mg	7
Copper	(2.0–3.0)	mg	0.8	mg	2

AMOUNT PER SERVING		CALORIES PER SERVING	% OF MEAL
Fat	3 grams	29	33
Proteins	4 grams	15	16
Carbohydrates	11 grams	46	51
Cholesterol	20 mg		
Amino acid (essential)			19–45
Fiber	2 grams		

Key: USRDA = Recommended Dietary Allowance

     IU = International Unit

     mg = milligrams

     μg = micrograms

NOTE: The numbers with arrows exceed 100 percent of required USRDA.

VEGETABLES RANKED IN THE HIGHEST ORDER FOR VITAMIN C PERCENTAGES GIVEN EQUAL ½ CUP

	VITAMIN C (MILLIGRAMS)	PERCENTAGE OF USRDA
Peppers, chili, raw	109.0	181.7
Peppers, raw	94.7	157.8
Peppers, cooked	76.0	126.7
Broccoli, cooked	49.0	81.7
Brussels sprouts, cooked	48.4	80.7
Cauliflower, with cheese	42.0	70.0
Broccoli, raw	41.0	68.3
Peas, cooked	38.0	63.3
Broccoli, frozen	36.9	61.5
Cauliflower, raw	36.0	60.0
Broccoli, with cheese sauce	36.0	60.0
Brussels sprouts, frozen	35.6	59.3
Beans, kidney, canned	35.0	58.3
Cauliflower, cooked	34.3	57.2
Cauliflower, frozen	28.2	47.0
Potato, sweet	28.0	46.7
Potato, baked, with skin	26.0	43.3
Scallions, raw	22.0	36.7
Tomato, raw	21.6	36.0
Spinach, frozen	21.0	35.0
Cabbage, red, raw	20.0	33.3
Cabbage, cooked	18.2	30.3
Asparagus, cooked	18.2	30.3
Asparagus, canned	18.2	30.3
Tomato, canned	18.2	30.3
Peas, frozen	17.6	29.3
Sauerkraut, canned	17.4	29.0
Cabbage, raw	16.5	27.5
Spinach, canned	15.0	25.0
Asparagus, frozen	14.7	24.5
Turnip, raw	13.7	22.8
Okra, cooked	13.1	21.8
Potato, scalloped	13.0	21.7
Potato, au gratin	12.0	20.0
Peas, canned	12.0	20.0
Parsnips, raw	11.4	19.0

CHAPTER TWO

Healing and Preventive Recipes for Stroke

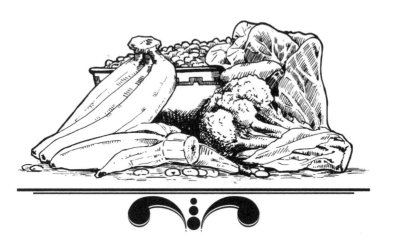

He who has health has hope, and he
who has hope has everything.
—Arabian proverb

Research shows that strokes are preventable and treatable. The best diets that protect against strokes caused by blockages of the arteries are those that are low in fat and low in cholesterol.

Government studies over a 12-year period indicate that potassium seems to protect against strokes. Eating just one banana or one serving of green leafy vegetables or beans daily was found to cut the risk of dying of a stroke by 40 percent.

Of course, smoking does not help. As a matter of fact, smoking is considered to be a major cause of stroke. It is also a matter of record that high blood pressure is one of the most important causes of stroke, so the recipes in this chapter include little or no salt or foods with high levels of sodium.

Since nutritionists and medical studies believe that daily intake of potassium-rich foods is of considerable importance in the prevention of strokes, the recipes here feature foods with very high content of potassium. This mineral is also known to lower blood pressure.

Getting lots of potassium in your diet isn't difficult when you know what foods contain how much. You can simply check the chart to determine exactly how much of the USRDA each meal is providing of this terrific mineral.

RECOMMENDED DIETARY ALLOWANCES
FOR POTASSIUM

GROUP/AGE	POTASSIUM (MILLIGRAMS)
Infants 0–6 months	350– 925
Infants 7–12 months	425–1,275
Children 1–3 years	550–1,650
Children 4–6 years	775–2,325
Children 7–10 years	1,000–3,000
Males 11–18 years	1,525–4,575
Males 19+ years	1,875–5,625
Females 11–18 years	1,525–4,575
Females 19+ years	1,875–5,625

Spaghetti, Potato, and Onion Round

Ingredients:

1 lb new potatoes, sliced
1 cup skim milk
1 lb whole wheat
   spaghetti
1 cup onions, sliced
1 tsp marjoram
½ tsp allspice
1 tsp safflower oil
6 cloves garlic, chopped
   finely
2 Tbs Parmesan cheese
1 tsp cinnamon
   juice of one lime
½ tsp caraway seeds
   chili powder

Preparation: Boil and saute

Time: 30 minutes

Calories: 413 per serving

Serves: 4

Directions

Put potatoes in a large saucepan, pour in milk, and add marjoram and allspice. Cover and simmer over medium heat until potatoes are tender enough for fork to pierce easily. Stir in caraway seeds, cinnamon, and chili powder to taste. Set aside. Cook pasta according to package instructions. Heat oil in skillet over medium heat. Stir in onion and saute until golden brown, about 3 minutes. Add onion to reserved potatoes. Add garlic to skillet and saute over medium heat. Stir in lime juice. Put low heat under potatoes. Stir in pasta and Parmesan cheese and cook until cheese melts. Check your chart to see the bonanza of potassium percentages, selenium, and essential amino acids.

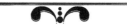

TIP: A study in the *New England Journal of Medicine* suggested that if people were to eat just a single additional serving of fresh vegetables or fruit a day, they might realize a 40 percent reduction in the risk of having a fatal stroke. That study followed 859 people in California for 12 years. After all the statistics were considered, potassium emerged as the antistroke power-house, independent of all other foods and factors.

MYTH: Hay fever is caused by exposure to stacks of hay.

FACT: The name is misleading. Hay fever is not caused by hay and does not cause fever. Ragweed is said to be the chief culprit in hay fever.

Nutrients Contained in: Spaghetti, Potato, and Onion Round

VITAMINS USRDA			ONE SERVING GIVES YOU APPROXIMATELY		APPROXIMATE PERCENTAGE OF USRDA
A	5,000	IU	144	IU	2
B₁	1.4	mg	0.44	mg	36
B₂	1.6	mg	0.21	mg	14
B₃	16	mg	4	mg	27
B₅	10	mg	2	mg	16
B₆	2.2	mg	0.82	mg	37
B₁₂	3	μg	0.24	μg	8
C	60	mg	29	mg	48
D	400	IU	25	IU	6
E	15	IU	2	IU	10
K	500	μg	0	μg	0
Folic Acid	400	μg	37	μg	9

MINERALS USRDA			ONE SERVING GIVES YOU APPROXIMATELY		APPROXIMATE PERCENTAGE OF USRDA
Sodium	(1,100–3,000)	mg	96	mg	9
Calcium	1,000	mg	154	mg	19
Phosphorus	(800–1,000)	mg	255	mg	31
Potassium	(1,875–5,625)	mg	1,152	mg	144◄
Magnesium	400	μg	78	μg	22
Selenium	200	μg	16	μg	7
Iodine	150	mg	3	mg	2
Zinc	15	mg	1	mg	8
Iron	10	mg	2	mg	17
Manganese	(2.5–5.0)	mg	0.43	mg	8
Copper	(2.0–3.0)	mg	0.53	mg	17

AMOUNT PER SERVING		CALORIES PER SERVING	% OF MEAL
Fat	5 grams	45	11
Proteins	12 grams	46	11
Carbohydrates	81 grams	322	78
Cholesterol	3 mg		
Amino acid (essential)			128–145
Fiber	1 gram		

Key: USRDA = Recommended Dietary Allowance

    IU = International Unit

    mg = milligrams

    μg = micrograms

NOTE: The numbers with arrows exceed 100 percent of required USRDA.

A Different Cabbage and Pork

Ingredients:

4 boneless pork loin cutlets, about 3.5 ounces each
1 Tbs vegetable oil
½ cup onion, chopped
1 tsp garlic, chopped
½ head of cabbage
½ cup low-sodium chicken broth
½ tsp coriander
¼ cup yogurt
1 tsp chili powder
black pepper

Preparation: Saute, simmer, boil

Time: 45 minutes

Calories: 435 per serving

Serves: 4

Directions

Sprinkle the cutlets with black pepper and a little garlic powder. Heat oil in a large iron skillet. When oil is hot, add the cutlets and cook over medium high heat for about 5 minutes. Turn the slices and cook until second side is brown. Sprinkle onion, coriander, garlic, and chili powder around the pork in the pan. Cook and stir for a few minutes. Add the chicken broth and bring to a boil. Simmer for 10 minutes. Stir in the yogurt and serve immediately.

TIP: Avocados' bad fat rap may have a good aspect. One avocado has about 300 calories, most of it coming from fat, but it also has a good amount of potassium. Bananas have less. Avocados also contain vitamins A, B$_6$, and C; copper; and 30 grams of fat. That means you wouldn't want to eat them very often.

MYTH: Sour milk will make you sick.

FACT: Slightly sour milk will not make you sick. For duration and taste, milk is at its best when kept at 45° F or below.

Nutrients Contained in: A Different Cabbage and Pork

VITAMINS USRDA			ONE SERVING GIVES YOU APPROXIMATELY		APPROXIMATE PERCENTAGE OF USRDA
A	5,000	IU	171	IU	3
B_1	1.4	mg	1	mg	86
B_2	1.6	mg	0.40	mg	28
B_3	16	mg	6	mg	38
B_5	10	mg	1	mg	11
B_6	2.2	mg	0.61	mg	27
B_{12}	3	μg	1	μg	35
C	60	mg	56	mg	92
D	400	IU	28	IU	6
E	15	IU	3	IU	17
K	500	μg	50	μg	10
Folic Acid	400	μg	76	μg	18

MINERALS USRDA			ONE SERVING GIVES YOU APPROXIMATELY		APPROXIMATE PERCENTAGE OF USRDA
Sodium	(1,100–3,000)	mg	202	mg	20
Calcium	1,000	mg	119	mg	14
Phosphorus	(800–1,000)	mg	303	mg	37
Potassium	(1,875–5,625)	mg	765	mg	95
Magnesium	400	μg	46	μg	13
Selenium	200	μg	19	μg	9
Iodine	150	mg	13	mg	8
Zinc	15	mg	3	mg	17
Iron	10	mg	2	mg	16
Manganese	(2.5–5.0)	mg	0.22	mg	4
Copper	(2.0–3.0)	mg	0.12	mg	3

AMOUNT PER SERVING		CALORIES PER SERVING	% OF MEAL
Fat	33 grams	297	68
Proteins	24 grams	96	22
Carbohydrates	11 grams	42	10
Cholesterol	83 mg		
Amino acid (essential)			272–490
Fiber	1 gram		

Key: USRDA = Recommended Dietary Allowance
    IU = International Unit
    mg = milligrams
    μg = micrograms
NOTE: The numbers with arrows exceed 100 percent of required USRDA.

Pork and Prunes

Ingredients:
- 2 lb boneless pork loin roast
- 2 tsp cornstarch
- $\frac{1}{4}$ tsp cinnamon
- 2 Tbs orange juice
- 2 cups prunes
- 1 tsp allspice
- cayenne pepper

Preparation: Roast

Time: 1 hour, 15 minutes

Calories: 324 per serving

Serves: 8

Directions

Preheat oven to 325° F. In a saucepan stir together all the ingredients except the pork and prunes. Cook stirring over medium heat until thickened. Set aside. Place roast in a baking dish with the prunes surrounding it and on top. Roast for about 45 minutes. Spoon $\frac{1}{2}$ cup of mixture over roast and continue roasting for 35 to 45 minutes more. Let stand about 10 minutes before slicing and serve with remaining sauce.

TIP: Potassium is one of the aids protecting against stroke and other diseases. You don't have to worry about overdosing when potassium is obtained from food, as the body flushes away excess amounts. Potassium can be toxic to people with diseases of heart, kidney, or liver. Check with your physician before taking supplements.

MYTH: Spinach is the best source of iron, except meat.

FACT: Popeye, to the contrary, the largest source of iron is from grain products. Such items as pasta, fortified cereal, and breads give more.

Nutrients Contained in: Pork and Prunes

VITAMINS USRDA			ONE SERVING GIVES YOU APPROXIMATELY		APPROXIMATE PERCENTAGE OF USRDA
A	5,000	IU	178	IU	3
B_1	1.4	mg	1	mg	120◄
B_2	1.6	mg	0.44	mg	31
B_3	16	mg	6	mg	35
B_5	10	mg	0.97	mg	9
B_6	2.2	mg	0.62	mg	28
B_{12}	3	μg	0.79	μg	26
C	60	mg	5	mg	8
D	400	IU	28	IU	7
E	15	IU	0.68	IU	4
K	500	μg	12	μg	2
Folic Acid	400	μg	34	μg	3

MINERALS USRDA			ONE SERVING GIVES YOU APPROXIMATELY		APPROXIMATE PERCENTAGE OF USRDA
Sodium	(1,100–3,000)	mg	63	mg	6
Calcium	1,000	mg	18	mg	2
Phosphorus	(800–1,000)	mg	358	mg	44
Potassium	(1,875–5,625)	mg	765	mg	95
Magnesium	400	μg	41	μg	11
Selenium	200	μg	53	μg	26
Iodine	150	mg	0	mg	0
Zinc	15	mg	2	mg	10
Iron	10	mg	6	mg	58
Manganese	(2.5–5.0)	mg	0.07	mg	1
Copper	(2.0–3.0)	mg	0.12	mg	4

AMOUNT PER SERVING		CALORIES PER SERVING	% OF MEAL
Fat	14 grams	123	38
Proteins	35 grams	140	43
Carbohydrates	16 grams	61	19
Cholesterol	101 mg		
Amino acid (essential)			216–538
Fiber	1 gram		

Key: USRDA = Recommended Dietary Allowance
  IU = International Unit
  mg = milligrams
  μg = micrograms
NOTE: The numbers with arrows exceed 100 percent of required USRDA.

Turkey Breast, Wheat Germ, and Shiitake

Ingredients:

1 ½ lb turkey breast, sliced
12 shiitake mushrooms, fresh if possible
2 Tbs wheat germ
2 Tbs vegetable oil
4 cloves garlic, minced
½ cup spring onion, coarsely chopped
½ cup low-sodium chicken broth
1 Tbs prepared mustard
1 Tbs horseradish
⅓ cup apple cider
pepper

Preparation: Saute

Time: 25 minutes

Calories: 366 per serving

Serves: 4

Directions

If turkey slices are too thick, pound them with a mallet to a thickness of about ¼ inch. Chop mushrooms. Season the wheat germ with pepper and dredge the slices on all sides. Heat 1 tablespoon of oil in a skillet and add turkey slices to skillet. Cook over medium-high heat until done on one side and then turn and repeat on other side, about 6 minutes all told. Remove slices to a warm platter, add remaining oil to skillet, and repeat if there are still slices to cook. Remove and place with other slices on platter. In the same skillet, add mushrooms and cook for about 3 minutes. Add garlic and spring onion and cook briefly. Add cider and cook, stirring, for about 5 minutes. Add broth and mustard. Blend well. Bring to a simmer and cook stirring for about 1 minute. Add juices from turkey slices if any has accumulated and mix. Pour over slices.

TIP: Researchers at the Cooper Institute for Aerobics in Dallas say a benefit of walking, even if you only amble rather than walk quickly, is that it raises "good" HDL cholesterol. This was the result of a group of women walkers who took up to a one-hour walk five days a week at a pace of under 3 miles an hour.

MYTH: New mothers should drink a glass of wine or beer before breast-feeding to boost the amount of milk they can produce.

FACT: Scientists at the Monell Chemical Senses Center in Philadelphia researching this say that this is an old wives' tale and such advice is not based on scientific fact.

Nutrients Contained in: Turkey Breast, Wheat Germ, and Shiitake

VITAMINS USRDA			ONE SERVING GIVES YOU APPROXIMATELY		APPROXIMATE PERCENTAGE OF USRDA
A	5,000	IU	746	IU	14
B$_1$	1.4	mg	0.41	mg	34
B$_2$	1.6	mg	0.31	mg	21
B$_3$	16	mg	8	mg	52
B$_5$	10	mg	5	mg	51
B$_6$	2.2	mg	0.56	mg	25
B$_{12}$	3	μg	0.32	μg	10
C	60	mg	7	mg	11
D	400	IU	0	IU	0
E	15	IU	0.23	IU	1
K	500	μg	3	μg	0
Folic Acid	400	μg	127	μg	31

MINERALS USRDA			ONE SERVING GIVES YOU APPROXIMATELY		APPROXIMATE PERCENTAGE OF USRDA
Sodium	(1,100–3,000)	mg	181	mg	18
Calcium	1,000	mg	35	mg	4
Phosphorus	(800–1,000)	mg	378	mg	47
Potassium	(1,875–5,625)	mg	715	mg	89
Magnesium	400	μg	118	μg	33
Selenium	200	μg	0	μg	0
Iodine	150	mg	0	mg	0
Zinc	15	mg	8	mg	50
Iron	10	mg	3	mg	31
Manganese	(2.5–5.0)	mg	4	mg	84
Copper	(2.0–3.0)	mg	0.20	mg	6

AMOUNT PER SERVING		CALORIES PER SERVING	% OF MEAL
Fat	10 grams	93	25
Proteins	25 grams	100	27
Carbohydrates	43 grams	173	47
Cholesterol	64 mg		
Amino acid (essential)			250–365
Fiber	0 gram		

Key: USRDA = Recommended Dietary Allowance
     IU = International Unit
     mg = milligrams
     μg = micrograms
NOTE: The numbers with arrows exceed 100 percent of required USRDA.

Black Fungus Lima Bean Soup

Ingredients:

2 cups cooked lima beans
2 cups carrots, sliced
1 Tbs olive oil
4 cloves of garlic, chopped
18 black fungus mushrooms, dried
½ cup skim milk
¼ cup half and half cream
½ tsp chili powder
½ tsp cumin
   cayenne pepper

Preparation: Steam and saute

Time: 35 minutes

Calories: 265 per serving

Serves: 6

Directions

Boil water, place mushrooms in water and let soak until tender, about 15 minutes. Steam carrots until tender. Reserve 1 cup of cooking water. Heat oil in skillet and saute garlic and mushrooms for about 8 to 10 minutes. Combine all the other ingredients (except milk and cream) along with the beans and carrot cooking water. Process in a blender until smooth. Pour mixture into a large pot and add milk and cream. Cook over medium heat for about 15 minutes. Your chart will show high percentages of vitamin A and potassium.

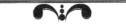

TIP: You can easily figure out your percentage of fat calories by multiplying the number of grams of fat per serving by 9 (1 gram of fat = 9 calories.) To check the percentage of calories from fat, divide by the total number of calories per serving. Let's take the 3 grams of fat from this recipe and the 262 total calories per serving. Multiply 3 (grams) by 9 (calories) and you get 27 calories from fat. Divide this by 262 (total calories), and you get 10 percent. These figures may vary by one or two percentage points.

MYTH: Placing aspirin directly on an aching gum gets fast relief.

FACT: Dr. Jerry F. Taintor of the University of Tennessee College of Dentistry says this process can cause an aspirin burn. He advises the old-fashioned way for aspirin intake—swallow it.

Nutrients Contained in: Black Fungus Lima Bean Soup

VITAMINS USRDA			ONE SERVING GIVES YOU APPROXIMATELY		APPROXIMATE PERCENTAGE OF USRDA
A	5,000	IU	13,585	IU	271◄
B$_1$	1.4	mg	0.14	mg	11
B$_2$	1.6	mg	0.14	mg	10
B$_3$	16	mg	4	mg	27
B$_5$	10	mg	0.31	mg	3
B$_6$	2.2	mg	0.22	mg	9
B$_{12}$	3	μg	.08	μg	2
C	60	mg	10	mg	17
D	400	IU	8	IU	2
E	15	IU	1	IU	7
K	500	μg	67	μg	13
Folic Acid	400	μg	126	μg	31

MINERALS USRDA			ONE SERVING GIVES YOU APPROXIMATELY		APPROXIMATE PERCENTAGE OF USRDA
Sodium	(1,100–3,000)	mg	47	mg	4
Calcium	1,000	mg	63	mg	7
Phosphorus	(800–1,000)	mg	122	mg	15
Potassium	(1,875–5,625)	mg	783	mg	97
Magnesium	400	μg	82	μg	23
Selenium	200	μg	1	μg	0
Iodine	150	mg	1	mg	0
Zinc	15	mg	4	mg	24
Iron	10	mg	2	mg	17
Manganese	(2.5–5.0)	mg	0.78	mg	15
Copper	(2.0–3.0)	mg	0.21	mg	7

AMOUNT PER SERVING		CALORIES PER SERVING	% OF MEAL
Fat	3 grams	27	9
Proteins	9 grams	34	13
Carbohydrates	51 grams	204	78
Cholesterol	0 mg		
Amino acid (essential)			52–86
Fiber	2 grams		

Key: USRDA = Recommended Dietary Allowance
     IU = International Unit
     mg = milligrams
     μg = micrograms
NOTE: The numbers with arrows exceed 100 percent of required USRDA.

Spear and Oval Salad

Ingredients:

16 spears of asparagus, trimmed
1 large red pepper
½ cup chopped onion
1 Tbs prepared mustard
1 Tbs vinegar
¼ tsp ground mint
¼ tsp dry chervil
   juice of one lime
4 tsp safflower oil

Preparation: Steam and broil

Time: 20 minutes

Calories: 148 per serving

Serves: 4

Directions

Put asparagus in hot steamer for about 6 minutes. Core pepper, discard seeds and cut into ¼ inch-wide rounds. Broil slices on both sides until well done. Combine broiled peppers and asparagus in a large salad bowl. Mix the mustard, vinegar, mint, chervil, and lime juice in a small bowl. Stir and gradually add the oil. Add this dressing to the vegetables and blend.

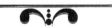

TIP: Using fruit and vegetable consumption as a marker for potassium, a British survey found a threefold variation in stroke rate across the population. The lowest rate was among people who ate the most fruits and vegetables. In the United States Dr. Louis Tobian, professor of medicine at the University of Minnesota at Minneapolis, said Americans could raise their potassium levels simply by cutting down on junk food and soft drinks.

MYTH: MSG (monosodium glutamate), commonly used to enhance the flavor of Chinese food, causes headaches.

FACT: Scientists say that nothing conclusively supporting this idea has been documented in human beings. The World Health Organization and the European Communities Scientific Committee for Food have concluded that MSG is safe.

Nutrients Contained in: Spear and Oval Salad

VITAMINS USRDA			ONE SERVING GIVES YOU APPROXIMATELY		APPROXIMATE PERCENTAGE OF USRDA
A	5,000	IU	1,194	IU	23
B$_1$	1.4	mg	0.08	mg	6
B$_2$	1.6	mg	0.10	mg	6
B$_3$	16	mg	0.72	mg	4
B$_5$	10	mg	0.12	mg	1
B$_6$	2.2	mg	0.10	mg	4
B$_{12}$	3	μg	0	μg	0
C	60	mg	42	mg	69
D	400	IU	0	IU	0
E	15	IU	8	IU	56
K	500	μg	40	μg	8
Folic Acid	400	μg	62	μg	15

MINERALS USRDA			ONE SERVING GIVES YOU APPROXIMATELY		APPROXIMATE PERCENTAGE OF USRDA
Sodium	(1,100–3,000)	mg	4	mg	0
Calcium	1,000	mg	23	mg	2
Phosphorus	(800–1,000)	mg	43	mg	5
Potassium	(1,875–5,625)	mg	242	mg	30
Magnesium	400	μg	15	μg	4
Selenium	200	μg	0.18	μg	0
Iodine	150	mg	0	mg	0
Zinc	15	mg	0.37	mg	2
Iron	10	mg	0.80	mg	7
Manganese	(2.5–5.0)	mg	0.14	mg	2
Copper	(2.0–3.0)	mg	0.08	mg	2

AMOUNT PER SERVING		CALORIES PER SERVING	% OF MEAL
Fat	14 grams	124	84
Proteins	2 grams	8	5
Carbohydrates	4 grams	16	11
Cholesterol	0 mg		
Amino acid (essential)			13–28*
Fiber	1 gram		

Key: USRDA = Recommended Dietary Allowance

IU = International Unit

mg = milligrams

μg = micrograms

NOTE: The numbers with arrows exceed 100 percent of required USRDA.

*Complementary food—1 cup of wheat berries raises EAA to 186–364%.

Open Sesame Turkey

Ingredients: 1 ½ lb skinless, boneless turkey breast
⅔ cup rolled oats
1 tsp canola oil
1 tsp thyme, dried
1 Tbs sesame seeds
1 Tbs prepared horseradish
1 tsp garlic powder
1 lemon, sliced
½ tsp sage
black pepper
noncaloric spray

Preparation: Bake

Time: 55 minutes

Calories: 207 per serving

Serves: 6

Directions

Preheat oven to 350° F. In a blender grind oats until fine. Mix oats with thyme, pepper, sesame seeds, garlic powder, and sage. Place mixture on a platter and roll turkey breasts to coat. Spray baking dish with noncaloric spray. Place turkey in the dish and cook for about 40 minutes. Serve with horseradish and lemon pieces.

TIP: Dark meat from turkey and chicken has a little more fat and cholesterol than white meat. A 3-ounce serving of skinless, roasted, dark turkey meat has about 7 grams of fat and 85 milligrams of cholesterol. The Mayo Clinic *Health Letter* recommends that you limit amounts of all types of meat to no more than 5 to 7 ounces daily.

MYTH: Eating a lot of high-fat almonds will increase your cholesterol levels.

FACT: A study in the *Journal of the American College of Nutrition* says that eating those almonds may *reduce* cholesterol levels. Researchers suggest that cholesterol levels dropped in participants because the fat in almonds is monounsaturated.

Nutrients Contained in: Open Sesame Turkey

VITAMINS USRDA			ONE SERVING GIVES YOU APPROXIMATELY		APPROXIMATE PERCENTAGE OF USRDA
A	5,000	IU	40	IU	0
B$_1$	1.4	mg	0.04	mg	3
B$_2$	1.6	mg	0.07	mg	5
B$_3$	16	mg	3	mg	16
B$_5$	10	mg	3	mg	33
B$_6$	2.2	mg	0.22	mg	10
B$_{12}$	3	μg	.19	μg	6
C	60	mg	0	mg	0
D	400	IU	0	IU	0
E	15	IU	0.43	IU	2
K	500	μg	0	μg	0
Folic Acid	400	μg	5	μg	0

MINERALS USRDA			ONE SERVING GIVES YOU APPROXIMATELY		APPROXIMATE PERCENTAGE OF USRDA
Sodium	(1,100–3,000)	mg	107	mg	10
Calcium	1,000	mg	70	mg	8
Phosphorus	(800–1,000)	mg	153	mg	19
Potassium	(1,875–5,625)	mg	159	mg	19
Magnesium	400	μg	25	μg	7
Selenium	200	μg	0	μg	0
Iodine	150	mg	0	mg	0
Zinc	15	mg	2	mg	10
Iron	10	mg	0.75	mg	7
Manganese	(2.5–5.0)	mg	0	mg	0
Copper	(2.0–3.0)	mg	0.15	mg	5

AMOUNT PER SERVING		CALORIES PER SERVING	% OF MEAL
Fat	11 grams	96	43
Proteins	15 grams	71	34
Carbohydrates	12 grams	4	23
Cholesterol	32 mg		
Amino acid (essential)			168–248
Fiber	1 gram		

Key: USRDA = Recommended Dietary Allowance
    IU = International Unit
    mg = milligrams
    μg = micrograms
NOTE: The numbers with arrows exceed 100 percent of required USRDA.

A Bean Bake

Ingredients:
- ½ cup navy beans, cooked
- 2 cups pinto beans, cooked
- 1 cup kidney beans, cooked
- 2 Tbs honey
- 1 tsp prepared mustard
- ½ cup chopped onions
- 2 cloves garlic, minced
- dash cayenne pepper
- ½ tsp chili powder
- ½ tsp chervil

Preparation: Bake

Time: 55 minutes

Calories: 152 per serving

Serves: 4-6

Directions

Preheat oven to 375° F. Combine all ingredients and place into large baking dish. Bake 45 minutes or until very hot. Stir and serve.

TIP: The National Stroke Association, a nonprofit education organization, offers materials on a wide range of topics from brochures on poststroke depression and home exercise for stroke patients. Free pamphlets on such subjects as stroke prevention also are available. Write 300 East Hampden Avenue, Suite 240, Englewood, CO 80110.

MYTH: Women who take vitamin A supplements benefit from lower rates of breast cancer.

FACT: Harvard researchers have found that women who eat foods rich in vitamin A have lower rates of breast cancer, but those who take vitamin A supplements do not. They do not know why this is so.

Nutrients Contained in: A Bean Bake

VITAMINS USRDA			ONE SERVING GIVES YOU APPROXIMATELY		APPROXIMATE PERCENTAGE OF USRDA
A	5,000	IU	3	IU	0
B_1	1.4	mg	0.14	mg	11
B_2	1.6	mg	0.07	mg	4
B_3	16	mg	0.57	mg	3
B_5	10	mg	0.02	mg	0
B_6	2.2	mg	0.09	mg	3
B_{12}	3	μg	0	μg	0
C	60	mg	2	mg	3
D	400	IU	0	IU	0
E	15	IU	0.76	IU	5
K	500	μg	0	μg	0
Folic Acid	400	μg	51	μg	12

MINERALS USRDA			ONE SERVING GIVES YOU APPROXIMATELY		APPROXIMATE PERCENTAGE OF USRDA
Sodium	(1,100–3,000)	mg	128	mg	12
Calcium	1,000	mg	46	mg	5
Phosphorus	(800–1,000)	mg	146	mg	18
Potassium	(1,875–5,625)	mg	395	mg	49
Magnesium	400	μg	27	μg	7
Selenium	200	μg	1	μg	0
Iodine	150	mg	0	mg	0
Zinc	15	mg	0.66	mg	4
Iron	10	mg	2	mg	22
Manganese	(2.5–5.0)	mg	0.02	mg	0
Copper	(2.0–3.0)	mg	0.22	mg	7

AMOUNT PER SERVING		CALORIES PER SERVING	% OF MEAL
Fat	0 gram	4	3
Proteins	8 grams	32	21
Carbohydrates	29 grams	116	76
Cholesterol	0 mg		
Amino acid (essential)			53–192
Fiber	5 grams		

Key: USRDA = Recommended Dietary Allowance

IU = International Unit

mg = milligrams

μg = micrograms

NOTE: The numbers with arrows exceed 100 percent of required USRDA.

Kidney Beans, Barley, and Wheat

Ingredients:

2 cups kidney beans, cooked
½ cup cracked wheat (groats)
½ cup pearl barley
1 onion, chopped fine
1 tsp margarine
2 cups low-sodium chicken broth
1 carrot, diced
2 stalks celery, cut in 1/4-inch slices
black pepper
½ tsp chili powder
1 bay leaf
½ tsp oregano

Preparation: Saute
Time: 60 minutes
Calories: 254 per serving
Serves: 4-6

Directions

Used large iron skillet. Heat margarine and cook onion and carrot until onion is lightly browned. Add broth, barley, and bay leaf. Let simmer; then cook, covered, over low heat until barley is tender, about 30 minutes. Stir in wheat, pepper, and celery and mix well. Cover and cook on low heat for about 15 minutes. Stir in drained beans and cook a few minutes more. Remove from heat and stir in oregano and chili powder. Let stand a few minutes then serve. This meal is high in EAA and potassium, as your chart will show.

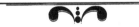

TIP: One cup of cooked beans provides almost half the federal government's Recommended Daily Allowance of iron for men and one-fourth of the USRDA for women. Beans are loaded with soluble and insoluble fiber and are an important asset in a cholesterol-lowering diet.

MYTH: All fats are equally harmful to eat.

FACT: Not so. Researchers at the Fred Hutchinson Cancer Research Center in Seattle, Washington, report that of the three basic fats—saturated, polyunsaturated, and monounsaturated—the real warning has been to avoid saturated fats. Meat and dairy products have large amounts of saturated fat.

Nutrients Contained in: Kidney, Barley, and Wheat

VITAMINS USRDA		ONE SERVING GIVES YOU APPROXIMATELY		APPROXIMATE PERCENTAGE OF USRDA
A	5,000 IU	5,004	IU	100
B_1	1.4 mg	0.25	mg	20
B_2	1.6 mg	0.12	mg	8
B_3	16 mg	3	mg	20
B_5	10 mg	0.28	mg	2
B_6	2.2 mg	0.17	mg	7
B_{12}	3 μg	0.11	μg	3
C	60 mg	5	mg	8
D	400 IU	0	IU	0
E	15 IU	2	IU	12
K	500 μg	25	μg	5
Folic Acid	400 μg	12	μg	3

MINERALS USRDA		ONE SERVING GIVES YOU APPROXIMATELY		APPROXIMATE PERCENTAGE OF USRDA
Sodium	(1,100–3,000) mg	301	mg	30
Calcium	1,000 mg	57	mg	7
Phosphorus	(800–1,000) mg	233	mg	29
Potassium	(1,875–5,625) mg	591	mg	73
Magnesium	400 μg	16	μg	4
Selenium	200 μg	1	μg	0
Iodine	150 mg	0	mg	0
Zinc	15 mg	0.20	mg	1
Iron	10 mg	3	mg	33
Manganese	(2.5–5.0) mg	0.34	mg	6
Copper	(2.0–3.0) mg	0.35	mg	11

AMOUNT PER SERVING		CALORIES PER SERVING	% OF MEAL
Fat	2 grams	14	6
Proteins	12 grams	47	18
Carbohydrates	48 grams	193	76
Cholesterol	0 mg		
Amino acid (essential)			128–362
Fiber	2 grams		

Key: USRDA = Recommended Dietary Allowance

IU = International Unit

mg = milligrams

μg = micrograms

NOTE: The numbers with arrows exceed 100 percent of required USRDA.

Celery, Pepper, and Lentil Refreshment

Ingredients:

- 1 lb new potatoes
- ½ lb lentils, clean and washed
- 1 tsp canola oil
- 1 cup onions, chopped
- 1 clove garlic, chopped finely
- 1 large green pepper, chopped
- ½ cup celery, chopped
- 1 ½ cups canned tomatoes
- 1 tsp dried chervil
- ½ tsp dried coriander
- ½ tsp dried basil
- juice of one lime
- black pepper

Preparation: Boil and saute

Time: 40 minutes

Calories: 350 per serving

Serves: 4

Directions

Cut potatoes in small pieces; do not peel. Boil for about 10 minutes or until fork easily pierces potato. Put lentils in a pot covering them with water. Cover pot and bring to a boil. Reduce heat, uncover, and cook 20–25 minutes. Don't let them get mushy. Heat the oil in a skillet and saute the onion and garlic for about 2 minutes. Add the green pepper, celery, and tomatoes and cook about 5 minutes. Drain the cooked potatoes and add to the skillet. Add the cooked lentils as well, drain off excess liquid. In last minute or so of cooking, add all the spices. Season with black pepper and sprinkle with lime juice. Potassium content is very high.

TIP: A high intake of dietary potassium protects individuals against stroke and stroke-related deaths, and as little as one extra serving of a potassium-rich food per day may reduce the risk of stroke death by up to 40 percent. This is from Dr. Kay-Tee Khaw, a professor of clinical gerontology at the University of Cambridge in England, reporting the results of her 12-year study of 589 men and women.

MYTH: Certain foods contain high HDL cholesterol, the good kind.

FACT: Food does not contain either HDL cholesterol or the bad kind, LDL cholesterol. These forms of cholesterol are made by the body from the foods you eat.

Nutrients Contained in: Celery, Pepper and Lentil Refreshment

VITAMINS USRDA			ONE SERVING GIVES YOU APPROXIMATELY		APPROXIMATE PERCENTAGE OF USRDA
A	5,000	IU	708	IU	14
B$_1$	1.4	mg	0.28	mg	23
B$_2$	1.6	mg	0.14	mg	9
B$_3$	16	mg	4	mg	23
B$_5$	10	mg	2	mg	16
B$_6$	2.2	mg	0.85	mg	38
B$_{12}$	3	μg	0	μg	0
C	60	mg	65	mg	108◄
D	400	IU	0	IU	0
E	15	IU	2	IU	13
K	500	μg	2	μg	0
Folic Acid	400	μg	38	μg	9

MINERALS USRDA			ONE SERVING GIVES YOU APPROXIMATELY		APPROXIMATE PERCENTAGE OF USRDA
Sodium	(1,100–3,000)	mg	206	mg	20
Calcium	1,000	mg	80	mg	10
Phosphorus	(800–1,000)	mg	170	mg	21
Potassium	(1,875–5,625)	mg	1,155	mg	144◄
Magnesium	400	μg	83	μg	23
Selenium	200	μg	4	μg	2
Iodine	150	mg	0	mg	0
Zinc	15	mg	1	mg	8
Iron	10	mg	4	mg	43
Manganese	(2.5–5.0)	mg	0.51	mg	10
Copper	(2.0–3.0)	mg	0.65	mg	21

AMOUNT PER SERVING		CALORIES PER SERVING	% OF MEAL
Fat	4 grams	36	12
Proteins	9 grams	37	12
Carbohydrates	57 grams	277	76
Cholesterol	0 mg		
Amino acid (essential)			93–231
Fiber	10 grams		

Key: USRDA = Recommended Dietary Allowance
　　　　IU = International Unit
　　　mg = milligrams
　　　μg = micrograms
NOTE: The numbers with arrows exceed 100 percent of required USRDA.

On Guard with Swordfish

Ingredients:

4 3.5-ounce pieces of swordfish
2 onions, quartered
1 red pepper, seeded and cut in pieces
12 cherry tomatoes
2 cloves of garlic, crushed
1 Tbs prepared mustard
2 Tbs horseradish
juice of one lemon
cayenne pepper

Preparation: Grill on skewer

Time: 20 minutes

Calories: 151 per serving

Serves: 4

Directions

Brush fish with a mixture of horseradish, prepared mustard, garlic, a bit of cayenne pepper, and lemon juice. Place fish on presoaked wooden or metal skewers alternating red pepper pieces, cherry tomatoes, and onion quarters. Cook quickly on either a grill or in broiler. Cook until fish is done through. Contains good levels of potassium and vitamin A.

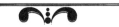

TIP: According to a University of Washington–Seattle report, older or postmenopausal women, especially former smokers, should consider estrogen replacement therapy as a stroke preventive. That finding reinforces a government report that indicated estrogen reduces all stroke risk by 24 percent.

MYTH: Scallops, shrimp, and other shellfish have no place as part of a low-fat, low-cholesterol diet.

FACT: The most recent report on this subject says that more accurate testing methods reveal that shellfish generally contain less cholesterol than was once thought. Their levels can be only slightly more than half that of some lean red meats. The National Center for Nutrition and Dietetics reports that shellfish offers some advantages taken in moderation. The majority are lower in total fat, and most are much lower in saturated fat than are most cuts of meat, including chicken.

Nutrients Contained in: On Guard with Swordfish

VITAMINS USRDA			ONE SERVING GIVES YOU APPROXIMATELY		APPROXIMATE PERCENTAGE OF USRDA
A	5,000	IU	2,004	IU	40
B_1	1.4	mg	0.11	mg	9
B_2	1.6	mg	0.08	mg	5
B_3	16	mg	8	mg	51
B_5	10	mg	0.35	mg	3
B_6	2.2	mg	0.11	mg	4
B_{12}	3	μg	1	μg	33
C	60	mg	37	mg	61
D	400	IU	0	IU	0
E	15	IU	0.82	IU	5
K	500	μg	3	μg	0
Folic Acid	400	μg	22	μg	5

MINERALS USRDA			ONE SERVING GIVES YOU APPROXIMATELY		APPROXIMATE PERCENTAGE OF USRDA
Sodium	(1,100–3,000)	mg	12	mg	1
Calcium	1,000	mg	41	mg	5
Phosphorus	(800–1,000)	mg	224	mg	28
Potassium	(1,875–5,625)	mg	649	mg	81
Magnesium	400	μg	19	μg	5
Selenium	200	μg	4	μg	2
Iodine	150	mg	0	mg	0
Zinc	15	mg	0.93	mg	6
Iron	10	mg	1	mg	14
Manganese	(2.5–5.0)	mg	0.11	mg	2
Copper	(2.0–3.0)	mg	0.07	mg	2

AMOUNT PER SERVING		CALORIES PER SERVING	% OF MEAL
Fat	4 grams	39	26
Proteins	20 grams	82	54
Carbohydrates	7 grams	30	20
Cholesterol	0 mg		
Amino acid (essential)			119–392
Fiber	1 gram		

Key: USRDA = Recommended Dietary Allowance

IU = International Unit

mg = milligrams

μg = micrograms

NOTE: The numbers with arrows exceed 100 percent of required USRDA.

Spaghetti, Asparagus, and Beetgreens with Almonds

Ingredients:

1	lb spaghetti
16	spears asparagus
1	cup beetgreens
1	tsp safflower oil
$\frac{1}{4}$	cup water
$\frac{1}{4}$	cup slivered almonds
2	tomatoes, chopped
4	cloves garlic, sliced
	chili powder
	sage
	crushed red pepper flakes

Preparation: Boil and saute

Time: 25 minutes

Calories: 185 per serving

Serves: 4

Directions

Cook spaghetti according to package instructions. Bring a large pot of water to boil. While that is taking place, cook the beetgreens in skillet with $\frac{1}{4}$ cup water for 1 minute, or until the stems are tender. Drain and save the liquid. Chop the greens in good-sized pieces. Warm the oil over medium heat in a large skillet, add the garlic, and saute until lightly colored. Reserve. Remove and add the almonds and saute to the same degree. Reserve almonds. Steam asparagus for about 5 minutes. Now add the beetgreens, asparagus, tomatoes, and $\frac{1}{2}$ cup of the reserved beet liquid to the oil. Season with chili powder, sage, and crushed red pepper flakes. Drain spaghetti and toss with the vegetables. Divide spaghetti among bowls and pour any remaining liquid over them. Sprinkle with the garlic and the almonds and serve.

TIP: Smoking is said to be a major cause of strokes. Swedish medical investigators report that smokers are up to 11 times more likely to have hemorrhage-type strokes than are nonsmokers, and they make up a large share of the 25 percent of stroke victims under age 65. Additional studies show that the stroke risk is cut nearly to that of a nonsmoker in about five years for men and two years for women who quit smoking.

MYTH: Snuff is a safe form of taking tobacco.

FACT: According to Dr. Jerome Goldstein of the American Academy of Otolaryngology, no form of tobacco is safe. Snuff is known to lead to mouth and nasal cancers. Chemicals in snuff are absorbed through the membranes lining the nose or mouth or through the intestinal tract, report physicians.

Nutrients Contained in: Spaghetti, Asparagus, and Beetgreens with Almonds

VITAMINS USRDA			ONE SERVING GIVES YOU APPROXIMATELY		APPROXIMATE PERCENTAGE OF USRDA
A	5,000	IU	1,272	IU	25
B_1	1.4	mg	0.20	mg	16
B_2	1.6	mg	0.17	mg	11
B_3	16	mg	2	mg	9
B_5	10	mg	0.20	mg	1
B_6	2.2	mg	0.08	mg	3
B_{12}	3	μg	0	μg	0
C	60	mg	14	mg	23
D	400	IU	0	IU	0
E	15	IU	2	IU	15
K	500	μg	5	μg	1
Folic Acid	400	μg	6	μg	1

MINERALS USRDA			ONE SERVING GIVES YOU APPROXIMATELY		APPROXIMATE PERCENTAGE OF USRDA
Sodium	(1,100–3,000)	mg	26	mg	2
Calcium	1,000	mg	35	mg	4
Phosphorus	(800–1,000)	mg	94	mg	11
Potassium	(1,875–5,625)	mg	286	mg	35
Magnesium	400	μg	42	μg	11
Selenium	200	μg	20	μg	10
Iodine	150	mg	0	mg	0
Zinc	15	mg	0. 26	mg	1
Iron	10	mg	2	mg	16
Manganese	(2.5–5.0)	mg	0.16	mg	3
Copper	(2.0–3.0)	mg	0.11	mg	3

AMOUNT PER SERVING		CALORIES PER SERVING	% OF MEAL
Fat	6 grams	56	30
Proteins	5 grams	22	12
Carbohydrates	27 grams	107	58
Cholesterol	0 mg		
Amino acid (essential)			39–71
Fiber	1 gram		

Key: USRDA = Recommended Dietary Allowance

  IU = International Unit

  mg = milligrams

  μg = micrograms

NOTE: The numbers with arrows exceed 100 percent of required USRDA.

Peas, Potatoes, and Tomatoes

Ingredients:

- 4 potatoes, peeled and cut into half-inch cubes
- 2 cloves garlic, minced
- 1 ½ cup fresh green peas
- 6 ripe tomatoes, chopped
- 1 tsp turmeric
- 1 tsp chili powder
- 1 Tbs margarine
- 1 tsp chervil
- juice of one lime
- 1 cup zucchini

Preparation: Saute

Time: 30 minutes

Calories: 166 per serving

Serves: 6

Directions

Heat half the margarine and add the garlic. Saute the potato cubes in the same skillet until potatoes are tender enough for a fork to pierce. Add peas and zucchini and cook for 3 minutes. Set these ingredients aside on a large platter. Add the remaining margarine to the pan with the spices and lime juice. Stir in tomatoes, potatoes, peas, and zucchini and cook over low heat until hot and well blended. Add pepper, thyme, and some rosemary. Chart shows high potassium level and high vitamin A.

TIP: Dr. Louis Tobian of the University of Minnesota School of Medicine says if you add one baked potato to what you normally eat each day (with a glass of orange juice and half a melon), you could help lower your stroke rate by 40 percent. You will find the recipes in this chapter have been selected for high potassium content.

MYTH: Drinking coffee can cause cancer and fibrocystic breast disease.

FACT: Delia A. Hammock, director of the Institute/Nutrition, Diet & Fitness Center, of Good Housekeeping writes in a report that no link has been established between coffee and cancer; early reports linking coffee to these diseases were not confirmed by later studies.

Nutrients Contained in:
Peas, Potatoes, and Tomatoes

VITAMINS USRDA			ONE SERVING GIVES YOU APPROXIMATELY		APPROXIMATE PERCENTAGE OF USRDA
A	5,000	IU	1,783	IU	35
B$_1$	1.4	mg	0.28	mg	23
B$_2$	1.6	mg	0.15	mg	10
B$_3$	16	mg	3	mg	17
B$_5$	10	mg	0.86	mg	8
B$_6$	2.2	mg	0.41	mg	18
B$_{12}$	3	μg	0	μg	0
C	60	mg	35	mg	58
D	400	IU	0	IU	0
E	15	IU	0.78	IU	5
K	500	μg	120	μg	24
Folic Acid	400	μg	50	μg	12

MINERALS USRDA			ONE SERVING GIVES YOU APPROXIMATELY		APPROXIMATE PERCENTAGE OF USRDA
Sodium	(1,100–3,000)	mg	39	mg	3
Calcium	1,000	mg	31	mg	3
Phosphorus	(800–1,000)	mg	129	mg	16
Potassium	(1,875–5,625)	mg	745	mg	93
Magnesium	400	μg	54	μg	15
Selenium	200	μg	0.77	μg	0
Iodine	150	mg	0	mg	0
Zinc	15	mg	0.93	mg	6
Iron	10	mg	2	mg	15
Manganese	(2.5–5.0)	mg	0.54	mg	10
Copper	(2.0–3.0)	mg	0.35	mg	11

AMOUNT PER SERVING		CALORIES PER SERVING	% OF MEAL
Fat	2 grams	21	13
Proteins	5 grams	20	12
Carbohydrates	31 grams	125	75
Cholesterol	14 mg		
Amino acid (essential)			44–61*
Fiber	2 grams		

Key: USRDA = Recommended Dietary Allowance

IU = International Unit

mg = milligrams

μg = micrograms

NOTE: The numbers with arrows exceed 100 percent of required USRDA.

*Complementary food—1 large egg raises EAA to 92–148%.

Stir-Fry Tofu and Beans

Ingredients:

1	lb green beans
1	tsp corn oil
½	tsp sugar
3	4-inch squares of tofu
	water
	salt
	lite soy sauce or hot prepared mustard

Preparation: Stir-fry

Time: 15 minutes

Calories: 102 per serving

Serves: 4

Directions

Prepare beans by snapping off the ends. Wash and drain. Heat a skillet or a wok until hot and add the oil. Stir-fry the green beans over high heat for 3 to 4 minutes. Add the sugar and a little salt and about ¼ cup of water. Mix and cover. Cook for about 3 minutes. Add the tofu and cook for another minute or two. Use a little lite soy sauce for flavor or add some hot prepared mustard. The fact that tofu is high in potassium and low in sodium makes it a good contender for stroke protection.

TIP: Dr. Kay-Tee Khaw, a professor of clinical gerontology at the University of Cambridge in England, reported that a 15-year study with several thousand participants showed about 25 percent reduction in stroke mortality among those with the greatest potassium intake.

MYTH: Shampoos can "nourish your hair" and make it healthy.

FACT: According to information in the *Wellness Letter* of the University of California at Berkeley, no shampoo can nourish your hair. The hair shaft is dead tissue, and the only real cure is to cut off the damaged parts.

Nutrients Contained in: Stir-Fry Tofu and Beans

VITAMINS USRDA			ONE SERVING GIVES YOU APPROXIMATELY		APPROXIMATE PERCENTAGE OF USRDA
A	5,000	IU	417	IU	8
B$_1$	1.4	mg	0.10	mg	8
B$_2$	1.6	mg	0.09	mg	6
B$_3$	16	mg	0.47	mg	2
B$_5$	10	mg	0.05	mg	0
B$_6$	2.2	mg	0.04	mg	1
B$_{12}$	3	μg	0	μg	0
C	60	mg	6	mg	10
D	400	IU	0	IU	0
E	15	IU	3	IU	18
K	500	μg	163	μg	32
Folic Acid	400	μg	21	μg	5

MINERALS USRDA			ONE SERVING GIVES YOU APPROXIMATELY		APPROXIMATE PERCENTAGE OF USRDA
Sodium	(1,100–3,000)	mg	15	mg	1
Calcium	1,000	mg	146	mg	18
Phosphorus	(800–1,000)	mg	143	mg	17
Potassium	(1,875–5,625)	mg	245	mg	30
Magnesium	400	μg	118	μg	33
Selenium	200	μg	0.30	μg	0
Iodine	150	mg	0	mg	0
Zinc	15	mg	0.31	mg	2
Iron	10	mg	3	mg	26
Manganese	(2.5–5.0)	mg	0.19	mg	3
Copper	(2.0–3.0)	mg	0.08	mg	2

AMOUNT PER SERVING		CALORIES PER SERVING	% OF MEAL
Fat	7 grams	66	65
Proteins	1 gram	5	5
Carbohydrates	8 grams	31	30
Cholesterol	0 mg		
Amino acid (essential)			87–138
Fiber	2 grams		

Key: USRDA = Recommended Dietary Allowance
     IU = International Unit
     mg = milligrams
     μg = micrograms
NOTE: The numbers with arrows exceed 100 percent of required USRDA.

Double-Flavor Onion and Garlic

Ingredients:

6 onions, sliced
8 cloves garlic, chopped very fine
2 tsp canola oil
2 tsp flour
1 ½ cup okra
½ tsp allspice
¼ cup chopped parsley
½ tsp chili powder
dash soy sauce

Preparation: Saute

Time: 20 minutes

Calories: 166 per serving

Serves: 4 to 6

Directions

Saute onions and garlic in 1 tsp of oil. In a separate pan using the second tsp of oil add the flour, allspice, chili powder, and black pepper and cook until there is a rather thick sauce. Add this to the onion-garlic mixture. Add okra, parsley, and water to cover if necessary. Cover and simmer until the okra is done. You might want to steam the okra for a few minutes before this step.

TIP: A 12-year study by the University of California at San Diego tested three groups according to dietary potassium intake. After the 12-year period, no stroke-associated deaths had occurred in the group with the highest intake of potassium. (859 men and women participants were stratified into three groups.)

MYTH: Varicose veins are an inevitable result of aging.

FACT: Mayo Clinic vascular surgeon John W. Hallett says this is not true. He says that varicose veins are frequently an inherited trait and that medical treatment can relieve the discomfort and disfigurement.

Nutrients Contained in: Double-Flavor Onion and Garlic

VITAMINS USRDA			ONE SERVING GIVES YOU APPROXIMATELY		APPROXIMATE PERCENTAGE OF USRDA
A	5,000	IU	198	IU	3
B_1	1.4	mg	0.35	mg	29
B_2	1.6	mg	0.12	mg	8
B_3	16	mg	1	mg	6
B_5	10	mg	0.40	mg	3
B_6	2.2	mg	0.37	mg	16
B_{12}	3	μg	0	μg	0
C	60	mg	18	mg	29
D	400	IU	0	IU	0
E	15	IU	2	IU	11
K	500	μg	0	μg	0
Folic Acid	400	μg	92	μg	22

MINERALS USRDA			ONE SERVING GIVES YOU APPROXIMATELY		APPROXIMATE PERCENTAGE OF USRDA
Sodium	(1,100–3,000)	mg	11	mg	1
Calcium	1,000	mg	66	mg	8
Phosphorus	(800–1,000)	mg	201	mg	25
Potassium	(1,875–5,625)	mg	443	mg	55
Magnesium	400	μg	69	μg	19
Selenium	200	μg	3	μg	1
Iodine	150	mg	0	mg	0
Zinc	15	mg	2	mg	15
Iron	10	mg	2	mg	17
Manganese	(2.5–5.0)	mg	3	mg	54
Copper	(2.0–3.0)	mg	0.43	mg	14

AMOUNT PER SERVING		CALORIES PER SERVING	% OF MEAL
Fat	7 grams	63	38
Proteins	6 grams	24	14
Carbohydrates	20 grams	79	48
Cholesterol	0 mg		
Amino acid (essential)			49–81
Fiber	2 grams		

Key: USRDA = Recommended Dietary Allowance
   IU = International Unit
   mg = milligrams
   μg = micrograms
NOTE: The numbers with arrows exceed 100 percent of required USRDA.

VEGETABLES RANKED IN THE HIGHEST ORDER FOR POTASSIUM
PERCENTAGES GIVEN EQUAL ½ CUP

	POTASSIUM (MILLIGRAMS)	PERCENTAGE OF USRDA
Potato, baked, with skin	844.0	15.0
Beans, fava, canned	690.0	12.3
Potato, au gratin	483.0	8.6
Beans, lima, cooked	478.0	8.5
Potato, scalloped	461.0	8.2
Yam, cooked	455.0	8.1
Squash, winter, cooked	445.0	7.9
Potato, boiled without skin	443.0	7.9
Spinach, cooked	419.0	7.4
Potato, sweet	397.0	7.1
Beans, baked, pork/sauce	378.0	6.7
Beans, baked, plain	376.0	6.7
Beans, lima, frozen	371.0	6.6
Spinach, canned	370.0	6.6
Potato, french fries	366.0	6.5
Peas, blackeye, cooked	344.0	6.1
Potato, hashed browns	340.0	6.0
Parsnips, cooked	287.0	5.1
Tomato, canned	265.0	4.7

CHAPTER THREE

Healing and Preventive Recipes for High Blood Pressure

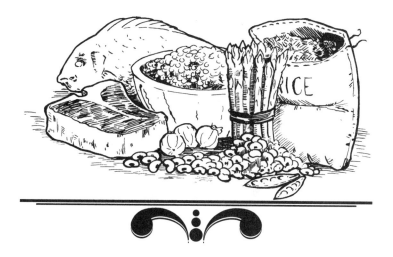

Health is that choice seasoning which gives
us relish to all our enjoyments.
—John Morgan (1735–1789)

Nutritional safeguards against the disease known as a "silent killer," or hypertension, include a variety of dietary factors. The recipes and information contained in this chapter feature foods with high levels of potassium, calcium, and fatty acids found in fish oil; low sodium; and low fat. These are the same diet guidelines that can be followed for a healthy heart.

You will find a simple recipe for helping the liver control cholesterol output using blackeye peas, a broccoli meal that will give you high levels of potassium, and a dish of garlic and lean pork—garlic being a good aid for the cardiovascular system. With information from several studies giving positive reports on the effectiveness of shiitake mushrooms, you will find numerous recipes including this vegetable.

When you cook any one of these meals, you won't have to check the food labels for milligrams of sodium per serving; just look at your nutritional chart, and you will know in an instant how much sodium, potassium, and calcium your delicious meal contains.

You will find tasty recipes for beans, rice, garlic, fish, asparagus, peas, and other foods that have been studied for their nutritional effectiveness by scientists at the National Heart, Lung and Blood Institute of the National Institutes of Health as well as university research centers throughout the world.

As with potassium, members of the Committee on Dietary Allowances set what they call a "safe and adequate" intake range for sodium as well as potassium with the idea that a good diet would include about equal intake of both minerals. Although the potassium table for the USRDA range is listed in Chapter 2 on stroke, the tables for sodium and potassium are listed together here for the convenience of comparison.

RECOMMENDED SAFE AND ADEQUATE RANGE FOR SODIUM AND POTASSIUM

GROUP/AGE	(MILLIGRAMS)	
	SODIUM	POTASSIUM
Infants 0–6 months	115– 350	350– 925
Infants 7–12 months	250– 750	425–1,275
Children 1–3 years	325– 975	550–1,650
Children 4–6 years	450–1,350	755–2,325
Children 7–10 years	600–1,800	1,000–3,000
Males 11–18 years	900–2,700	1,525–4,575
Males 19+ years	1,100–3,300	1,875–5,625
Females 11–18 years	900–2,700	1,525–4,575
Females 19+ years	1,100–3,300	1,875–5,625

Blackeyes

Ingredients:

- 1 16-oz can blackeye peas
- 3 cups fresh spinach
- 1 tsp olive oil
- 1 large onion, chopped
- 4 cloves garlic, diced in small bits
- 1 tsp paprika

Preparation: Saute

Time: 10 minutes

Calories: 136 per serving

Serves: 4

Directions

Saute onion and garlic in the oil in a large pan until soft. Add peas and spinach and saute for about 3 minutes or until spinach is done to taste and peas are hot. Check the chart to see levels of potassium, calcium, and vitamin A.

TIP: Blackeye peas are not peas but, rather, beans that contain a lot of iron and other nutrients that help protect the heart. Beans help the liver to control cholesterol output and clear away the bad LDL cholesterol.

MYTH: For exercise to benefit you, it must be done for 30 continuous minutes.

FACT: A Stanford University study shows an easier way. Their researchers found that 10 minutes of exercise three times a day is about just as good.

Nutrients Contained in: Blackeyes

VITAMINS USRDA			ONE SERVING GIVES YOU APPROXIMATELY		APPROXIMATE PERCENTAGE OF USRDA
A	5,000	IU	11,189	IU	223◄
B_1	1.4	mg	0.19	mg	16
B_2	1.6	mg	0.37	mg	26
B_3	16	mg	1	mg	7
B_5	10	mg	0.25	mg	2
B_6	2.2	mg	0.41	mg	18
B_{12}	3	μg	0	μg	0
C	60	mg	17	mg	28
D	400	IU	0	IU	0
E	15	IU	5	IU	1
K	500	μg	135	μg	27
Folic Acid	400	μg	248	μg	61

MINERALS USRDA			ONE SERVING GIVES YOU APPROXIMATELY		APPROXIMATE PERCENTAGE OF USRDA
Sodium	(1,100–3,000)	mg	99	mg	9
Calcium	1,000	mg	206	mg	25
Phosphorus	(800–1,000)	mg	93	mg	11
Potassium	(1,875–5,625)	mg	879	mg	109◄
Magnesium	400	μg	143	μg	40
Selenium	200	μg	14	μg	7
Iodine	150	mg	0	mg	0
Zinc	15	mg	1	mg	9
Iron	10	mg	6	mg	55
Manganese	(2.5–5.0)	mg	1	mg	26
Copper	(2.0–3.0)	mg	0.26	mg	8

AMOUNT PER SERVING		CALORIES PER SERVING	% OF MEAL
Fat	4 grams	38	28
Proteins	8 grams	32	24
Carbohydrates	16 grams	66	48
Cholesterol	0 mg		
Amino acid (essential)			54–64
Fiber	4 grams		

Key: USRDA = Recommended Dietary Allowance
    IU = International Unit
    mg = milligrams
    μg = micrograms
NOTE: The numbers with arrows exceed 100 percent of required USRDA.

Reliable Broccoli

Ingredients:

1 bunch broccoli
5 cloves garlic, chopped
1 tsp safflower oil
$\frac{1}{2}$ cup mushrooms
$\frac{1}{4}$ tsp crushed red pepper
juice of one lime

Preparation: Saute

Time: 10 minutes

Calories: 52 per serving

Serves: 4

Directions

Heat oil in a large skillet and add garlic and crushed red pepper. After cutting broccoli in pieces, add to pan and toss, Saute for about 7 minutes or more if you want them done more than al dente. Sprinkle with lime juice.

TIP: Remember, broccoli featured as a star in our cancer-fighting chapter of recipes. With its high content of potassium, it is also a heart protector, as potassium helps to control your blood pressure. You can always increase the amount for any recipe; I keep the amounts small because we need so little to achieve our USRDAs.

MYTH: Bananas have the highest potassium content of all fruits.

FACT: Try five dried figs. In addition to vitamins, fiber, and practically no fat, they have 48 percent more potassium than a banana. They also give you some iron and protein.

Nutrients Contained in: Reliable Broccoli

VITAMINS USRDA			ONE SERVING GIVES YOU APPROXIMATELY		APPROXIMATE PERCENTAGE OF USRDA
A	5,000	IU	339	IU	6
B$_1$	1.4	mg	0.04	mg	3
B$_2$	1.6	mg	0.08	mg	6
B$_3$	16	mg	1	mg	6
B$_5$	10	mg	0.54	mg	5
B$_6$	2.2	mg	0.05	mg	2
B$_{12}$	3	μg	0	μg	0
C	60	mg	21	mg	35
D	400	IU	0	IU	0
E	15	IU	1	IU	9
K	500	μg	77	μg	15
Folic Acid	400	μg	19	μg	4

MINERALS USRDA			ONE SERVING GIVES YOU APPROXIMATELY		APPROXIMATE PERCENTAGE OF USRDA
Sodium	(1,100–3,000)	mg	11	mg	1
Calcium	1,000	mg	15	mg	1
Phosphorus	(800–1,000)	mg	40	mg	5
Potassium	(1,875–5,625)	mg	172	mg	21
Magnesium	400	μg	11	μg	3
Selenium	200	μg	3	μg	1
Iodine	150	mg	0	mg	0
Zinc	15	mg	0.35	mg	2
Iron	10	mg	0.56	mg	5
Manganese	(2.5–5.0)	mg	0.07	mg	1
Copper	(2.0–3.0)	mg	0.12	mg	4

AMOUNT PER SERVING		CALORIES PER SERVING	% OF MEAL
Fat	4 grams	32	62
Proteins	1 gram	5	10
Carbohydrates	4 grams	15	28
Cholesterol	0 mg		
Amino acid (essential)			10–18*
Fiber	19 grams		

Key: USRDA = Recommended Dietary Allowance
IU = International Unit
mg = milligrams
μg = micrograms

NOTE: The numbers with arrows exceed 100 percent of required USRDA.

*Complementary food—1 cup of peas raises EAA to 88–131%.

Favorite Fava Beans

Ingredients:
    1 16-oz can fava beans
    1 large onion
    ⅛ lb sliced ham, diced
    1 celery stalk, diced
    1 can okra
    1 tsp olive oil
    ¼ tsp paprika

Preparation: Saute

Time: 40 minutes

Calories: 146 per serving

Serves: 4

Directions

Saute diced onion and ham pieces in the oil until soft and brown. Add the beans, okra, and celery. Mix well. Cover and cook for 5 to 10 minutes. Add the paprika and pepper to taste. Notice high fiber count on chart.

TIP: It's the soluble fiber in beans that makes it a good food for the heart and reduces levels of blood cholesterol. Physicians at the University of Kentucky and researchers elsewhere have conducted tests where they have documented the beneficial effects beans have on lowering blood cholesterol levels. They say it doesn't matter much which beans you eat as they all are about the same nutritionally.

MYTH: Frozen tofu has less fat than sherbet.

FACT: The fat in tofu is highly unsaturated, but frozen tofu has six times the fat of sherbet.

Nutrients Contained in: Favorite Fava Beans

VITAMINS USRDA			ONE SERVING GIVES YOU APPROXIMATELY		APPROXIMATE PERCENTAGE OF USRDA
A	5,000	IU	178	IU	3
B_1	1.4	mg	0.34	mg	28
B_2	1.6	mg	0.11	mg	7
B_3	16	mg	2	mg	10
B_5	10	mg	0.19	mg	1
B_6	2.2	mg	0.27	mg	12
B_{12}	3	µg	0.12	µg	3
C	60	mg	10	mg	17
D	400	IU	4	IU	0
E	15	IU	0.32	IU	2
K	500	µg	0	µg	0
Folic Acid	400	µg	121	µg	30

MINERALS USRDA			ONE SERVING GIVES YOU APPROXIMATELY		APPROXIMATE PERCENTAGE OF USRDA
Sodium	(1,100–3,000)	mg	283	mg	28
Calcium	1,000	mg	95	mg	11
Phosphorus	(800–1,000)	mg	65	mg	8
Potassium	(1,875–5,625)	mg	558	mg	69
Magnesium	400	µg	66	µg	18
Selenium	200	µg	8	µg	4
Iodine	150	mg	0	mg	0
Zinc	15	mg	1	mg	8
Iron	10	mg	2	mg	23
Manganese	(2.5–5.0)	mg	0.32	mg	6
Copper	(2.0–3.0)	mg	0.26	mg	8

AMOUNT PER SERVING		CALORIES PER SERVING	% OF MEAL
Fat	2 grams	19	13
Proteins	11 grams	42	29
Carbohydrates	21 grams	85	58
Cholesterol	8 mg		
Amino acid (essential)			40–58
Fiber	30 grams		

Key: USRDA = Recommended Dietary Allowance
     IU = International Unit
     mg = milligrams
     µg = micrograms
NOTE: The numbers with arrows exceed 100 percent of required USRDA.

Garlic and Pork Combine

Ingredients:

- 1 lb lean boneless, pork loin
- 6 cloves garlic, sliced very thin
- 1 Tbs horseradish
- 2 cups water
- 1 ½ cups strawberries, hulled
- ⅛ tsp cayenne pepper
- 1 tsp thyme
- juice of one lime
- black pepper

Preparation: Bake

Time: 1 ½ hours

Calories: 295 per serving

Serves: 4

Directions

Preheat oven to 350° F. Trim all fat from the pork and make a few incisions in the meat. Combine garlic and thyme and insert in meat. Rub pork with lime juice and pepper and place in a shallow roasting pan filled with the water. Roast for about 1 ½ hours. Baste with liquid occasionally. Add strawberries to pork last 5 minutes of baking and let stand 10 minutes after removing from oven. Pork is a great source of B vitamins, zinc, protein, and iron. Just make sure you buy the leanest cut available.

TIP: Dr. R. C. Jain of the University of LBenghazi in Libya, Drs. Sainani and Desai of India, Professor Hans Reuter of Germany, Dr. Tarig Abdullah of Florida's Akbar Clinic, and Chinese, Japanese, and Russian physicians have all touted garlic as good for the cardiovascular system. Can they all be wrong?

MYTH: Drinking tea causes iron deficiencies.

FACT: Research indicates this could happen only in extreme cases. The word is that tea in moderation can be part of a healthy diet, and there's no evidence that it can lead to iron-deficiency anemia.

Nutrients Contained in:
Garlic and Pork Combine

VITAMINS USRDA			ONE SERVING GIVES YOU APPROXIMATELY		APPROXIMATE PERCENTAGE OF USRDA
A	5,000	IU	0	IU	0
B$_1$	1.4	mg	2	mg	133◄
B$_2$	1.6	mg	0.43	mg	30
B$_3$	16	mg	6	mg	35
B$_5$	10	mg	1	mg	10
B$_6$	2.2	mg	0.56	mg	25
B$_{12}$	3	μg	0.88	μg	29
C	60	mg	15	mg	25
D	400	IU	31	IU	7
E	15	IU	0.75	IU	5
K	500	μg	14	μg	2
Folic Acid	400	μg	10	μg	2

MINERALS USRDA			ONE SERVING GIVES YOU APPROXIMATELY		APPROXIMATE PERCENTAGE OF USRDA
Sodium	(1,100–3,000)	mg	70	mg	7
Calcium	1,000	mg	8	mg	0
Phosphorus	(800–1,000)	mg	385	mg	48
Potassium	(1,875–5,625)	mg	660	mg	82
Magnesium	400	μg	34	μg	9
Selenium	200	μg	59	μg	29
Iodine	150	mg	0	mg	0
Zinc	15	mg	2	mg	11
Iron	10	mg	6	mg	58
Manganese	(2.5–5.0)	mg	0.02	mg	0
Copper	(2.0–3.0)	mg	0.03	mg	0

AMOUNT PER SERVING		CALORIES PER SERVING	% OF MEAL
Fat	15 grams	136	46
Proteins	39 grams	154	52
Carbohydrates	1 gram	5	2
Cholesterol	113 mg		
Amino acid (essential)			239–714*
Fiber	0 grams		

Key: USRDA = Recommended Dietary Allowance
     IU = International Unit
    mg = milligrams
    μg = micrograms
NOTE: The numbers with arrows exceed 100 percent of required USRDA.

*A bonanza of EAA.

Rice, Garlic, Carrots, and Curry

Ingredients:

1 cup rice
6 cloves of garlic
1 Tbs margarine
2 tsp curry powder
1 carrot, scraped and
    cut into strips
1 ½ cups low-sodium
    chicken broth
    bay leaf
¼ cup spring onions cut
    in small pieces

Preparation: Boil

Time: 25 minutes

Calories: 231 per serving

Serves: 4

Directions

Melt the margarine in a skillet and add the spring onions and sliced garlic. Cook for a minute or two and add the bay leaf. Sprinkle with curry powder. Add the rice and carrot strips. Stir and add the broth; cover. Bring to a boil and then simmer for 15 to 20 minutes.

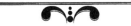

TIP: Do not overeat with large portions. The medically approved serving of meat, for example, is 3 ounces, similar in size to a deck of playing cards. A medium piece of fruit is one serving.

MYTH: Vegetable fats have less calories than animal fats.

FACT: Animal fats contain more saturated fats which raises blood cholesterol, but both fats provide 9 calories per gram, which is about 260 calories per ounce.

Nutrients Contained in:
Rice, Garlic, Carrots, and Curry

VITAMINS USRDA			ONE SERVING GIVES YOU APPROXIMATELY		APPROXIMATE PERCENTAGE OF USRDA
A	5,000	IU	5,429	IU	108◄
B_1	1.4	mg	0.21	mg	17
B_2	1.6	mg	0.07	mg	4
B_3	16	mg	4	mg	23
B_5	10	mg	0.57	mg	5
B_6	2.2	mg	0.29	mg	12
B_{12}	3	μg	0.12	μg	3
C	60	mg	4	mg	7
D	400	IU	0	IU	0
E	15	IU	0.92	IU	6
K	500	μg	25	μg	5
Folic Acid	400	μg	5	μg	1

MINERALS USRDA			ONE SERVING GIVES YOU APPROXIMATELY		APPROXIMATE PERCENTAGE OF USRDA
Sodium	(1,100–3,000)	mg	336	mg	33
Calcium	1,000	mg	30	mg	3
Phosphorus	(800–1,000)	mg	128	mg	15
Potassium	(1,875–5,625)	mg	283	mg	35
Magnesium	400	μg	49	μg	14
Selenium	200	μg	20	μg	9
Iodine	150	mg	0	mg	0
Zinc	15	mg	1	mg	7
Iron	10	mg	1	mg	11
Manganese	(2.5–5.0)	mg	0.83	mg	16
Copper	(2.0–3.0)	mg	0.13	mg	4

AMOUNT PER SERVING		CALORIES PER SERVING	% OF MEAL
Fat	4 grams	39	17
Proteins	6 grams	25	11
Carbohydrates	42 grams	167	72
Cholesterol	21 mg		
Amino acid (essential)			32–66
Fiber	1 gram		

Key: USRDA = Recommended Dietary Allowance

IU = International Unit

mg = milligrams

μg = micrograms

NOTE: The numbers with arrows exceed 100 percent of required USRDA.

Asparagus with Shiitake Mushrooms

Ingredients:

- 8 pieces of shiitake mushrooms
- 16 spears asparagus, stems peeled
- 1 tsp corn oil
- 1 onion, sliced
- ½ cup pea pods
  Parmesan cheese
  juice of one lemon
  black pepper

Preparation: Saute

Time: 30 minutes

Calories: 101 per serving

Serves: 4

Directions

In a large pan, heat the corn oil. Add the mushrooms, sprinkle with black pepper, and cook until tender, about 5 minutes or so. Remove mushrooms from pan to a warm platter and replace with onions, pea pods, and asparagus spears. Cook for about 8 minutes or until al dente; sprinkle with lemon juice and stir in the mushrooms. Transfer to platter and sprinkle with Parmesan cheese.

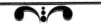

TIP: Shiitake mushrooms have been under study for over three decades in this country although the Japanese have long used mushrooms for therapeutic purposes. As little as 3 ounces of shiitakes a day may lower blood cholesterol, according to reports of tests conducted with a small group of healthy women.

MYTH: Your blood pressure should equal your age plus 100.

FACT: Really not true. The rule runs off course as one approaches the midcentury mark. A 60-year-old with repeated readings of 160/90 is considered to have high, not normal, blood pressure, and might consider ways to lower it. At age 40, a reading of 140/80 would seem to be normal, but things change as one ages.

Nutrients Contained in:
Asparagus with Shiitake Mushrooms

VITAMINS USRDA		ONE SERVING GIVES YOU APPROXIMATELY		APPROXIMATE PERCENTAGE OF USRDA
A	5,000 IU	548	IU	10
B$_1$	1.4 mg	0.11	mg	8
B$_2$	1.6 mg	0.12	mg	8
B$_3$	16 mg	1	mg	8
B$_5$	10 mg	0.40	mg	4
B$_6$	2.2 mg	0.17	mg	7
B$_{12}$	3 μg	0	μg	0
C	60 mg	27	mg	44
D	400 IU	0	IU	0
E	15 IU	6	IU	39
K	500 μg	40	μg	8
Folic Acid	400 μg	74	μg	18

MINERALS USRDA		ONE SERVING GIVES YOU APPROXIMATELY		APPROXIMATE PERCENTAGE OF USRDA
Sodium	(1,100–3,000) mg	7	mg	0
Calcium	1,000 mg	44	mg	5
Phosphorus	(800–1,000) mg	66	mg	8
Potassium	(1,875–5,625) mg	359	mg	44
Magnesium	400 μg	28	μg	8
Selenium	200 μg	0.80	μg	0
Iodine	150 mg	0	mg	0
Zinc	15 mg	1	mg	6
Iron	10 mg	1	mg	12
Manganese	(2.5–5.0) mg	0.18	mg	3
Copper	(2.0–3.0) mg	0.08	mg	2

AMOUNT PER SERVING		CALORIES PER SERVING	% OF MEAL
Fat	4 grams	34	34
Proteins	4 grams	14	14
Carbohydrates	13 grams	53	52
Cholesterol	0 mg		
Amino acid (essential)			24–41
Fiber	2 grams		

Key: USRDA = Recommended Dietary Allowance
    IU = International Unit
    mg = milligrams
    μg = micrograms
NOTE: The numbers with arrows exceed 100 percent of required USRDA.

Spicy Curried Rice

Ingredients:
2 cups brown rice
1 tsp curry powder
1 onion, chopped
1 tsp cinnamon
1 tsp ground cumin
3 ½ cups low-sodium
    chicken broth
canola oil

Preparation: Boil

Time: 1 hour

Calories: 417 per serving

Serves: 4

Directions

Bring chicken broth to a boil and add rice, cinnamon, cumin, and curry powder. Cover, reduce the heat, and simmer for about 45 to 50 minutes, or until the rice is done and the broth has been absorbed. Saute onion in a drop of canola oil. Add the cooked rice. Heat and blend for a few minutes.

TIP: Reducing your daily intake to between 1,500 and 2,500 milligrams of sodium may be all the sodium restriction you need to control mild or moderate high blood pressure according to the Mayo Clinic. That's roughly the same amount of sodium contained in a teaspoon of table salt.

MYTH: The human body works better when eating six small meals daily rather than three large ones.

FACT: The University of California at Berkeley School of Public Health says no. It's what you eat that matters, not when you eat it. It's one's culture that influences eating patterns; the body really doesn't care when it gets it due as long as it gets it.

Nutrients Contained in: Spicy Curried Rice

VITAMINS USRDA			ONE SERVING GIVES YOU APPROXIMATELY		APPROXIMATE PERCENTAGE OF USRDA
A	5,000	IU	0.38	IU	31
B$_1$	1.4	mg	0.11	mg	7
B$_2$	1.6	mg	8	mg	47
B$_3$	16	mg	1	mg	11
B$_5$	10	mg	0.58	mg	26
B$_6$	2.2	mg	0.26	mg	8
B$_{12}$	3	μg	0	μg	0
C	60	mg	3	mg	5
D	400	IU	0	IU	0
E	15	IU	2	IU	10
K	500	μg	0	μg	0
Folic Acid	400	μg	12	μg	3

MINERALS USRDA			ONE SERVING GIVES YOU APPROXIMATELY		APPROXIMATE PERCENTAGE OF USRDA
Sodium	(1,100–3,000)	mg	689	mg	68
Calcium	1,000	mg	79	mg	10
Phosphorus	(800–1,000)	mg	232	mg	29
Potassium	(1,875–5,625)	mg	510	mg	64
Magnesium	400	μg	93	μg	26
Selenium	200	μg	39	μg	19
Iodine	150	mg	0	mg	0
Zinc	15	mg	2	mg	14
Iron	10	mg	2	mg	21
Manganese	(2.5–5.0)	mg	2	mg	33
Copper	(2.0–3.0)	mg	0.22	mg	7

AMOUNT PER SERVING		CALORIES PER SERVING	% OF MEAL
Fat	3 grams	28	7
Proteins	12 grams	49	12
Carbohydrates	80 grams	340	81
Cholesterol	1 mg		
Amino acid (essential)			64–128
Fiber	1 gram		

Key: USRDA = Recommended Dietary Allowance

    IU = International Unit

    mg = milligrams

    μg = micrograms

NOTE: The numbers with arrows exceed 100 percent of required USRDA.

Quick Beans and Spinach

Ingredients:

1 cup canned chick peas
3 cloves garlic
2 cups fresh spinach
1 tsp olive oil
black pepper

Preparation: Saute
Time: 15 minutes
Calories: 244 per serving
Serves: 4

Directions

Heat olive oil in large skillet. Add the garlic and saute for a minute or two. Add the spinach and saute about 3 minutes. Add the beans, sprinkle black pepper over mixture, and cover and cook for a few minutes more, until the spinach is just tender. You get a lot of nourishment for the little work involved. Notice the high amounts of vitamin A, potassium, and 100 percent plus listing of all essential amino acids.

TIP: Researchers at Arizona State University cite skim milk, dairy products, and fortified orange juice as helping to reduce high blood pressure. Associate Professor of Nutrition Melinda Manore says high calcium intake may help those whose blood pressure won't fall with a low-sodium diet.

MYTH: Milk is a mucus maker and should be avoided when you have a cold.

FACT: University of Southern California researcher Branton Lachman says milk is not a mucus maker, and in a study of people with colds, there was no difference in the mucus of those who drank milk and those who did not.

Nutrients Contained in: Quick Beans and Spinach

VITAMINS USRDA			ONE SERVING GIVES YOU APPROXIMATELY		APPROXIMATE PERCENTAGE OF USRDA
A	5,000	IU	7,396	IU	147◄
B$_1$	1.4	mg	0.25	mg	20
B$_2$	1.6	mg	0.29	mg	20
B$_3$	16	mg	1	mg	9
B$_5$	10	mg	0.78	mg	7
B$_6$	2.2	mg	0.47	mg	21
B$_{12}$	3	μg	0.0	μg	0
C	60	mg	9	mg	14
D	400	IU	0	IU	0
E	15	IU	3	IU	20
K	500	μg	90	μg	18
Folic Acid	400	μg	131	μg	32

MINERALS USRDA			ONE SERVING GIVES YOU APPROXIMATELY		APPROXIMATE PERCENTAGE OF USRDA
Sodium	(1,100–3,000)	mg	77	mg	7
Calcium	1,000	mg	198	mg	24
Phosphorus	(800–1,000)	mg	220	mg	27
Potassium	1,875–5,625)	mg	830	mg	103◄
Magnesium	400	μg	153	μg	43
Selenium	200	μg	9	μg	4
Iodine	150	mg	0	mg	0
Zinc	15	mg	2	mg	13
Iron	10	mg	7	mg	66
Manganese	(2.5–5.0)	mg	1	mg	29
Copper	(2.0–3.0)	mg	0.56	mg	18

AMOUNT PER SERVING		CALORIES PER SERVING	% OF MEAL
Fat	6 grams	54	22
Proteins	13 grams	52	22
Carbohydrates	35 grams	138	56
Cholesterol	0 mg		
Amino acid (essential)			127–202
Fiber	3 grams		

Key: USRDA = Recommended Dietary Allowance
    IU = International Unit
    mg = milligrams
    μg = micrograms
NOTE: The numbers with arrows exceed 100 percent of required USRDA.

Lentil Mushroom Powerhouse

Ingredients:

2 cups lentils
1 cup onions, diced
3 carrots, diced
2 stalks celery, diced
4 shiitake mushrooms, diced
½ lb cooked ham, diced
½ cup spring onions, chopped
2 Tbs parsley, chopped
2 Tbs lime juice
1 tsp allspice
6 cups water
chervil
black pepper

Preparation: Boil

Time: 40 minutes

Calories: 272 per serving

Serves: 4

Directions

Place lentils, onions, carrots, celery, and mushrooms in a large pot with the water. Bring to a boil and then reduce the heat. Simmer for 25–30 minutes. Keep a check on the lentils and the water to make certain the water does not boil away before the lentils are done. When the lentils are chewy, stir in the lime juice and the allspice. Stir in the meat and let it heat. Add some chervil and black pepper for seasoning. Sprinkle chopped parsley when serving.

TIP: Many studies indicate that a high-fiber intake will help lower blood pressure. High-fiber foods include barley, lentils, sweet potatoes, asparagus, and carrots. Popcorn and fresh fruit fiber are particularly effective in lowering blood pressure, according to the Baltimore Longitudinal Study on Aging.

MYTH: People with high blood pressure shouldn't lift weights.

FACT: The facts show that weight-lifting exercises can reduce blood pressure. None of the long-term studies on weight lifting and blood pressure showed any adverse effects.

Nutrients Contained in:
Lentil Mushroom Powerhouse

VITAMINS USRDA			ONE SERVING GIVES YOU APPROXIMATELY		APPROXIMATE PERCENTAGE OF USRDA
A	5,000	IU	16,308	IU	326◄
B_1	1.4	mg	0.66	mg	54
B_2	1.6	mg	0.28	mg	20
B_3	16	mg	5	mg	28
B_5	10	mg	2	mg	18
B_6	2.2	mg	0.65	mg	29
B_{12}	3	μg	0.47	μg	15
C	60	mg	28	mg	46
D	400	IU	16	IU	3
E	15	IU	2	IU	15
K	500	μg	75	μg	15
Folic Acid	400	μg	43	μg	10

MINERALS USRDA			ONE SERVING GIVES YOU APPROXIMATELY		APPROXIMATE PERCENTAGE OF USRDA
Sodium	(1,100–3,000)	mg	789	mg	78
Calcium	1,000	mg	80	mg	9
Phosphorus	(800–1,000)	mg	309	mg	38
Potassium	(1,875–5,625)	mg	839	mg	104◄
Magnesium	400	μg	73	μg	20
Selenium	200	μg	37	μg	18
Iodine	150	mg	0	mg	0
Zinc	15	mg	3	mg	18
Iron	10	mg	4	mg	38
Manganese	(2.5–5.0)	mg	0.24	mg	4
Copper	(2.0–3.0)	mg	0.38	mg	12

AMOUNT PER SERVING		CALORIES PER SERVING	% OF MEAL
Fat	6 grams	57	21
Proteins	20 grams	79	29
Carbohydrates	34 grams	136	50
Cholesterol	32 mg		
Amino acid (essential)			276–555*
Fiber	2 grams		

Key: USRDA = Recommended Dietary Allowance
    IU = International Unit
    mg = milligrams
    μg = micrograms
NOTE: The numbers with arrows exceed 100 percent of required USRDA.

*Powerhouse of EAA.

Barley and Mushroom Casserole

Ingredients:

- 1 cup barley
- 1 cup low-sodium chicken broth
- 8 pieces shiitake mushroom
- 1 tsp margarine
- ¼ cup cilantro
- cayenne pepper
- chili pepper

Preparation: Bake and saute

Time: 1 ½ hours

Calories: 263 per serving

Serves: 4

Directions

Heat oven to 375° F and combine barley with the chicken broth in a baking dish. Cover and bake for 1 hour stirring once or twice. Heat margarine in a small pan and saute mushrooms until tender. Add to the cooked barley with the cilantro, a bit of cayenne pepper, and a dash of chili pepper. Notice the high amounts of potassium, phosphorus, and dietary fiber in this meal.

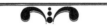

TIP: Several studies have suggested that taking extra potassium may help lower blood pressure. George Webb, associate professor of physiology and biophysics at the University of Vermont College of Medicine, says there is strong evidence that diets low in potassium may lead to high blood pressure. This mineral is plentiful in most diets.

MYTH: Beans are fattening.

FACT: Not according to the American Dry Bean Board. They say beans are one of nature's near-perfect foods—low in fat, calories, and sodium and full of muscle-building protein and vitamins.

Nutrients Contained in:
Barley and Mushroom Casserole

VITAMINS USRDA			ONE SERVING GIVES YOU APPROXIMATELY		APPROXIMATE PERCENTAGE OF USRDA
A	5,000	IU	58	IU	1
B$_1$	1.4	mg	2	mg	175◄
B$_2$	1.6	mg	0.56	mg	39
B$_3$	16	mg	8	mg	52
B$_5$	10	mg	2	mg	15
B$_6$	2.2	mg	0.31	mg	14
B$_{12}$	3	μg	2	μg	0
C	60	mg	0.01	mg	25
D	400	IU	0	IU	0
E	15	IU	0.02	IU	2
K	500	μg	3	μg	0
Folic Acid	400	μg	459	μg	114◄

MINERALS USRDA			ONE SERVING GIVES YOU APPROXIMATELY		APPROXIMATE PERCENTAGE OF USRDA
Sodium	(1,100–3,000)	mg	239	mg	23
Calcium	1,000	mg	47	mg	5
Phosphorus	(800–1,000)	mg	365	mg	45
Potassium	(1,875–5,625)	mg	469	mg	58
Magnesium	400	μg	52	μg	14
Selenium	200	μg	0	μg	0
Iodine	150	mg	0	mg	0
Zinc	15	mg	2	mg	12
Iron	10	mg	3	mg	34
Manganese	(2.5–5.0)	mg	0.05	mg	1
Copper	(2.0–3.0)	mg	0.65	mg	21

AMOUNT PER SERVING		CALORIES PER SERVING	% OF MEAL
Fat	2 grams	22	8
Proteins	12 grams	46	18
Carbohydrates	49 grams	195	74
Cholesterol	10 mg		
Amino acid (essential)			118–177
Fiber	19 grams		

Key: USRDA = Recommended Dietary Allowance
   IU = International Unit
   mg = milligrams
   μg = micrograms
NOTE: The numbers with arrows exceed 100 percent of required USRDA.

Simple Lentils with Garlic

Ingredients:

1 cup lentils
3 cups water
4 cloves garlic, mashed
1 Tbs olive oil
10 iceberg lettuce leaves
1 lemon
6 spring onions, chopped
1 tsp chervil
1 tsp basil
juice of one lemon

Preparation: Boil

Time: 1 hour and 15 minutes

Calories: 134 per serving

Serves: 4 to 6

Directions

Add lentils to 3 cups of water. Add chervil and cook for about 25 to 30 minutes. Drain and let cool. Add mashed cloves of garlic, the lemon juice, and the olive oil, and blend with lentils. Arrange lettuce leaves on salad plates and place $\frac{1}{4}$ cup of the mixture in each (more when serving only 4). Garnish with spring onions. Very high in the important blood pressure regulator potassium and low in calories.

TIP: Some may not like this news much, but researchers have found that talking too much can raise your blood pressure. A University of Maryland study reports that speaking can cause blood pressure to increase from 10 to 50 percent. The report claims that just about any form of communication can cause your pressure to rise, even sign language.

MYTH: Vegetarians have to combine proteins at every meal.

FACT: Researchers at the University of California at Berkeley say that contrary to popular belief, you don't have to combine complementary proteins at the same meal. Eating a wide variety of foods will give you enough of a variety of amino acids on any given day. So it's not necessary to consume complementary proteins at the same meal.

Nutrients Contained in:
Simple Lentils with Garlic

VITAMINS USRDA			ONE SERVING GIVES YOU APPROXIMATELY		APPROXIMATE PERCENTAGE OF USRDA
A	5,000	IU	751	IU	15
B_1	1.4	mg	0.07	mg	6
B_2	1.6	mg	0.06	mg	4
B_3	16	mg	0.40	mg	2
B_5	10	mg	0.76	mg	7
B_6	2.2	mg	0.18	mg	8
B_{12}	3	μg	0	μg	0
C	60	mg	15	mg	24
D	400	IU	0	IU	0
E	15	IU	2	IU	13
K	500	μg	65	μg	13
Folic Acid	400	μg	31	μg	7

MINERALS USRDA			ONE SERVING GIVES YOU APPROXIMATELY		APPROXIMATE PERCENTAGE OF USRDA
Sodium	(1,100–3,000)	mg	5	mg	0
Calcium	1,000	mg	31	mg	3
Phosphorus	(800–1,000)	mg	79	mg	9
Potassium	(1,875–5,625)	mg	246	mg	30
Magnesium	400	μg	34	μg	9
Selenium	200	μg	6	μg	2
Iodine	150	mg	0	mg	0
Zinc	15	mg	0.68	mg	4
Iron	10	mg	2	mg	15
Manganese	(2.5–5.0)	mg	0.05	mg	1
Copper	(2.0–3.0)	mg	0.17	mg	5

AMOUNT PER SERVING		CALORIES PER SERVING	% OF MEAL
Fat	7 grams	62	46
Proteins	5 grams	19	14
Carbohydrates	13 grams	53	40
Cholesterol	0 mg		
Amino acid (essential)			45–191
Fiber	1 gram		

Key: USRDA = Recommended Dietary Allowance
     IU = International Unit
     mg = milligrams
     μg = micrograms
NOTE: The numbers with arrows exceed 100 percent of required USRDA.

Garlic Straight

Ingredients: 4 heads garlic
                     fresh basil leaves
                     juice of one lemon

Preparation: Bake

Time: 1 hour

Calories: 76 per serving

Serves: 4

Directions

Preheat oven to 325° F. Place garlic and basil leaves on aluminum foil on baking tin and sprinkle with lemon juice. Fold foil around garlic heads fairly tightly. Bake for about 1 hour.

TIP: The results of many studies seem to confirm garlic has a definite therapeutic effect in reducing cholesterol which leads to high blood pressure. At the University of Geneva, in one of numerous studies, Dr. F. G. Piotrowski used garlic on 100 patients with abnormally high blood pressure. The blood pressure was effectively lowered in 40 percent of his hypertensive patients.

MYTH: Mayonnaise is a villain with high cholesterol counts.

FACT: The American Heart Association recommends 300 milligrams of cholesterol a day. Mayonnaise contains only 5 milligrams of cholesterol per tablespoon. That gives you a lot of leeway if you want mayonnaise on your sandwiches without being concerned about high levels of cholesterol.

Nutrients Contained in: Garlic Straight

VITAMINS USRDA			ONE SERVING GIVES YOU APPROXIMATELY		APPROXIMATE PERCENTAGE OF USRDA
A	5,000	IU	1	IU	0
B$_1$	1.4	mg	0.16	mg	13
B$_2$	1.6	mg	0	mg	0
B$_3$	16	mg	0.02	mg	0
B$_5$	10	mg	0.02	mg	0
B$_6$	2.2	mg	0	mg	0
B$_{12}$	3	μg	0	μg	0
C	60	mg	2	mg	3
D	400	IU	0	IU	0
E	15	IU	0.19	IU	1
K	500	μg	0	μg	0
Folic Acid	400	μg	0.75	μg	0

MINERALS USRDA			ONE SERVING GIVES YOU APPROXIMATELY		APPROXIMATE PERCENTAGE OF USRDA
Sodium	(1,100–3,000)	mg	18	mg	1
Calcium	1,000	mg	17	mg	2
Phosphorus	(800–1,000)	mg	99	mg	13
Potassium	(1,875–5,625)	mg	264	mg	33
Magnesium	400	μg	23	μg	4
Selenium	200	μg	0	μg	0
Iodine	150	mg	0	mg	0
Zinc	15	mg	0.61	mg	4
Iron	10	mg	0	mg	0
Manganese	(2.5–5.0)	mg	0	mg	0
Copper	(2.0–3.0)	mg	0.20	mg	4

AMOUNT PER SERVING		CALORIES PER SERVING	% OF MEAL
Fat	0 grams	3	4
Proteins	4 grams	13	17
Carbohydrates	15 grams	60	79
Cholesterol	0 mg		
Amino acid (essential)			3–4
Fiber	1 gram		

Key: USRDA = Recommended Dietary Allowance

IU = International Unit

mg = milligrams

μg = micrograms

NOTE: The numbers with arrows exceed 100 percent of required USRDA.

Rice and Greenery

Ingredients:

- 1 bunch scallions, cut in 1-inch pieces
- ½ lb mustard greens, cut in small pieces
- ½ lb Swiss chard, cut into small pieces
- 1 bunch watercress
- 1 whole tomato
- 1 cup rice (brown or white)
- ¼ cup almond slivers
  low-sodium chicken broth
  cayenne pepper
  juice of one lime

Preparation: Saute

Time: 50 minutes

Calories: 156 per serving

Serves: 6

Directions

Cut tomato in chunks and place in large skillet. Add a little chicken broth to start cooking. After a minute add scallions, mustard greens, chard, and watercress broken into small pieces. Add enough water to cover vegetables; then add rice. Cover tightly and simmer until rice is done, about 20 minutes for white rice, 60 minutes for brown. Add almonds and season with cayenne pepper and lime juice.

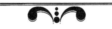

TIP: Brown rice has an edge over white rice in providing a bit more fiber. A half cup of cooked brown rice has about 1.7 grams of dietary fiber. You can get your fiber when using white rice by adding vegetables and beans. Rice is also low in sodium for those who want or need to keep sodium low.

MYTH: Drink milk to relieve ulcer pain.

FACT: Health experts say that food has little to do with either causing ulcers or treating ulcers. Milk stimulates gastric acid production, and acid irritates any type of wound, including an ulcer, so milk doesn't offer any help.

Nutrients Contained in: Rice and Greenery

VITAMINS USRDA			ONE SERVING GIVES YOU APPROXIMATELY		APPROXIMATE PERCENTAGE OF USRDA
A	5,000	IU	3197	IU	63
B$_1$	1.4	mg	0.17	mg	14
B$_2$	1.6	mg	0.13	mg	9
B$_3$	16	mg	2	mg	11
B$_5$	10	mg	0.52	mg	5
B$_6$	2.2	mg	0.21	mg	9
B$_{12}$	3	μg	0	μg	0
C	60	mg	29	mg	48
D	400	IU	0	IU	0
E	15	IU	2	IU	13
K	500	μg	2	μg	0
Folic Acid	400	μg	4	μg	1

MINERALS USRDA			ONE SERVING GIVES YOU APPROXIMATELY		APPROXIMATE PERCENTAGE OF USRDA
Sodium	(1,100–3,000)	mg	24	mg	2
Calcium	1,000	mg	78	mg	9
Phosphorus	(800–1,000)	mg	110	mg	13
Potassium	(1,875–5,625)	mg	274	mg	34
Magnesium	400	μg	56	μg	16
Selenium	200	μg	13	μg	6
Iodine	150	mg	0	mg	0
Zinc	15	mg	0.78	mg	5
Iron	10	mg	2	mg	17
Manganese	(2.5–5.0)	mg	0.69	mg	13
Copper	(2.0–3.0)	mg	0.14	mg	4

AMOUNT PER SERVING		CALORIES PER SERVING	% OF MEAL
Fat	2 grams	22	14
Proteins	4 grams	17	11
Carbohydrates	29 grams	117	75
Cholesterol	0 mg		
Amino acid (essential)			37–63
Fiber	1 gram		

Key: USRDA = Recommended Dietary Allowance
    IU = International Unit
    mg = milligrams
    μg = micrograms
NOTE: The numbers with arrows exceed 100 percent of required USRDA.

Garlic and Trout

Ingredients:
    4 pieces trout,
        3.5 ounces each
    4 cloves garlic, chopped
    2 tsp safflower oil
    1 cup onions, chopped
    1 tsp rosemary
    1 tsp oregano
    1 lemon quartered

Preparation: Bake

Time: 20 minutes

Calories: 276 per serving

Serves: 4

Directions

Preheat oven to 375° F. Saute chopped garlic in oil. Add chopped onions, rosemary, and oregano; saute for a few minutes. Mix all ingredients and spread on top of the trout pieces. Bake for about 10 minutes. If desired, broil trout 6 inches from flame to brown pieces. Remove from oven/broiler and serve with parsley and lemon quarters.

    Although trout is not as good as salmon or mackerel for the fish oils that help the heart, it is still relatively good. Mixing it with the garlic gives it an edge and taste. Notice the tremendous amount of essential amino acids and high levels of calcium and phosphorus.

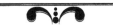

TIP: The medical term for high blood pressure is hypertension. Doctors say it doesn't mean you're under stress, although anxiety can raise blood pressure temporarily. Hyper means high and tension describes the pressure inside your arteries. High blood pressure is linked to many problems that affect older adults, and becomes even more common as you age say heart experts.

MYTH: Nuts contain cholesterol.

FACT: Not being an animal food, you won't find cholesterol in nuts. Cholesterol can be found only in meat, eggs, cheese, and other animal products.

Nutrients Contained in: Garlic and Trout

VITAMINS USRDA			ONE SERVING GIVES YOU APPROXIMATELY		APPROXIMATE PERCENTAGE OF USRDA
A	5,000	IU	319	IU	6
B_1	1.4	mg	0.15	mg	12
B_2	1.6	mg	0.06	mg	4
B_3	16	mg	3	mg	15
B_5	10	mg	0.05	mg	0
B_6	2.2	mg	0.06	mg	2
B_{12}	3	μg	0	μg	0
C	60	mg	4	mg	7
D	400	IU	0	IU	0
E	15	IU	3	IU	18
K	500	μg	0	μg	0
Folic Acid	400	μg	8	μg	2

MINERALS USRDA			ONE SERVING GIVES YOU APPROXIMATELY		APPROXIMATE PERCENTAGE OF USRDA
Sodium	(1,100–3,000)	mg	2	mg	0
Calcium	1,000	mg	229	mg	28
Phosphorus	(800–1,000)	mg	290	mg	36
Potassium	(1,875–5,625)	mg	78	mg	9
Magnesium	400	μg	40	μg	11
Selenium	200	μg	0.80	μg	0
Iodine	150	mg	0	mg	0
Zinc	15	mg	0.11	mg	0
Iron	10	mg	1	mg	12
Manganese	(2.5–5.0)	mg	0.05	mg	1
Copper	(2.0–3.0)	mg	0.02	mg	0

AMOUNT PER SERVING		CALORIES PER SERVING	% OF MEAL
Fat	18 grams	162	59
Proteins	24 grams	97	35
Carbohydrates	4 grams	17	6
Cholesterol	0 mg		
Amino acid (essential)			116–389
Fiber	0 grams		

Key: USRDA = Recommended Dietary Allowance
IU = International Unit
mg = milligrams
μg = micrograms
NOTE: The numbers with arrows exceed 100 percent of required USRDA.

Miracle Chicken Livers

Ingredients:

12 chicken livers
1 cup onions, chopped
1 tsp olive oil
2 Tbs horseradish
½ cup dry red wine
½ cup mushrooms, sliced
½ tsp thyme
½ tsp black pepper

Preparation: Saute

Time: 30 minutes

Calories: 173 per serving

Serves: 4

Directions

Saute onion and mushrooms in oil until golden. Add livers, wine, thyme, and black pepper and saute until livers are cooked, about 12 minutes. Serve with horseradish. One chicken liver contains large amounts of vitamin A, potassium, and phosphorus.

This recipe allocates three livers for each person. Even though livers are high in cholesterol, they offer so much in iron and other nutrients that you can indulge every now and then.

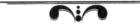

TIP: Folic acid may protect against cervical cancer and certain birth defects according to papers presented at a New York Academy of Sciences conference. Folic acid is contained in dark green leafy vegetables, dried beans and peas, kidneys, and liver. Again notice the high amount of folic acid on your chart for chicken livers.

MYTH: Ghee is healthier than butter in your diet.

FACT: Not according to researchers at the School for Public Health, University of California at Berkeley. They say it's even higher in fat than conventional butter. Ghee is clarified butter with a rich nutty flavor. Because of the process in making it, ghee is a more concentrated source of fat than butter.

Nutrients Contained in: Miracle Chicken Livers

VITAMINS USRDA			ONE SERVING GIVES YOU APPROXIMATELY		APPROXIMATE PERCENTAGE OF USRDA
A	5,000	IU	19,728	IU	394◄
B₁	1.4	mg	0.17	mg	14
B₂	1.6	mg	2	mg	139◄
B₃	16	mg	10	mg	60
B₅	10	mg	6	mg	64
B₆	2.2	mg	0.80	mg	36
B₁₂	3	μg	22	μg	735◄
C	60	mg	37	mg	61
D	400	IU	15	IU	3
E	15	IU	3	IU	19
K	500	μg	86	μg	17
Folic Acid	400	μg	720	μg	179◄

MINERALS USRDA			ONE SERVING GIVES YOU APPROXIMATELY		APPROXIMATE PERCENTAGE OF USRDA
Sodium	(1,100–3,000)	mg	84	mg	8
Calcium	1,000	mg	25	mg	3
Phosphorus	(800–1,000)	mg	292	mg	36
Potassium	(1,875–5,625)	mg	372	mg	46
Magnesium	400	μg	27	μg	7
Selenium	200	μg	3	μg	1
Iodine	150	mg	0	mg	0
Zinc	15	mg	0.62	mg	4
Iron	10	mg	9	mg	87
Manganese	(2.5–5.0)	mg	0.32	mg	6
Copper	(2.0–3.0)	mg	0.50	mg	16

AMOUNT PER SERVING		CALORIES PER SERVING	% OF MEAL
Fat	7 grams	65	38
Proteins	18 grams	73	42
Carbohydrates	9 grams	35	20
Cholesterol	420 mg		
Amino acid (essential)			240–311
Fiber	0 grams		

Key: USRDA = Recommended Dietary Allowance
     IU = International Unit
    mg = milligrams
    μg = micrograms
NOTE: The numbers with arrows exceed 100 percent of required USRDA.

VEGETABLES RANKED IN THE HIGHEST ORDER FOR SODIUM
PERCENTAGES GIVEN EQUAL ½ CUP

	SODIUM (MILLIGRAMS)	PERCENTAGE OF USRDA
Pepper, jalapeno, canned	995.0	30.2
Beans, baked, pork/sce	945.0	28.6
Sauerkraut, canned	780.0	23.6
Broccoli, with cheese sauce	530.0	16.1
Potato, au gratin	528.0	16.0
Beans, baked, plain	504.0	15.3
Asparagus, canned	450.0	13.6
Cauliflower, with cheese	415.0	12.6
Potato, scalloped	409.0	12.4
Spinach, creamed, frozen	395.0	12.0
Garbanzos, canned	359.0	10.9
Peas, blackeye, canned	359.0	10.9
Beans, green, canned	355.0	10.8
Beans, lima, canned	355.0	10.8
Corn, canned	355.0	10.8
Peas, canned	355.0	10.8
Spinach, canned	341.0	10.3
Vegetables, mixed, canned	330.0	10.0
Beets, canned	324.0	9.8
Corn, cream of, canned	320.0	9.7
Potato, mashed	315.0	9.5
Beets, pickled, canned	301.0	9.1
Carrots, canned	265.0	8.0
Mushrooms, canned	260.0	7.9
Tomato, canned	220.0	6.7

CHAPTER FOUR

Healing and Preventive Recipes for Heart Disease

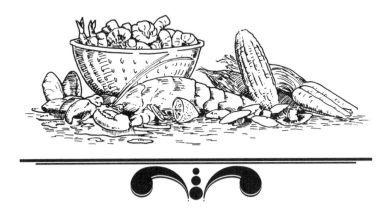

To know that we know what we know, and that we do not know what we do not know, that is true knowledge.
—Henry David Thoreau

Research has made eating for a healthy heart a relatively easy task. A variety of nutritional assets have been studied, and these are included in the recipes in this chapter. The recipes also take into account two key factors that scientists have reported to be most effective in maintaining a healthy heart:—cutting back on fat and cholesterol.

One study reported a reduction in death rate by 30 percent in 2,000 previous heart attack patients when they included in their diet omega-3 fatty acids from eating fish. Studies from Montana State University found that barley fiber can lower cholesterol levels as much as 15 percent. Additional research shows that such foods as potatoes, beans, deep green leafy vegetables, and seafood are good sources of magnesium, a mineral that regulates the heartbeat and may protect men against heart disease.

A number of studies have shown that adding garlic to the diet daily dramatically reduces blood cholesterol. Other foods that have had a positive effect for heart disease include apples, carrots, Chinese mushrooms, corn, fruit, and shellfish.

Look for imaginative easy recipes such as Minced and Mashed Chicken with Bean Curd, which is loaded with magnesium and features low sodium and cholesterol; broiled mackerel, loaded with vitamin B_{12} and vitamin D; and Tofu with Asparagus, also high in magnesium. You will notice that the recipes use little or no salt and very little oil. You can, of course, always add seasonings and more oil if you wish, but remember, any additional oil or fat or sodium will raise the fat percentages.

RECOMMENDED DIETARY ALLOWANCES FOR MAGNESIUM

GROUP/AGE	MAGNESIUM (MILLIGRAMS)
Infants 0–6 months	50
Infants 6–12 months	70
Children 1–3 years	150
Children 4–6 years	200
Children 7–10 years	250
Males 11–14 years	350
Males 15–18 years	400
Males 19+ years	350
Females 11+ years	300
Pregnant and nursing women	450

Minced and Mashed Chicken with Bean Curd

Ingredients:

1 cup chicken meat (white), minced
2 cups bean curd, mashed
2 whole large white eggs
½ tsp lime juice
1 tsp olive oil
1 tsp allspice
½ tsp curry powder
½ tsp chili powder
4 iceberg lettuce leaves
1 whole cucumber

Preparation: Steam
Time: 60 minutes
Calories: 90 per serving
Serves: 4

Directions

Mince chicken and mash the bean curd in a food processor. Use a bowl to combine the eggs, oil, lime juice, allspice powder, chili powder, and curry powder; stir and blend. Steam chicken and bean curd for about 40 minutes at medium boil. The mixture should be very smooth and firm. Do not overcook at this point as the mixture will become too dry and hard. Add cooked chicken and bean curd to the mixture combined in the bowl and mix well. Place lettuce leaves on a platter. Arrange cucumber slices on leaves, top with chicken mixture, and serve. If you have a favorite sauce that is simple to make, prepare it and pour over the meal when ready to serve. This attractive dish is low in calories and high in potassium and phosphorus.

TIP: Chicken, being relatively low in fat and sodium and high in protein, with the cholesterol-lowering power of bean curd, and the storehouse of amino acids, make this combination a powerful heart supporter. White meat has less fat and fewer calories than dark meat.

MYTH: If you don't eat red meat, your cholesterol count will not go up.

FACT: The major contributor to high levels of cholesterol is saturated fat. And if you eat cheese, butter, whole milk, and other items with saturated fat, you will find your dietary cholesterol levels rising like a good stock investment (without the profit).

Nutrients Contained in: Minced and Mashed Chicken with Bean Curd

VITAMINS USRDA			ONE SERVING GIVES YOU APPROXIMATELY		APPROXIMATE PERCENTAGE OF USRDA
A	5,000	IU	93	IU	1
B_1	1.4	mg	.07	mg	6
B_2	1.6	mg	.10	mg	6
B_3	16	mg	1	mg	9
B_5	10	mg	.33	mg	3
B_6	2.2	mg	.11	mg	4
B_{12}	3	μg	.05	μg	1
C	60	mg	4	mg	7
D	400	IU	0	IU	0
E	15	IU	1	IU	8
K	500	μg	34	μg	6
Folic Acid	400	μg	23	μg	5

MINERALS USRDA			ONE SERVING GIVES YOU APPROXIMATELY		APPROXIMATE PERCENTAGE OF USRDA
Sodium	(1,100–3,000)	mg	40	mg	3
Calcium	1,000	mg	92	mg	11
Phosphorus	(800–1,000)	mg	116	mg	14
Potassium	(1,875–5,625)	mg	211	mg	26
Magnesium	400	μg	80	μg	22
Selenium	200	μg	.97	μg	0
Iodine	150	mg	0	mg	0
Zinc	15	mg	.32	mg	2
Iron	10	mg	2	mg	15
Manganese	(2.5–5.0)	mg	.08	mg	1
Copper	(2.0–3.0)	mg	.05	mg	1

AMOUNT PER SERVING		CALORIES PER SERVING	% OF MEAL
Fat	69 grams	56	62
Proteins	5 grams	19	21
Carbohydrates	4 grams	15	17
Cholesterol	10 mg		
Amino acid (essential)			113–146˙
Fiber	1 gram		

Key: USRDA = Recommended Dietary Allowance
     IU = International Unit
     mg = milligrams
     μg = micrograms
NOTE: The numbers with arrows exceed 100 percent of required USRDA.
˙Very high EAA.

Broiled Mackerel

Ingredients:

4 mackerel pieces, 3 ounces each
1 lemon, quartered
$\frac{1}{4}$ cup chopped parsley
1 Tbs horseradish
juice of one lemon or lime

Preparation: Broil

Time: 15 minutes

Calories: 182 per serving

Serves: 4

Directions

Broiling is suitable for almost all seafood. Preheat the oven to 550° F. Since mackerel is an oily fish, you need only dust it lightly with flour. Place fish on a broiling rack and put it under the flame 2 to 6 inches away. Broil 5 to 8 minutes or until slightly brown. Baste with lemon or lime juice. Turn and repeat the process. Serve on a hot platter and garnish with chopped parsley, horseradish, and lemon quarters.

TIP: Large fatty fish such as salmon and mackerel contain the highest amount of the omega-3 fatty acids. In a recent study of a group of Eskimos from Greenland, the virtual absence of coronary heart disease was linked to eating 14 ounces of fatty fish per day. Dr. Daan Kromhout of the University of Leiden in the Netherlands says one to two fish dishes per week can be beneficial.

MYTH: The omega-3 fatty acids are depleted when fish is canned.

FACT: It happens that canned fish has just as much omega-3 fatty acids as fresh fish. You get additional benefits by eating the bones of canned fish and raising your intake of calcium, which helps to prevent osteoporosis and colon cancer.

Nutrients Contained in: Broiled Mackerel

VITAMINS USRDA			ONE SERVING GIVES YOU APPROXIMATELY		APPROXIMATE PERCENTAGE OF USRDA
A	5,000	IU	573	IU	11
B_1	1.4	mg	.14	mg	10
B_2	1.6	mg	.05	mg	3
B_3	16	mg	5	mg	35
B_5	10	mg	0	mg	01
B_6	2.2	mg	.04	mg	20
B_{12}	3	μg	16	μg	550◄
C	60	mg	14	mg	23
D	400	IU	595	IU	149◄
E	15	IU	1	IU	10
K	500	μg	0	μg	0
Folic Acid	400	μg	16	μg	4

MINERALS USRDA			ONE SERVING GIVES YOU APPROXIMATELY		APPROXIMATE PERCENTAGE OF USRDA
Sodium	(1,100–3,000)	mg	76	mg	6
Calcium	1,000	mg	14	mg	1
Phosphorus	(800–1,000)	mg	6	mg	0
Potassium	(1,875–5,625)	mg	399	mg	18
Magnesium	400	μg	93	μg	22
Selenium	200	μg	3	μg	1
Iodine	150	mg	0	mg	0
Zinc	15	mg	.08	mg	5
Iron	10	mg	1	mg	10
Manganese	(2.5–5.0)	mg	.04	mg	0
Copper	(2.0–3.0)	mg	.03	mg	0

AMOUNT PER SERVING		CALORIES PER SERVING	% OF MEAL
Fat	15 grams	69	40
Proteins	20 grams	113	60
Carbohydrates	0 grams	0	0
Cholesterol	64 mg		
Amino acid (essential)			Very high
Fiber	0 grams		

Key: USRDA = Recommended Dietary Allowance

IU = International Unit

mg = milligrams

μg = micrograms

NOTE: The numbers with arrows exceed 100 percent of required USRDA.

Potato, Pepper, and Onion Gathering

Ingredients:

4 medium potatoes with skins
1 tsp olive oil
1 ½ cup onions, chopped
2 cloves garlic, sliced
4 green and/or red peppers, seeded and cut in strips
3 large red tomatoes, coarsely chopped

Preparation: Saute

Time: 30 minutes

Calories: 311 per serving

Serves: 4

Directions

Slice the potatoes into thin pieces and saute them in the oil in a large skillet. Add the onions and the garlic once potatoes begin to brown. After they have softened sufficiently, add the peppers and finally the tomatoes. Cover and cook over medium heat until all the ingredients are well blended, about 10 minutes. If you want a side dish, try a modest serving of Italian sausages cooked separately, but remember the fat and calories.

TIP: The American Heart Association recommends that daily fat consumption be reduced to 30 percent of total calories and that only 10 percent come from saturated fat sources. Saturated fat, found primarily in meats and dairy products, contributes to raising cholesterol levels.

MYTH: Headstands increase blood supply to the brain and provide health benefits.

FACT: University of California *Wellness Letter* researchers report no evidence that this activity is good for you and, indeed, that it can involve some risks to your eyes and associated blood vessels and can cause other injuries.

Nutrients Contained in: Potato, Pepper, and Onion Gathering

VITAMINS USRDA			ONE SERVING GIVES YOU APPROXIMATELY		APPROXIMATE PERCENTAGE OF USRDA
A	5,000	IU	1258	IU	25
B$_1$	1.4	mg	0.34	mg	28
B$_2$	1.6	mg	0.14	mg	9
B$_3$	16	mg	4	mg	25
B$_5$	10	mg	1	mg	14
B$_6$	2.2	mg	0.90	mg	40
B$_{12}$	3	μg	0	μg	0
C	60	mg	108	mg	179◄
D	400	IU	0	IU	0
E	15	IU	2	IU	12
K	500	μg	11	μg	2
Folic Acid	400	μg	23	μg	2

MINERALS USRDA			ONE SERVING GIVES YOU APPROXIMATELY		APPROXIMATE PERCENTAGE OF USRDA
Sodium	(1,100–3,000)	mg	27	mg	2
Calcium	1,000	mg	44	mg	5
Phosphorus	(800–1,000)	mg	165	mg	20
Potassium	(1,875–5,625)	mg	1,206	mg	150◄
Magnesium	400	μg	77	μg	22
Selenium	200	μg	3	μg	1
Iodine	150	mg	0	mg	0
Zinc	15	mg	0.94	mg	6
Iron	10	mg	4	mg	38
Manganese	(2.5–5.0)	mg	0.73	mg	14
Copper	(2.0–3.0)	mg	0.75	mg	25

AMOUNT PER SERVING		CALORIES PER SERVING	% OF MEAL
Fat	4 grams	37	12
Proteins	7 grams	26	8
Carbohydrates	62 grams	248	80
Cholesterol	0 mg		
Amino acid (essential)			58–100
Fiber	3 grams		

Key: USRDA = Recommended Dietary Allowance
   IU = International Unit
   mg = milligrams
   μg = micrograms
NOTE: The numbers with arrows exceed 100 percent of required USRDA.

Kerstin's Tomato Spinach

Ingredients:

6 cups spinach, chopped
12 cloves garlic, peeled and minced
2 tomatoes, chopped fine
1 onion, chopped
   juice of one lemon
1 tsp chervil
1 tsp vegetable oil

Preparation: Steam and saute

Time: 20 minutes

Calories: 157 per serving

Serves: 4

Directions

Steam spinach until wilted and then allow to sit. In the meantime, heat oil in a large skillet. Saute garlic and onion in the oil. When onions are transparent, place the spinach in the pan and mix all ingredients together, saving the tomatoes for last. Heat for a few minutes and serve.

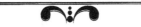

TIP: Researchers from the Veterans Affairs Medical Center in Houston say that emotional stress may be dangerous to the heart. In a study conducted with men with mild heart disease who were asked to describe an incident that made them angry, the pumping efficiency of the men's hearts dropped significantly in response. The study results suggested that anger was sending the diseased arteries into spasm.

MYTH: The majority of vegan vegetarians are subject to anemia because they eat no animal foods and have a vitamin B_{12} deficiency.

FACT: Doctors who have studied diets of vegans say that because so little B_{12} is needed, most vegans are getting enough. The USRDA of 3 micrograms (μg) is three times more than most people need, they say. They also report that B_{12} is recycled by the body and uses it more than once. Research also indicates that people who eat less protein need less B_{12}.

Nutrients Contained in:
Kerstin's Tomato Spinach

VITAMINS USRDA			ONE SERVING GIVES YOU APPROXIMATELY		APPROXIMATE PERCENTAGE OF USRDA
A	5,000	IU	22,814	IU	456◀
B$_1$	1.4	mg	0.35	mg	29
B$_2$	1.6	mg	0.68	mg	48
B$_3$	16	mg	2	mg	10
B$_5$	10	mg	0.62	mg	6
B$_6$	2.2	mg	0.76	mg	34
B$_{12}$	3	μg	0	μg	0
C	60	mg	48	mg	80
D	400	IU	0	IU	0
E	15	IU	12	IU	79
K	500	μg	275	μg	55
Folic Acid	400	μg	408	μg	102◀

MINERALS USRDA			ONE SERVING GIVES YOU APPROXIMATELY		APPROXIMATE PERCENTAGE OF USRDA
Sodium	(1,100–3,000)	mg	198	mg	19
Calcium	1,000	mg	387	mg	48
Phosphorus	(800–1,000)	mg	196	mg	24
Potassium	(1,875–5,625)	mg	1,514	mg	189◀
Magnesium	400	μg	257	μg	73
Selenium	200	μg	31	μg	15
Iodine	150	mg	0	mg	0
Zinc	15	mg	2	mg	15
Iron	10	mg	10	mg	101◀
Manganese	(2.5–5.0)	mg	3	mg	52
Copper	(2.0–3.0)	mg	0.56	mg	18

AMOUNT PER SERVING		CALORIES PER SERVING	% OF MEAL
Fat	4 grams	39	25
Proteins	10 grams	39	25
Carbohydrates	20 grams	79	50
Cholesterol	0 mg		
Amino acid (essential)			108–122
Fiber	3 grams		

Key: USRDA = Recommended Dietary Allowance

　　IU　= International Unit

　　mg　= milligrams

　　μg　= micrograms

NOTE: The numbers with arrows exceed 100 percent of required USRDA.

Sweet Potato Smoothie

Ingredients:
2 cups sweet potato
8 shiitake mushrooms
1 red pepper, seeded
    and sliced crosswise
    into ¼-inch pieces
1 cantaloupe
1 Tbs soy sauce
1 large onion, sliced
1 tsp lime juice
1 tsp lemon juice

Preparation: Broil

Time: 25 minutes

Calories: 341 per serving

Serves: 4

Direction

Turn on broiler. Cut sweet potatoes into slices about ½-inch thick. Brush lemon juice over them and place on broiler. Place onion slices on broiler and red pepper slices with the mushrooms on the broiler. Sprinkle soy sauce over them and broil all ingredients about 5 minutes on each side or until sweet potatoes are done. Cut up cantaloupe into thin slices and serve with meal. Notice the large amounts of vitamin C and A contained in this delicious preparation.

TIP: Dr. Bryant Stamford, director of the Health Promotion Center at the University of Louisville in Kentucky, says that sports and recreation provide a moderate amount of exercise and you'll live longer if you get regular, moderate exercise. To reduce the risk of heart disease, researchers say that you have to burn at least 285 calories a day.

MYTH: Flavored coffees are higher in fat and calories than regular coffee.

FACT: Flavoring in fresh coffee adds only taste and aroma. The Long Beach, California, Specialty Coffee Association says that one 6-fluid-ounce serving of brewed, flavored coffee, taken without milk or sugar, has no fat and only 4 calories.

Nutrients Contained in: Sweet Potato Smoothie

VITAMINS USRDA			ONE SERVING GIVES YOU APPROXIMATELY		APPROXIMATE PERCENTAGE OF USRDA
A	5,000	IU	32,375	IU	647◀
B$_1$	1.4	mg	0.17	mg	14
B$_2$	1.6	mg	0.29	mg	20
B$_3$	16	mg	4	mg	26
B$_5$	10	mg	1	mg	11
B$_6$	2.2	mg	0.66	mg	30
B$_{12}$	3	μg	0	μg	0
C	60	mg	108	mg	179◀
D	400	IU	0	IU	0
E	15	IU	3	IU	23
K	500	μg	0	μg	0
Folic Acid	400	μg	81	μg	20

MINERALS USRDA			ONE SERVING GIVES YOU APPROXIMATELY		APPROXIMATE PERCENTAGE OF USRDA
Sodium	(1,100–3,000)	mg	298	mg	29
Calcium	1,000	mg	65	mg	8
Phosphorus	(800–1,000)	mg	90	mg	11
Potassium	(1,875–5,625)	mg	985	mg	123◀
Magnesium	400	μg	58	μg	16
Selenium	200	μg	1	μg	0
Iodine	150	mg	0	mg	
Zinc	15	mg	3	mg	18
Iron	10	mg	2	mg	16
Manganese	(2.5–5.0)	mg	0.68	mg	13
Copper	(2.0–3.0)	mg	0.35	mg	11

AMOUNT PER SERVING		CALORIES PER SERVING	% OF MEAL
Fat	1 gram	10	3
Proteins	7 grams	28	8
Carbohydrates	76 grams	303	89
Cholesterol	0 mg		
Amino acid (essential)			40–50*
Fiber	2 grams		

Key: USRDA = Recommended Dietary Allowance

    IU = International Unit

    mg = milligrams

    μg = micrograms

NOTE: The numbers with arrows exceed 100 percent of required USRDA.

*1 ounce of Brie cheese raises EAA to 124–142%.

Steamy Greens

Ingredients:

1 cup bok choy
1 cup turnip greens
1 cup mustard greens
½ cup cooked chick peas
½ cup nonfat plain yogurt
1 Tbs lemon juice
1 Tbs chervil

Preparation: Steam

Time: 15 minutes

Calories: 136 per serving

Serves: 4

Directions

Prepare water in steamer and bring to a boil. Place greens in steamer and cover. Steam for about 5 minutes or until greens are tender. Mix lemon juice and chick peas into yogurt. Top greens with mixture of yogurt and chervil. Serve while hot. High amounts of vitamin A and potassium are recorded.

TIP: Studies reveal that too much iron may increase the risk of a heart attack. A five-year study at the University of Kuopio's Research Institute of Public Health in Finland monitored the iron intake of 1,931 healthy men ages 42 to 60 and linked iron overload in the blood to an increased heart attack risk. Their intake was 19 milligrams a day, 9 milligrams more than the USRDA in the United States.

MYTH: Nuts that are known to be high in fat are not good foods to eat for a healthy heart.

FACT: According to researchers at Loma Linda University in California, people who eat any kind of nuts five times a week could lower their cardiac risk by 50 percent. The blood lipids may be altered in a positive way is the suggested reason. Of course, your weight may be altered also, as nuts are fattening.

Nutrients Contained in: Steamy Greens

VITAMINS USRDA			ONE SERVING GIVES YOU APPROXIMATELY		APPROXIMATE PERCENTAGE OF USRDA
A	5,000	IU	5,068	IU	101◄
B_1	1.4	mg	0.15	mg	12
B_2	1.6	mg	0.21	mg	14
B_3	16	mg	0.84	mg	5
B_5	10	mg	0.65	mg	6
B_6	2.2	mg	0.18	mg	8
B_{12}	3	μg	0.16	μg	5
C	60	mg	45	mg	74
D	400	IU	13	IU	3
E	15	IU	2	IU	11
K	500	μg	93	μg	18
Folic Acid	400	μg	30	μg	7

MINERALS USRDA			ONE SERVING GIVES YOU APPROXIMATELY		APPROXIMATE PERCENTAGE OF USRDA
Sodium	(1,100–3,000)	mg	56	mg	5
Calcium	1,000	mg	225	mg	28
Phosphorus	(800–1,000)	mg	158	mg	19
Potassium	(1,875–5,625)	mg	578	mg	72
Magnesium	400	μg	64	μg	18
Selenium	200	μg	0	μg	0
Iodine	150	mg	13	mg	8
Zinc	15	mg	0.96	mg	6
Iron	10	mg	3	mg	32
Manganese	(2.5–5.0)	mg	0.39	mg	7
Copper	(2.0–3.0)	mg	0.25	mg	8

AMOUNT PER SERVING		CALORIES PER SERVING	% OF MEAL
Fat	2 grams	18	13
Proteins	9 grams	34	25
Carbohydrates	21 grams	84	62
Cholesterol	2 mg		
Amino acid (essential)			82–136
Fiber	2 grams		

Key: USRDA = Recommended Dietary Allowance
   IU = International Unit
   mg = milligrams
   μg = micrograms
NOTE: The numbers with arrows exceed 100 percent of required USRDA.

Lemon, Lettuce, and Chicken Breasts

Ingredients:
1 ½ lb boned chicken breasts, sliced
½ head iceberg lettuce leaves
1 lemon, cut in slices
½ cup apple juice
¼ cup apricot nectar
⅓ cup rice bran
1 Tbs lemon juice
1 Tbs horseradish

Preparation: Broil
Time: 20 minutes
Calories: 107 per serving
Serves: 4

Directions

Preheat broiler. Spread lemon juice, horseradish, apricot nectar, rice bran, and apple juice over chicken breasts. Broil about 15 minutes 4 to 6 inches from flame, turning pieces until meat is done. Serve on lettuce leaves with sliced lemons.

TIP: Many studies have indicated that beta-carotene found in fruits and leafy green vegetables can protect against cancer and disease in the male heart. Based on a study at Boston's Brigham and Women's Hospital carried out on 87,245 women, women who eat a cup of beta-carotene-rich food a day have 40 percent fewer strokes and 22 percent fewer heart attacks than do those who eat a quarter cupful a day.

MYTH: For vitamins to be effective, they must be taken in exactly prescribed amounts and ratios to each other.

FACT: The U.S. Department of Health and Human Services report that intake should be adequate but not excessive for each. No precise or exact ratios are required.

Nutrients Contained in: Lemon, Lettuce, and Chicken Breasts

VITAMINS USRDA			ONE SERVING GIVES YOU APPROXIMATELY		APPROXIMATE PERCENTAGE OF USRDA
A	5,000	IU	443	IU	8
B$_1$	1.4	mg	0.26	mg	21
B$_2$	1.6	mg	0.08	mg	5
B$_3$	16	mg	6	mg	38
B$_5$	10	mg	0.33	mg	3
B$_6$	2.2	mg	0.52	mg	23
B$_{12}$	3	μg	0.13	μg	4
C	60	mg	12	mg	20
D	400	IU	0	IU	0
E	15	IU	1	IU	8
K	500	μg	130	μg	26
Folic Acid	400	μg	46	μg	11

MINERALS USRDA			ONE SERVING GIVES YOU APPROXIMATELY		APPROXIMATE PERCENTAGE OF USRDA
Sodium	(1,100–3,000)	mg	31	mg	3
Calcium	1,000	mg	28	mg	3
Phosphorus	(800–1,000)	mg	81	mg	10
Potassium	(1,875–5,625)	mg	368	mg	45
Magnesium	400	μg	79	μg	22
Selenium	200	μg	3	μg	1
Iodine	150	mg	0	mg	0
Zinc	15	mg	0.93	mg	6
Iron	10	mg	2	mg	21
Manganese	(2.5–5.0)	mg	0.14	mg	2
Copper	(2.0–3.0)	mg	0.06	mg	1

AMOUNT PER SERVING		CALORIES PER SERVING	% OF MEAL
Fat	2 grams	20	19
Proteins	10 grams	38	36
Carbohydrates	12 grams	49	45
Cholesterol	29 mg		
Amino acid (essential)			97–147
Fiber	1 gram		

Key: USRDA = Recommended Dietary Allowance
    IU = International Unit
    mg = milligrams
    μg = micrograms
NOTE: The numbers with arrows exceed 100 percent of required USRDA.

Tore's Turnips

Ingredients:

4 cups yellow turnips, peeled and cut into pieces
1 white potato, diced
½ cup skim milk
½ cup low-sodium chicken broth
½ tsp ground ginger
¼ cup fresh chopped parsley
1 Tbs dried chervil
1 tsp lime juice

Preparation: Boil

Time: 25 minutes

Calories: 102 per serving

Serves: 4

Directions

Boil turnips and potatoes until tender. Pour off water and mash turnips and potatoes. Add chicken broth and milk to vegetable mixture a little at a time. Mix and add the ginger, chervil, parsley, and lime juice. This is a simple and tasty way of eating turnips, which are extremely low in calories, for a healthy heart and a trimmer profile.

TIP: Scientists at the University of Pittsburgh report that the amount of alcohol contained in three to six glasses of wine per week boosts levels of estrogen, the hormone that protects against cardiovascular problems and osteoporosis in women. Dr. Judith Gavaler, professor of medicine at the university, says that the decrease in the risk of heart disease and bone loss from the wine applies only to women who have undergone menopause.

MYTH: Organic food is more nutritious than nonorganic food.

FACT: The former director of the Center for Science in the Public Interest's Americans for Safe Food project (ASF), Roger Blobaum, says researchers have not found any good evidence that organically grown produce has more vitamins or minerals, as studies of that kind have never been done.

Nutrients Contained in: Tore's Turnips

VITAMINS USRDA			ONE SERVING GIVES YOU APPROXIMATELY		APPROXIMATE PERCENTAGE OF USRDA
A	5,000	IU	763	IU	15
B1	1.4	mg	0.12	mg	9
B2	1.6	mg	0.17	mg	12
B3	16	mg	2	mg	12
B5	10	mg	0.66	mg	6
B6	2.2	mg	0.25	mg	11
B12	3	μg	0.32	μg	10
C	60	mg	43	mg	72
D	400	IU	25	IU	6
E	15	IU	0.25	IU	1
K	500	μg	0	μg	0
Folic Acid	400	μg	26	μg	6

MINERALS USRDA			ONE SERVING GIVES YOU APPROXIMATELY		APPROXIMATE PERCENTAGE OF USRDA
Sodium	(1,100-3,000)	mg	319	mg	31
Calcium	1,000	mg	135	mg	16
Phosphorus	(800-1,000)	mg	115	mg	14
Potassium	(1,875-5,625)	mg	567	mg	70
Magnesium	400	μg	31	μg	8
Selenium	200	μg	1	μg	2
Iodine	150	mg	3	mg	0
Zinc	15	mg	0.46	mg	3
Iron	10	mg	1	mg	11
Manganese	(2.5-5.0)	mg	12	mg	2
Copper	(2.0-3.0)	mg	0.12	mg	3

AMOUNT PER SERVING		CALORIES PER SERVING	% OF MEAL
Fat	1 gram	6	6
Proteins	5 grams	21	21
Carbohydrates	19 grams	75	73
Cholesterol	1 mg		
Amino acid (essential)			45-60*
Fiber	1 gram		

Key: USRDA = Recommended Dietary Allowance

IU = International Unit

mg = milligrams

μg = micrograms

NOTE: The numbers with arrows exceed 100 percent of required USRDA.

*1 large egg white raises EAA to 94-144%.

Stir-Fry Tofu with Asparagus

Ingredients:

16 oz package tofu
2 cups asparagus pieces
$\frac{1}{2}$ cup cucumbers, sliced
1 tsp oregano
1 Tbs soy sauce
$\frac{1}{2}$ tsp chili spice

Preparation: Stir-fry

Time: 25 minutes

Calories: 79 per serving

Serves: 4

Directions

Drain tofu and cut into cubes. Add soy sauce to skillet, heat, and then add the tofu pieces. Stir-fry until tofu takes up the soy sauce flavors; then add asparagus pieces and cucumbers. Sprinkle with oregano and chili spice; stir-fry for a few minutes. Serve hot. Notice the high amount of magnesium and potassium and the low amount of calories in this meal.

TIP: Scientists report that magnesium is an important mineral in regulating the heartbeat. U.S. Department of Agriculture Human Nutrition Research Center studies suggest that eating enough of it may protect men against heart disease and possibly bring down high blood pressure.

MYTH: Fingernails continue to grow after one dies.

FACT: Fingernails do not continue to grow after death, but it is reported that the cuticle retracts in death. This can make it appear that the nail is growing according to the Mayo Clinic *Health Letter*.

Nutrients Contained in:
Stir-Fry Tofu with Asparagus

VITAMINS USRDA			ONE SERVING GIVES YOU APPROXIMATELY		APPROXIMATE PERCENTAGE OF USRDA
A	5,000	IU	345	IU	6
B$_1$	1.4	mg	0.13	mg	11
B$_2$	1.6	mg	0.10	mg	7
B$_3$	16	mg	0.89	mg	5
B$_5$	10	mg	0.26	mg	2
B$_6$	2.2	mg	0.10	mg	4
B$_{12}$	3	μg	0	μg	0
C	60	mg	13	mg	22
D	400	IU	0	IU	0
E	15	IU	2	IU	16
K	500	μg	26	μg	5
Folic Acid	400	μg	48	μg	11

MINERALS USRDA			ONE SERVING GIVES YOU APPROXIMATELY		APPROXIMATE PERCENTAGE OF USRDA
Sodium	(1,100-3,000)	mg	269	mg	26
Calcium	1,000	mg	171	mg	21
Phosphorus	(800-1,000)	mg	200	mg	24
Potassium	(1,875-5,625)	mg	292	mg	36
Magnesium	400	μg	149	μg	42
Selenium	200	μg	0	μg	0
Iodine	150	mg	0	mg	0
Zinc	15	mg	0.36	mg	2
Iron	10	mg	3	mg	29
Manganese	(2.5-5.0)	mg	0.12	mg	2
Copper	(2.0-3.0)	mg	0.07	mg	2

AMOUNT PER SERVING		CALORIES PER SERVING	% OF MEAL
Fat	5 grams	47	59
Proteins	2 grams	7	10
Carbohydrates	6 grams	25	31
Cholesterol	0 mg		
Amino acid (essential)			108-177[*]
Fiber	1 gram		

Key: USRDA = Recommended Dietary Allowance
     IU = International Unit
    mg = milligrams
    μg = micrograms
NOTE: The numbers with arrows exceed 100 percent of required USRDA.
[*]Very high levels of EAA.

Pearly Barley with Okra, Zucchini, and Tomatoes

Ingredient:

- 2 cups cooked barley
- 2 cups zucchini, sliced and quartered
- 2 fresh tomatoes
- ½ cup onion, chopped
- 1 cup canned okra
- ¼ celery, chopped
- ¼ tsp allspice

Preparation: Saute, steam, boil

Time: 1 hour, 10 minutes

Calories: 272 per serving

Serves: 6

Directions

Use a 4-quart saucepan and combine barley and 8 cups of water. Bring to a boil and then simmer uncovered for 20 minutes. Steam the okra until al dente, about 3 to 5 minutes. Saute onion and zucchini for about 3 minutes in a little water. Drain the barley and discard the water. Combine okra with all remaining ingredients and saute for about 3 minutes until all ingredients are blended. Don't overcook. In addition to its cholesterol-lowering power, notice the high content of phosphorus and potassium on your chart.

TIP: Barley is known as "medicine for the heart" in Pakistan. U.S. Department of Agriculture researchers say there are three constituents in barley that hamper the liver's ability to produce bad LDL-type cholesterol. This is a big boost for the cardiovascular system.

MYTH: Wild rice is equal to white or brown rice.

FACT: Wild rice is not a rice at all. It is a grass seed and is known to have more protein and fewer calories than rice. It produces double the volume of rice when cooked.

Nutrients Contained in: Pearly Barley with Okra, Zucchini, and Tomatoes

VITAMINS USRDA			ONE SERVING GIVES YOU APPROXIMATELY		APPROXIMATE PERCENTAGE OF USRDA
A	5,000	IU	736	IU	14
B$_1$	1.4	mg	0.23	mg	19
B$_2$	1.6	mg	0.11	mg	7
B$_3$	16	mg	3	mg	20
B$_5$	10	mg	0.25	mg	2
B$_6$	2.2	mg	0.12	mg	5
B$_{12}$	3	μg	0	μg	0
C	60	mg	15	mg	25
D	400	IU	0	IU	0
E	15	IU	0.44	IU	2
K	500	μg	3	μg	0
Folic Acid	400	μg	32	μg	8

MINERALS USRDA			ONE SERVING GIVES YOU APPROXIMATELY		APPROXIMATE PERCENTAGE OF USRDA
Sodium	(1,100–3,000)	mg	20	mg	2
Calcium	1,000	mg	55	mg	6
Phosphorus	(800–1,000)	mg	245	mg	30
Potassium	(1,875–5,625)	mg	543	mg	67
Magnesium	400	μg	53	μg	15
Selenium	200	μg	0.55	μg	0
Iodine	150	mg	0	mg	0
Zinc	15	mg	0.30	mg	1
Iron	10	mg	2	mg	24
Manganese	(2.5–5.0)	mg	0.36	mg	7
Copper	(2.0–3.0)	mg	0.25	mg	8

AMOUNT PER SERVING		CALORIES PER SERVING	% OF MEAL
Fat	1 gram	8	3
Proteins	8 grams	31	11
Carbohydrates	58 grams	233	86
Cholesterol	0 mg		
Amino acid (essential)			67–126
Fiber	2 grams		

Key: USRDA = Recommended Dietary Allowance
IU = International Unit
mg = milligrams
μg = micrograms
NOTE: The numbers with arrows exceed 100 percent of required USRDA.

Tuna Stuffed Tomatoes

Ingredients:

10 ounces canned tuna
4 large tomatoes
2 spring onions
½ cup romaine lettuce
1 Tbs horseradish
¼ cup parsley
2 Tbs margarine
4 Tbs wheat germ
1 tsp dill

Preparation: No cooking required

Time: 20 minutes

Calories: 204 per serving

Serves: 4

Directions

Cut away the top of each tomato and scoop out the pulp, leaving enough so the tomatoes retain their roundness. Drain the pulp and chop coarsely. Mix the pulp, scallion, lettuce, and tuna in a bowl. In another bowl, combine the margarine, horseradish, parsley, dill, and wheat germ and gently toss with the tuna mixture. Spoon into tomato shells.

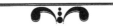

TIP: Another soldier in the fight against increased blood levels of the bad cholesterol HDL is olive oil. Dutch scientists of the De Dreijen Agricultural University report that a study carried out with a diet rich in olive oil reduced the level of cholesterol and fats in all the 57 people given this diet.

MYTH: Most of a potato's vitamin C is just under the skin.

FACT: Not so according to researchers who have determined that peeling potatoes has almost no effect on their vitamin C content. With or without skin they say a large potato supplies about 30 milligrams of the vitamin. As you know from your nutrient chart, this is half of your daily requirement.

Nutrients Contained in: Tuna Stuffed Tomatoes

VITAMINS USRDA			ONE SERVING GIVES YOU APPROXIMATELY		APPROXIMATE PERCENTAGE OF USRDA
A	5,000	IU	2,468	IU	49
B$_1$	1.4	mg	0.23	mg	19
B$_2$	1.6	mg	0.18	mg	13
B$_3$	16	mg	10	mg	61
B$_5$	10	mg	0.49	mg	4
B$_6$	2.2	mg	0.39	mg	17
B$_{12}$	3	μg	0.98	μg	32
C	60	mg	33	mg	54
D	400	IU	6	IU	1
E	15	IU	2	IU	15
K	500	μg	17	μg	3
Folic Acid	400	μg	49	μg	12

MINERALS USRDA			ONE SERVING GIVES YOU APPROXIMATELY		APPROXIMATE PERCENTAGE OF USRDA
Sodium	(1,100–3,000)	mg	407	mg	40
Calcium	1,000	mg	33	mg	4
Phosphorus	(800–1,000)	mg	272	mg	34
Potassium	(1,875–5,625)	mg	578	mg	72
Magnesium	400	μg	63	μg	18
Selenium	200	μg	44	μg	21
Iodine	150	mg	0	mg	0
Zinc	15	mg	2	mg	11
Iron	10	mg	3	mg	25
Manganese	(2.5–5.0)	mg	2	mg	32
Copper	(2.0–3.0)	mg	0.21	mg	7

AMOUNT PER SERVING		CALORIES PER SERVING	% OF MEAL
Fat	8 grams	73	36
Proteins	23 grams	91	44
Carbohydrates	10 grams	40	20
Cholesterol	65 mg		
Amino acid (essential)			143–420
Fiber	1 gram		

Key: USRDA = Recommended Dietary Allowance
IU = International Unit
mg = milligrams
μg = micrograms
NOTE: The numbers with arrows exceed 100 percent of required USRDA.

Stir-Fry Variation with Zucchini, Carrots, and Leeks

Ingredients:

2 medium zucchini, cut in 2 " strips
3 carrots, scraped and cut in 2 " sticks
2 leeks, cut in 2 " sticks
3 cloves garlic, peeled
1 tsp olive oil
1 tsp parsley, chopped
various seasonings
pepper to taste

Preparation: Stir-fry
Time: 15 minutes
Calories: 99 per serving
Serves: 4

Directions

Make certain that the carrots are thinly cut so that they can cook faster. Trim the leeks and cut similarly. Cut the peeled garlic into thin slices. Heat the oil in a wok preferably but a good skillet will work just as well. Stir-fry the garlic, parsley, and pepper for about 30 to 40 seconds. Add carrots and continue to stir-fry for equal time. Sprinkle with various seasonings such as thyme, marjoram, and basil. The idea is to be creative with the spices that you like, tossing the ingredients as you sprinkle. Then serve on warm platter.

TIP: Of the many strategies for reducing heart disease, a six-year study by Dr. Charles Hennekens at Brigham and Women's Hospital in Boston found that a form of vitamin A common in carrots and many other vegetables appears to reduce substantially the risk of heart trouble in people who have coronary artery disease.

MYTH: Vitamins provide energy and build parts of the body.

FACT: The U.S. Department of Health and Human Services says vitamins do not provide energy, nor do they construct or build any part of the body. They are needed for transforming foods into energy and body maintenance. There are 13 or more of them, and the FDA says that if any one is missing, a deficiency disease can result.

Nutrients Contained in: Stir-Fry Variation with Zucchini, Carrots, and Leeks

VITAMINS USRDA			ONE SERVING GIVES YOU APPROXIMATELY		APPROXIMATE PERCENTAGE OF USRDA
A	5,000	IU	15,108	IU	302◄
B_1	1.4	mg	0.08	mg	6
B_2	1.6	mg	0.05	mg	3
B_3	16	mg	0.69	mg	4
B_5	10	mg	0.16	mg	1
B_6	2.2	mg	0.11	mg	5
B_{12}	3	μg	0	μg	0
C	60	mg	10	mg	18
D	400	IU	0	IU	0
E	15	IU	0.92	IU	6
K	500	μg	75	μg	15
Folic Acid	400	μg	17	μg	4

MINERALS USRDA			ONE SERVING GIVES YOU APPROXIMATELY		APPROXIMATE PERCENTAGE OF USRDA
Sodium	(1,100–3,000)	mg	25	mg	2
Calcium	1,000	mg	26	mg	3
Phosphorus	(800–1,000)	mg	45	mg	5
Potassium	(1,875–5,625)	mg	344	mg	42
Magnesium	400	μg	25	μg	7
Selenium	200	μg	0.88	μg	0
Iodine	150	mg	2	mg	0
Zinc	15	mg	0.20	mg	1
Iron	10	mg	1	mg	9
Manganese	(2.5–5.0)	mg	0.07	mg	2
Copper	(2.0–3.0)	mg	0.37	mg	12

AMOUNT PER SERVING		CALORIES PER SERVING	% OF MEAL
Fat	4 grams	32	48
Proteins	1 gram	4	6
Carbohydrates	15 grams	63	46
Cholesterol	0 mg		
Amino acid (essential)			7–9
Fiber	1 gram		

Key: USRDA = Recommended Dietary Allowance
IU = International Unit
mg = milligrams
μg = micrograms
NOTE: The numbers with arrows exceed 100 percent of required USRDA.

Heart-Rending Potatoes, Tomatoes, and Peas

Ingredients:

4 medium-sized white potatoes, unpeeled
3 bunches green spring onions
3 large tomatoes
12 ounces peas (preferably fresh)
1 tsp curry
¼ tsp cayenne pepper
1 tsp ground ginger
1 tsp chopped chile pepper
1 tsp vegetable oil

Preparation: Boil and saute

Time: 50 minutes

Calories: 198 per serving

Serves: 4

Directions

Cut potatoes into cubes and cover with water in a deep pot. Cover pot and boil until potatoes are tender—from 15 to 20 minutes. Heat the oil in an iron skillet. Add the onions, chile pepper, curry, cayenne pepper, and ginger and saute until onions are soft. Ingredients should be lightly browned. Add the tomatoes and peas and cook until they are evenly heated through. Drain the cooked potatoes and add to the vegetables. You should not need any further seasoning. Observe the high amounts of potassium and vitamin A on your chart.

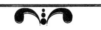

TIP: Heart researchers consider the potato a good food to help the heart stay healthy. Potatoes have large amounts of potassium, and researchers at the University of Minnesota are convinced that a low-potassium intake is linked to heart disease and stroke. This vegetable is also a good source of the fiber that aids in lowering cholesterol.

MYTH: Eating chocolate will raise your cholesterol levels.

FACT: Penn State researchers indicate it does not. Chocolate is high in saturated fat that comes mainly from cocoa butter. But this type of fat, which is stearic acid, does not raise the levels as dairy butter fat does.

Nutrients Contained in: Heart-Rending Potatoes, Tomatoes, and Peas

VITAMINS USRDA			ONE SERVING GIVES YOU APPROXIMATELY		APPROXIMATE PERCENTAGE OF USRDA
A	5,000	IU	2654	IU	53
B_1	1.4	mg	0.36	mg	30
B_2	1.6	mg	0.20	mg	14
B_3	16	mg	4	mg	22
B_5	10	mg	1	mg	10
B_6	2.2	mg	0.54	mg	24
B_{12}	3	μg	0	μg	0
C	60	mg	46	mg	76
D	400	IU	0	IU	0
E	15	IU	0.67	IU	4
K	500	μg	173	μg	34
Folic Acid	400	μg	62	μg	15

MINERALS USRDA			ONE SERVING GIVES YOU APPROXIMATELY		APPROXIMATE PERCENTAGE OF USRDA
Sodium	(1,100–3,000)	mg	17	mg	1
Calcium	1,000	mg	48	mg	5
Phosphorus	(800–1,000)	mg	154	mg	19
Potassium	(1,875–5,625)	mg	860	mg	107◄
Magnesium	400	μg	65	μg	18
Selenium	200	μg	0.64	μg	1
Iodine	150	mg	0	mg	0
Zinc	15	mg	1	mg	8
Iron	10	mg	2	mg	22
Manganese	(2.5–5.0)	mg	0.62	mg	12
Copper	(2.0–3.0)	mg	0.41	mg	13

AMOUNT PER SERVING		CALORIES PER SERVING	% OF MEAL
Fat	8 grams	4	2
Proteins	7 grams	27	14
Carbohydrates	42 grams	167	84
Cholesterol	0 mg		
Amino acid (essential)			64–86
Fiber	3 grams		

Key: USRDA = Recommended Dietary Allowance

IU = International Unit

mg = milligrams

μg = micrograms

NOTE: The numbers with arrows exceed 100 percent of required USRDA.

Turnip, Carrot, and Squash Free-for-All

Ingredients:

1 cup firm white turnips, scraped and cubed

3 large carrots, scraped and cubed

1 cup summer squash, sliced

1 tsp olive oil

2 Tbs chopped onions

2 Tbs fresh chopped parsley

juice of one lemon

Preparation: Saute

Time: 15 minutes

Calories: 79 per serving

Serves: 4

Directions

Cut the carrots into cubes to the same size as the turnip cubes. Slice the summer squash in ¼-inch slices. Heat the oil in an iron skillet if you have one and add the cubed turnips and carrots and squash. Cook for about 1 minute. Then add the onions and cook until soft, about another minute. Add lemon juice and the parsley and cook until all vegetables are tender but not overcooked. Stir and serve. Look at the chart and notice the high amounts of vitamin A and potassium you get from this meal.

TIP: More than 40 epidemiological studies have shown a correlation between taking in too low levels of vitamin C and being at risk for a wide range of malignancies, including oral, esophageal, cervical, and lung cancers.

MYTH: Aging people need a lot of rest.

FACT: The U.S. Department of Agriculture's Human Nutrition Research Center on Aging at Tuft's University says just the opposite is true. People in their 90s and those starting in middle age need exercise to avoid physically retarding and also to reverse the aging process or to avoid what researchers call the "disability zone."

Nutrients Contained in: Turnip, Carrot, and Squash Free-for-All

VITAMINS USRDA			ONE SERVING GIVES YOU APPROXIMATELY		APPROXIMATE PERCENTAGE OF USRDA
A	5,000	IU	15,289	IU	305◄
B_1	1.4	mg	0.09	mg	7
B_2	1.6	mg	0.07	mg	4
B_3	16	mg	0.89	mg	5
B_5	10	mg	0.25	mg	2
B_6	2.2	mg	0.15	mg	6
B_{12}	3	μg	0	μg	0
C	60	mg	18	mg	29
D	400	IU	0	IU	0
E	15	IU	1	IU	7
K	500	μg	75	μg	15
Folic Acid	400	μg	22	μg	5

MINERALS USRDA			ONE SERVING GIVES YOU APPROXIMATELY		APPROXIMATE PERCENTAGE OF USRDA
Sodium	(1,100–3000)	mg	42	mg	4
Calcium	1,000	mg	41	mg	5
Phosphorus	(800–1,000)	mg	53	mg	6
Potassium	(1,875–5,625)	mg	345	mg	43
Magnesium	400	μg	24	μg	6
Selenium	200	μg	4	μg	1
Iodine	150	mg	0	mg	0
Zinc	15	mg	0.31	mg	2
Iron	10	mg	0.66	mg	6
Manganese	(2.5–5.0)	mg	0.19	mg	3
Copper	(2.0–3.0)	mg	0.08	mg	2

AMOUNT PER SERVING		CALORIES PER SERVING	% OF MEAL
Fat	4 grams	33	42
Proteins	1 gram	6	6
Carbohydrates	10 grams	40	52
Cholesterol	0 mg		
Amino acid (essential)			10–15
Fiber	1 gram		

Key: USRDA = Recommended Dietary Allowance

IU = International Unit

mg = milligrams

μg = micrograms

NOTE: The numbers with arrows exceed 100 percent of required USRDA.

Salmon Steaks

Ingredients:

4 pieces of salmon,
    3.5 ounces each
1 cup mushrooms, sliced
1 garlic clove, chopped
½ cup onion, chopped
¼ cup parsley, chopped
½ cup dry white wine
   flour
   lemon juice
   chervil

Preparation: Bake

Time: 45 minutes

Calories: 204 per serving

Serves: 4

Directions

Preheat oven to 400° F. Dust salmon very lightly with flour and bake 5 minutes in oven. Baste with lemon juice frequently. Combine the mushrooms, onion, garlic, and wine and spoon onto the salmon. Add a bay leaf, cover and cook 15 minutes longer. Remove the salmon onto a heated platter. Season to taste with chervil and citrus juice and chopped parsley.

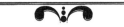

TIP: Five to 40 percent of the fat in seafood is omega-3 fatty acids. Only very small quantities of fish can be of help to the cardiovascular system. Eating only one or two fish dishes a week may help prevent coronary heart disease, report researchers in the Netherlands.

MYTH: The healthiest way to prepare chicken is to cook it without the skin.

FACT: University of Minnesota researchers disagree with this idea promoted by nutritionists. The researchers say that leaving the skin on poultry while it cooks—and removing it afterward—does not produce a fattier bird. An advantage is that it makes for a juicier bird.

Nutrients Contained in: Salmon Steaks

	VITAMINS USRDA		ONE SERVING GIVES YOU APPROXIMATELY		APPROXIMATE PERCENTAGE OF USRDA
A	5,000	IU	479	IU	9
B1	1.4	mg	0.21	mg	17
B2	1.6	mg	0.19	mg	13
B3	16	mg	12	mg	71
B5	10	mg	2	mg	21
B6	2.2	mg	0.77	mg	35
B12	3	μg	4	μg	133◄
C	60	mg	19	mg	31
D	400	IU	650	IU	162◄
E	15	IU	2	IU	14
K	500	μg	4	μg	0
Folic Acid	400	μg	37	μg	9

	MINERALS USRDA		ONE SERVING GIVES YOU APPROXIMATELY		APPROXIMATE PERCENTAGE OF USRDA
Sodium	(1,100–3,000)	mg	119	mg	11
Calcium	1,000	mg	429	mg	53
Phosphorus	(800–1,000)	mg	234	mg	29
Potassium	(1,875–5,625)	mg	644	mg	80
Magnesium	400	μg	38	μg	10
Selenium	200	μg	5	μg	2
Iodine	150	mg	0	mg	0
Zinc	15	mg	1	mg	8
Iron	10	mg	2	mg	21
Manganese	(2.5–5.0)	mg	0.11	mg	2
Copper	(2.0–3.0)	mg	0.42	mg	14

AMOUNT PER SERVING		CALORIES PER SERVING	% OF MEAL
Fat	8 grams	69	34
Proteins	28 grams	113	55
Carbohydrates	6 grams	22	11
Cholesterol	47 mg		
Amino acid (essential)			169-557*
Fiber	0 grams		

Key: USRDA = Recommended Dietary Allowance
    IU = International Unit
    mg = milligrams
    μg = micrograms
NOTE: The numbers with arrows exceed 100 percent of required USRDA.
*Chock full of all EAA.

Bean Insurance

Ingredients:

2 cups canned navy beans
1 onion, diced
3 cloves garlic, diced
¼ cup soy sauce
¼ cheddar cheese
¼ cup wheat germ

Preparation: Cook

Time: 10 minutes

Calories: 170 per serving

Serves: 4

Directions

Cook in a skillet the onions, diced garlic, wheat germ, and soy sauce for about 5 minutes. While this mixture is cooking, open the can of navy beans and heat in a saucepan until hot. After beans are hot, spoon into bowls and mix in the remaining ingredients. Sprinkle with cheese. Again, over 400 percent of essential amino acids and high amounts of potassium and phosphorus and low calories are in this dish.

TIP: Beans are known to lower harmful cholesterol levels. Researchers at the University of Kentucky found that eating a cup and a half of navy or pinto beans daily reduced one man's cholesterol from 274 to 190 and another's from 218 to 167.

MYTH: Cottage cheese is a good source of calcium.

FACT: According to the University of California School of Public Health, cottage cheese is only a modest source of calcium, giving just 60 to 70 milligrams in half a cup in contrast to 200 milligrams in a half a cup of yogurt.

Nutrients Contained in: Bean Insurance

VITAMINS USRDA			ONE SERVING GIVES YOU APPROXIMATELY		APPROXIMATE PERCENTAGE OF USRDA
A	5,000	IU	19	IU	0
B$_1$	1.4	mg	0.29	mg	23
B$_2$	1.6	mg	0.14	mg	9
B$_3$	16	mg	1	mg	7
B$_5$	10	mg	0.16	mg	1
B$_6$	2.2	mg	0.14	mg	6
B$_{12}$	3	µg	0.01	µg	0
C	60	mg	4	mg	6
D	400	IU	0	IU	0
E	15	IU	0.30	IU	1
K	500	µg	0	µg	0
Folic Acid	400	µg	33	µg	8

MINERALS USRDA			ONE SERVING GIVES YOU APPROXIMATELY		APPROXIMATE PERCENTAGE OF USRDA
Sodium	(1,100–3,000)	mg	84	mg	8
Calcium	1,000	mg	74	mg	9
Phosphorus	(800–1,000)	mg	249	mg	31
Potassium	(1,875–5,625)	mg	542	mg	67
Magnesium	400	µg	28	µg	8
Selenium	200	µg	8	µg	3
Iodine	150	mg	1	mg	0
Zinc	15	mg	2	mg	14
Iron	10	mg	3	mg	33
Manganese	(2.5–5.0)	mg	1	mg	29
Copper	(2.0–3.0)	mg	0.07	mg	2

AMOUNT PER SERVING		CALORIES PER SERVING	% OF MEAL
Fat	2 grams	18	11
Proteins	11 grams	42	25
Carbohydrates	27 grams	110	64
Cholesterol	2 mg		
Amino acid (essential)			145–405
Fiber	2 grams		

Key: USRDA = Recommended Dietary Allowance
     IU = International Unit
    mg = milligrams
    µg = micrograms
NOTE: The numbers with arrows exceed 100 percent of required USRDA.

Sweet Sweet Potatoes

Ingredients:
    4 fresh sweet potatoes
½ cup orange juice
1 orange

Preparation: Bake

Time: 40 minutes

Calories: 254 per serving

Serves: 6

Directions

Preheat oven to 350° F. Arrange sweet potatoes in baking dish and pour orange juice over them. Place orange slices on top. Bake for 30 minutes or until sweet potatoes can easily be pierced with a fork. (Do not substitute yams for this recipe as the vitamin A level of yams is much lower.)

You may sprinkle potatoes with ¼ cup of brown sugar and dot with a little butter. The fat, cholesterol, sodium, potassium, and vitamin A in the adjusted recipe are as follows:

Fat, 8 grams and 75 calories   Vitamin A, 37, 708 IU
Sodium, 110 mg   Potassium, 527 mg
Cholesterol, 21 mg   Total calories, 395

TIP: A half-cup serving of steamed carrots supplies almost two times a person's daily recommended intake of 1,000 IU of vitamin A. Other good sources are liver, tomatoes, apricots, and cantaloupe. Since vitamin A is easy to get from your diet and is extremely toxic in high doses, experts recommend avoiding supplements.

MYTH: You cannot get enough vitamins from the conventional foods you eat.

FACT: The U.S. Department of Health and Human Services says this is a myth, as anyone who eats a reasonably varied diet should normally never need supplemental vitamins.

Nutrients Contained in: Sweet Sweet Potatoes

VITAMINS USRDA			ONE SERVING GIVES YOU APPROXIMATELY		APPROXIMATE PERCENTAGE OF USRDA
A	5,000	IU	37,420	IU	748◄
B$_1$	1.4	mg	0.15	mg	12
B$_2$	1.6	mg	0.32	mg	22
B$_3$	16	mg	2	mg	9
B$_5$	10	mg	1	mg	12
B$_6$	2.2	mg	0.55	mg	26
B$_{12}$	3	μg	0	μg	0
C	60	mg	59	mg	98
D	400	IU	0	IU	0
E	15	IU	4	IU	27
K	500	μg	0.17	μg	0
Folic Acid	400	μg	42	μg	10

MINERALS USRDA			ONE SERVING GIVES YOU APPROXIMATELY		APPROXIMATE PERCENTAGE OF USRDA
Sodium	(1,100–3,000)	mg	28	mg	2
Calcium	1,000	mg	58	mg	7
Phosphorus	(800–1,000)	mg	65	mg	8
Potassium	(1,875–5,625)	mg	482	mg	60
Magnesium	400	μg	26	μg	7
Selenium	200	μg	0.88	μg	0
Iodine	150	mg	0	mg	0
Zinc	15	mg	0.61	mg	4
Iron	10	mg	1	mg	12
Manganese	(2.5–5.0)	mg	0.74	mg	14
Copper	(2.0–3.0)	mg	0.37	mg	12

AMOUNT PER SERVING		CALORIES PER SERVING	% OF MEAL
Fat	19 grams	6	3
Proteins	4 grams	16	6
Carbohydrates	58 grams	232	91
Cholesterol	0 mg		
Amino acid (essential)			45–60
Fiber	2 grams		

Key: USRDA = Recommended Dietary Allowance
　　　 IU = International Unit
　　　 mg = milligrams
　　　 μg = micrograms
NOTE: The numbers with arrows exceed 100 percent of required USRDA.

VEGETABLES RANKED IN THE HIGHEST ORDER FOR MAGNESIUM
PERCENTAGES GIVEN EQUAL ½ CUP

	MAGNESIUM (MILLIGRAMS)	PERCENTAGE OF USRDA
Tofu	127.0	45.4
Beans, fava, canned	85.0	30.4
Spinach, canned	81.0	28.9
Spinach, cooked	79.0	28.2
Potato, baked	55.0	19.6
Beans, mung, cooked	53.0	18.9
Beans, pinto, cooked	52.0	18.6
Broccoli, cooked	47.0	16.8
Artichoke, cooked	47.0	16.8
Okra, cooked	46.0	16.4
Beans, baked, pork/sauce	44.0	15.7
Beans, lima, canned	42.0	15.0
Beans, lima, cooked	41.0	14.6
Beans, baked, plain	41.0	14.6
Peas, blackeye, cooked	41.0	14.6
Beans, kidney, canned	40.0	14.3
Garbanzos, canned	35.0	12.5
Corn on the cob, cooked	34.0	12.1
Artichoke hearts	33.0	11.8
Beets, cooked	31.0	11.1

CHAPTER FIVE

Healing and Preventive Recipes for Diabetes

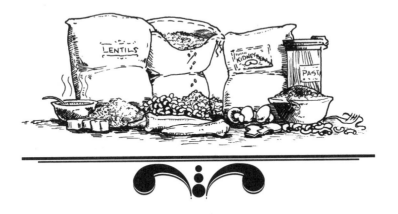

Read not to contradict and confute, nor to believe
and take for granted, but to weigh and consider.
—Francis Bacon

The recipes in this chapter will provide you with meals that contain high-complex-carbohydrate, low-sodium, low-fat nutrients. Since an overweight condition is one of the risks for adult-onset (type II) diabetes, you will want to eat those foods that help control weight.

Again, fish with a high omega-3 fatty acid content helps the diabetic as research has shown that these fatty acids help protect the heart. The American Diabetes Association (ADA) suggests that foods such as grains, pasta, beans, peas, fruits, and vegetables should make up half or more of your diet. Protein intake should be about 12 to 20 percent of your daily calorie intake according to ADA.

You will find the recipes here are very low in fat and high in fiber. You should use these recipes and information in this chapter to build your fiber intake gradually to 40 grams of dietary fiber a day, the amount recommended by ADA. You will discover a variety of meals meeting your needs such as Barley, Okra, and Mushroom Salad, Tofu and Friends, Kidney Beans with a Flair, and others.

The advice to avoid or limit sugar is valuable for the public at large as well as people with diabetes as is the idea of limiting fat to less than 30 percent of calories and to eat food with fiber.

Barley, Okra, and Mushroom Salad

Ingredients:

1 ½ cups cooked pearl barley
½ cup tomato, diced
½ cup plain yogurt
1 tsp honey
1 tsp lemon juice
¼ sliced scallions
2 Tbs balsamic vinegar
12 fresh shiitake mushrooms
½ tsp dill weed
¼ cup fresh parsley
¼ tsp chili powder
1 cup okra
¼ cup Parmesan cheese
¾ tsp mint leaves, fresh or dried

Preparation: Steam

Time: 30 minutes

Calories: 431 per serving

Serves: 4

Directions

Steam okra for 8 minutes and set aside. Whisk the yogurt, vinegar, honey, lemon juice, and ¼ tsp of curry powder together in a bowl and refrigerate until ready to serve over salad ingredients. Combine barley, cooked mushrooms, okra, parsley, scallions, tomatoes, and spices in a large bowl. Cover and refrigerate for an hour. Use dressing made earlier when ready to serve.

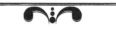

TIP: Pearl barley looks like small white pearls and cooks in about 30 or 40 minutes. A quick-cook type that's presteamed can be prepared in as little as 10 minutes. Barley contains plenty of soluble fiber and protein.

MYTH: Foods that are crunchy are high in fiber.

FACT: Bananas and green peas are not crunchy, and yet they offer more fiber than celery and crunchy cereals. Celery provides less than 1 gram of fiber per half cup. Green peas offer more than 4 grams of fiber a half cup when cooked.

Nutrients Contained in: Barley, Okra, and Mushroom Salad

VITAMINS USRDA			ONE SERVING GIVES YOU APPROXIMATELY		APPROXIMATE PERCENTAGE OF USRDA
A	5,000	IU	826	IU	16
B$_1$	1.4	mg	0.23	mg	19
B$_2$	1.6	mg	0.12	mg	8
B$_3$	16	mg	7	mg	41
B$_5$	10	mg	0.15	mg	1
B$_6$	2.2	mg	0.10	mg	4
B$_{12}$	3	μg	0	μg	0
C	60	mg	15	mg	24
D	400	IU	0	IU	0
E	15	IU	0.31	IU	2
K	500	μg	3	μg	0
Folic Acid	400	μg	76	μg	19

MINERALS USRDA			ONE SERVING GIVES YOU APPROXIMATELY		APPROXIMATE PERCENTAGE OF USRDA
Sodium	(1,100–3,000)	mg	17	mg	1
Calcium	1,000	mg	61	mg	7
Phosphorus	(800–1,000)	mg	243	mg	30
Potassium	(1,875–5,625)	mg	668	mg	83
Magnesium	400	μg	78	μg	22
Selenium	200	μg	0.18	μg	0
Iodine	150	mg	0	mg	0
Zinc	15	mg	3	mg	21
Iron	10	mg	3	mg	25
Manganese	(2.5–5.0)	mg	0.29	mg	5
Copper	(2.0–3.0)	mg	0.26	mg	8

AMOUNT PER SERVING		CALORIES PER SERVING	% OF MEAL
Fat	1 gram	9	2
Proteins	12 grams	46	11
Carbohydrates	94 grams	376	87
Cholesterol	0 mg		
Amino acid (essential)			70–135
Fiber	1 gram		

Key: USRDA = Recommended Dietary Allowance

IU = International Unit

mg = milligrams

μg = micrograms

NOTE: The numbers with arrows exceed 100 percent of required USRDA.

Tofu and Friends

Ingredients:

1 cup tofu, cut in small cubes

1 sweet red pepper, seeded and cut in strips

1 stalk celery, cut in thin slices

4 cloves garlic, chopped

1 tsp canola oil

1 tsp chili powder

12 shiitake mushrooms (fresh if available)

1 cup turnip greens

1/2 cup beet greens

1 cup zucchini slices

1 large onion, sliced

1/4 cup low-sodium chicken broth

8 oz canned fava beans

juice of one lemon

black pepper

Preparation: Saute

Time: 20 minutes

Calories: 265 per serving

Serves: 4

Directions

Use a large iron skillet and saute onions, red peppers, celery, and garlic for 5 minutes or so. Steam the turnip greens and beet greens for about 7 minutes. Add to the skillet the greens, mushrooms, zucchini, and chili powder. Stir and blend. Add the tofu, broth, and fava beans. Cover and cook for a few minutes. Add lemon juice and black pepper to season. Check the chart for the high percentages of vitamin A_1, potassium, magnesium, and fiber.

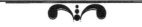

TIP: A report in the *Wellness Letter* of the University of California at Berkeley says that even after iron pots and skillets have been used many times, they still appear to be a good source of iron. Researchers cooked spaghetti sauce and applesauce 50 times in an iron skillet and found that the foods absorbed about as much iron the 50th time as earlier. The iron gets added to the foods cooked in them.

MYTH: There are four specific regions of the tongue that detect a primary flavor such as sweet, sour, or salty.

FACT: Scientists at the National Institutes of Health say any of these flavors can be tasted on any part of the tongue, although the whole taste perception itself involves very complex interactions with the oral and nasal senses.

Nutrients Contained in: Tofu and Friends

VITAMINS USRDA			ONE SERVING GIVES YOU APPROXIMATELY		APPROXIMATE PERCENTAGE OF USRDA
A	5,000	IU	1,537	IU	30
B_1	1.4	mg	0.21	mg	17
B_2	1.6	mg	0.14	mg	10
B_3	16	mg	4	mg	25
B_5	10	mg	0.21	mg	2
B_6	2.2	mg	0.25	mg	11
B_{12}	3	μg	0	μg	0
C	60	mg	37	mg	62
D	400	IU	0	IU	0
E	15	IU	0.87	IU	5
K	500	μg	93	μg	18
Folic Acid	400	μg	136	μg	33

MINERALS USRDA			ONE SERVING GIVES YOU APPROXIMATELY		APPROXIMATE PERCENTAGE OF USRDA
Sodium	(1,100–3,000)	mg	94	mg	9
Calcium	1,000	mg	206	mg	25
Phosphorus	(800–1,000)	mg	167	mg	20
Potassium	(1,875–5,625)	mg	803	mg	100
Magnesium	400	μg	178	μg	50
Selenium	200	μg	1	μg	0
Iodine	150	mg	0	mg	0
Zinc	15	mg	4	mg	24
Iron	10	mg	4	mg	36
Manganese	(2.5–5.0)	mg	0.24	mg	4
Copper	(2.0–3.0)	mg	0.14	mg	4

AMOUNT PER SERVING		CALORIES PER SERVING	% OF MEAL
Fat	4 grams	39	15
Proteins	8 grams	33	13
Carbohydrates	48 grams	193	72
Cholesterol	0 mg		
Amino acid (essential)			83–144
Fiber	16 grams		

Key: USRDA = Recommended Dietary Allowance
   IU = International Unit
   mg = milligrams
   μg = micrograms
NOTE: The numbers with arrows exceed 100 percent of required USRDA.

Kidney Beans with a Flair

Ingredients:
20 brussels sprouts
2 cups cooked kidney beans
1 large sweet onion, chopped
¼ cup wheat germ
½ cinnamon
½ tsp sesame seeds
2 cups skim milk
4 Tbs Romano cheese
1 tsp canola oil

Preparation: Steam and saute
Time: 30 minutes
Calories: 319 per serving
Serves: 4

Directions

Peel outer leaves of brussels sprouts, make an "X" in the stem end with a sharp knife, and steam about 8 minutes, until tender. Set aside. Saute onion in canola oil for about 5 minutes. Stir wheat germ and seasonings into the sauteed onion. Continue stirring while gradually adding milk. Cook on low heat for about 10 minutes. Remove from heat and add cheese and brussels sprouts. Top the sprouts with kidney beans that have been drained and heated. Notice percentages on the chart of vitamin K, C, calcium, phosphorus, potassium, and very high EAA range.

TIP: Most all beans are an excellent source of complex carbohydrates, fiber, and protein. They have large percentages of iron, calcium, and phosphorus and all-important soluble fiber. Swiss researchers showed that beans suppress the appetite for hours because they are digested very slowly, so they can control your weight as well.

MYTH: Eating a lot of sugar causes diabetes.

FACT: Dietitians report that the amount of sugar eaten has nothing to do with diabetes, but sugar can aggravate the disease. Diabetics need to keep the level of sugar in their blood stable so sugar is not a particularly friendly ingredient.

Nutrients Contained in:
Kidney Beans with a Flair

VITAMINS USRDA			ONE SERVING GIVES YOU APPROXIMATELY		APPROXIMATE PERCENTAGE OF USRDA
A	5,000	IU	932	IU	18
B$_1$	1.4	mg	0.39	mg	32
B$_2$	1.6	mg	0.27	mg	19
B$_3$	16	mg	2	mg	14
B$_5$	10	mg	0.51	mg	5
B$_6$	2.2	mg	0.35	mg	15
B$_{12}$	3	μg	0	μg	0
C	60	mg	85	mg	141◀
D	400	IU	0	IU	0
E	15	IU	3	IU	20
K	500	μg	750	μg	150◀
Folic Acid	400	μg	92	μg	22

MINERALS USRDA			ONE SERVING GIVES YOU APPROXIMATELY		APPROXIMATE PERCENTAGE OF USRDA
Sodium	(1,000–3,000)	mg	203	mg	20
Calcium	1,000	mg	249	mg	31
Phosphorus	(800–1,000)	mg	450	mg	56
Potassium	(1,875–5,625)	mg	852	mg	106◀
Magnesium	400	μg	64	μg	18
Selenium	200	μg	46	μg	22
Iodine	150	mg	0	mg	0
Zinc	15	mg	3	mg	17
Iron	10	mg	5	mg	45
Manganese	(2.5–5.0)	mg	2	mg	35
Copper	(2.0–3.0)	mg	0.60	mg	19

AMOUNT PER SERVING		CALORIES PER SERVING	% OF MEAL
Fat	10 grams	94	30
Proteins	19 grams	77	24
Carbohydrates	37 grams	148	46
Cholesterol	15 mg		
Amino acid (essential)			289–511
Fiber	3 grams		

Key: USRDA = Recommended Dietary Allowance
    IU = International Unit
    mg = milligrams
    μg = micrograms
NOTE: The numbers with arrows exceed 100 percent of required USRDA.

Six Who Passed While the Lentils Boiled

Ingredients:
- ½ cup lentils
- 2 cups water
- 1 tsp canola oil
- 1 onion, chopped
- 1 clove garlic, minced
- 16 asparagus spears, stalks peeled
- 1 red pepper, seeded and sliced crosswise
- ½ cup instant brown rice
- ½ tsp oregano
- ½ tsp cinnamon
- black pepper
- juice of one lemon

Preparation: Boil and saute

Time: 55 minutes

Calories: 184 per serving

Serves: 4

Directions

Put lentils in pan and bring to boil. Lower heat and simmer for 20 minutes. Saute onions, asparagus, and red pepper in oil until vegetables are soft, but don't overcook. Add lemon juice. In the meantime cook instant rice according to instructions on the package. Pour lentils and water over the sauteed mixture, bring to a boil, cover, and simmer for 15 minutes more. Serve with rice.

TIP: The ADA recommends that you eat no more than 300 milligrams of cholesterol daily. You should eat sparingly of organ meats, egg yolks, meat, and dairy fats. This recipe has zero cholesterol.

MYTH: Waffles are very high in fat.

FACT: According to a national survey conducted for the Kellogg Company, each waffle has only about 2 grams of fat (18 calories' worth). It's when you put all the good stuff on it that the fat builds.

Nutrients Contained in: Six Who Passed While the Lentils Boiled

VITAMINS USRDA			ONE SERVING GIVES YOU APPROXIMATELY		APPROXIMATE PERCENTAGE OF USRDA
A	5,000	IU	574	IU	11
B$_1$	1.4	mg	0.20	mg	16
B$_2$	1.6	mg	0.11	mg	7
B$_3$	16	mg	2	mg	12
B$_5$	10	mg	0.77	mg	7
B$_6$	2.2	mg	0.37	mg	16
B$_{12}$	3	μg	0	μg	0
C	60	mg	39	mg	65
D	400	IU	0	IU	0
E	15	IU	4	IU	29
K	500	μg	40	μg	8
Folic Acid	400	μg	73	μg	18

MINERALS USRDA			ONE SERVING GIVES YOU APPROXIMATELY		APPROXIMATE PERCENTAGE OF USRDA
Sodium	(1,100–3,000)	mg	7	mg	0
Calcium	1,000	mg	41	mg	5
Phosphorus	(800–1,000)	mg	137	mg	17
Potassium	(1,875–5,625)	mg	394	mg	49
Magnesium	400	μg	49	μg	13
Selenium	200	μg	12	μg	6
Iodine	150	mg	0	mg	0
Zinc	15	mg	1	mg	7
Iron	10	mg	2	mg	26
Manganese	(2.5–5.0)	mg	0.59	mg	11
Copper	(2.0–3.0)	mg	0.21	mg	7

AMOUNT PER SERVING		CALORIES PER SERVING	% OF MEAL
Fat	4 grams	38	20
Proteins	6 grams	24	14
Carbohydrates	31 grams	122	66
Cholesterol	0 mg		
Amino acid (essential)			57–136
Fiber	1 gram		

Key: USRDA = Recommended Dietary Allowance
     IU = International Unit
    mg = milligrams
    μg = micrograms
NOTE: The numbers with arrows exceed 100 percent of required USRDA.

Soybean Strength

Ingredients:

2 cups soybeans, cooked
1 cup ziti
1 spring onion, chopped
1 stalk celery, chopped coarse
1 cup mustard greens, chopped
½ cup low-sodium chicken broth
1 cup canned tomatoes
2 Tbs grated Romano cheese
various seasonings

Preparation: Steam and saute

Time: 30 minutes

Calories: 264 per serving

Serves: 4

Directions

Cook ziti according to package instructions. Steam mustard greens for about 5 minutes. Saute the onion and celery in chicken broth for about 5 minutes. Stir mustard greens with some seasonings to taste into the ingredients in the skillet. Add cooked ziti, soybeans, and tomatoes to the cooking vegetables. Bring to a simmer. Remove pan from heat, stir in the cheese, and sprinkle with oregano, paprika, and chili powder to taste. Note potassium, vitamin A, calcium, magnesium, and EAA percentages.

TIP: Soak soybeans in hot water and cover overnight. Drain and place in a large pan with water. Bring to a boil and simmer for about three hours or until tender. These excellent nutrients control fatty accumulations in the cells and help break down fat deposits.

MYTH: Fish oil supplements loaded with omega-3 fatty acids are a good source for a healthy diet.

FACT: Not according to the ADA. This type of supplement may be unhealthy for people with diabetes. Studies have shown that high amounts increase blood glucose levels.

Nutrients Contained in: Soybean Strength

VITAMINS USRDA			ONE SERVING GIVES YOU APPROXIMATELY		APPROXIMATE PERCENTAGE OF USRDA
A	5,000	IU	4,840	IU	96
B$_1$	1.4	mg	0.41	mg	34
B$_2$	1.6	mg	0.35	mg	25
B$_3$	16	mg	2	mg	14
B$_5$	10	mg	2	mg	18
B$_6$	2.2	mg	0.89	mg	40
B$_{12}$	3	μg	0	μg	0
C	60	mg	81	mg	135◄
D	400	IU	0	IU	0
E	15	IU	3	IU	20
K	500	μg	19	μg	38
Folic Acid	400	μg	189	μg	47

MINERALS USRDA			ONE SERVING GIVES YOU APPROXIMATELY		APPROXIMATE PERCENTAGE OF USRDA
Sodium	(1,100–3,000)	mg	215	mg	21
Calcium	1,000	mg	328	mg	41
Phosphorus	(800–1,000)	mg	255	mg	31
Potassium	(1,875–5,625)	mg	970	mg	121◄
Magnesium	400	μg	297	μg	84
Selenium	200	μg	41	μg	20
Iodine	150	mg	0	mg	0
Zinc	15	mg	2	mg	13
Iron	10	mg	5	mg	48
Manganese	(2.5–5.0)	mg	1	mg	28
Copper	(2.0–3.0)	mg	0.10	mg	3

AMOUNT PER SERVING		CALORIES PER SERVING	% OF MEAL
Fat	8 grams	75	28
Proteins	18 grams	72	27
Carbohydrates	29 grams	117	45
Cholesterol	7 mg		
Amino acid (essential)			158–224
Fiber	8 grams		

Key: USRDA = Recommended Dietary Allowance
     IU = International Unit
     mg = milligrams
     μg = micrograms
NOTE: The numbers with arrows exceed 100 percent of required USRDA.

Oysters Non-Rockefeller

Ingredients:

2 dozen fresh oysters in the shell
1 cup bok choy, finely chopped
4 cloves garlic, minced
½ cup low-sodium chicken broth
1 tsp mint
1 tsp basil
1 tsp Italian parsley, chopped
juice of one lemon
1 tsp hot sauce
½ tsp cayenne pepper
2 Tbs Parmesan cheese

Preparation: Saute and bake

Time: 20 minutes

Calories: 379 per serving

Serves: 4

Directions

Preheat oven to 375° F. Rinse shucked oysters with cold water and place them back in the shell. Blend the cheese, garlic, parsley, basil, pepper, and mint. Distribute the mixture evenly over the oysters. In a medium-sized pan, saute bok choy in a little chicken broth for about 5 minutes once the stove is very hot. Place oysters with shells and mixture in a heavy baking dish. Cover each oyster with the bok choy and sprinkle with lemon juice and hot sauce. Sprinkle cheese evenly on the oysters and bake for about 8 minutes. Your chart will show tremendous amounts of vitamins A, D, and C; potassium; magnesium; zinc; and iron.

TIP: Most registered dietitians advise against taking fiber pills and powders. The benefits that come with increased fiber intake, they say, comes from eating fiber-rich foods themselves (whole grains, fruits, and vegetables).

MYTH: Your taste perceptions tend to change with age.

FACT: Research from the National Institute on Aging indicates that this is untrue. Studies show taste sensitivity actually undergoes few changes in healthy older individuals.

Nutrients Contained in: Oysters Non-Rockefeller

VITAMINS USRDA			ONE SERVING GIVES YOU APPROXIMATELY		APPROXIMATE PERCENTAGE OF USRDA
A	5,000	IU	4,252	IU	85
B_1	1.4	mg	0.81	mg	67
B_2	1.6	mg	1	mg	80
B_3	16	mg	7	mg	42
B_5	10	mg	0.05	mg	0
B_6	2.2	mg	0.02	mg	0
B_{12}	3	μg	90	μg	3,000◄
C	60	mg	265	mg	442◄
D	400	IU	300	IU	75
E	15	IU	5	IU	34
K	500	μg	0	μg	0
Folic Acid	400	μg	53	μg	13

MINERALS USRDA			ONE SERVING GIVES YOU APPROXIMATELY		APPROXIMATE PERCENTAGE OF USRDA
Sodium	(1,100–3,000)	mg	628	mg	62
Calcium	1,000	mg	314	mg	39
Phosphorus	(800–1,000)	mg	43	mg	5
Potassium	(1,875–5,625)	mg	1,375	mg	171◄
Magnesium	400	μg	292	μg	83
Selenium	200	μg	3	μg	1
Iodine	150	mg	0	mg	0
Zinc	15	mg	456	mg	3,041◄
Iron	10	mg	34	mg	343◄
Manganese	(2.5–5.0)	mg	0.04	mg	0
Copper	(2.0–3.0)	mg	0.04	mg	1

AMOUNT PER SERVING		CALORIES PER SERVING	% OF MEAL
Fat	13 grams	116	31
Proteins	44 grams	177	47
Carbohydrates	21 grams	86	23
Cholesterol	278 mg		
Amino acid (essential)			23–33*
Fiber	0 grams		

Key: USRDA = Recommended Dietary Allowance
    IU = International Unit
    mg = milligrams
    μg = micrograms
NOTE: The numbers with arrows exceed 100 percent of required USRDA.

*Complementary food—substitute spinach for bok choy and EAA rises to 91–102%.

Okra and Cauliflower with Your Macaroni

Ingredients:

16 ounces macaroni
2 cups cauliflower pieces
1 ½ cups okra
4 cloves of garlic, minced
½ cup of tomato paste
    with ½ cup water
1 Spanish onion, diced
1 cup of chick peas
2 Tbs Parmesan cheese
1 tomato, cut into pieces
    noncaloric spray

Preparation: Saute and boil

Time: 20 minutes

Calories: 387 per serving

Serves: 4

Directions

Cook macaroni according to package instructions. Steam cauliflower and okra for about 5 minutes. Heat the noncaloric spray in a large skillet and saute the onion until it is lucid. Add the chick peas and garlic and heat. Add the tomato and tomato paste/water mixture, the cauliflower, and the okra. Sprinkle in some basil and chervil and a little cayenne pepper. Stir in the drained cooked macaroni. Use a teaspoonful of oregano to season and sprinkle with the cheese. Check your chart to see the large amounts of vitamin A, calcium, phosphorus, and potassium with an EAA range also tops.

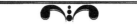

TIP: A Johns Hopkins University and University of Maryland study reports that type II diabetic, prediabetic, and normal men may improve sugar metabolism by lifting weights. The theory is that strength training helps build bigger muscles, which uses up more sugar from the bloodstream.

MYTH: Heart disease is only a man's disease.

FACT: Dr. Bernadine Healy, former director of the National Institutes of Health, indicates that studies now point out that women, after age 50, begin to develop cardiovascular disease at an increasing rate. And by the age of 60, women develop the disease at the same rate as men at 50. After age 75, heart disease is the chief killer of women.

Nutrients Contained in: Okra and Cauliflower with Your Macaroni

VITAMINS USRDA			ONE SERVING GIVES YOU APPROXIMATELY		APPROXIMATE PERCENTAGE OF USRDA
A	5,000	IU	1,728	IU	34
B_1	1.4	mg	0.52	mg	42
B_2	1.6	mg	0.27	mg	19
B_3	16	mg	4	mg	24
B_5	10	mg	0.96	mg	9
B_6	2.2	mg	0.52	mg	23
B_{12}	3	μg	0	μg	0
C	60	mg	68	mg	114◄
D	400	IU	0	IU	0
E	15	IU	0.29	IU	1
K	500	μg	1,803	μg	360◄
Folic Acid	400	μg	77	μg	19

MINERALS USRDA			ONE SERVING GIVES YOU APPROXIMATELY		APPROXIMATE PERCENTAGE OF USRDA
Sodium	(1,100–3,000)	mg	87	mg	8
Calcium	1,000	mg	184	mg	23
Phosphorus	(800–1,000)	mg	328	mg	40
Potassium	(1,875–5,625)	mg	1,171	mg	146◄
Magnesium	400	μg	126	μg	36
Selenium	200	μg	21	μg	10
Iodine	150	mg	0	mg	0
Zinc	15	mg	2	mg	12
Iron	10	mg	6	mg	63
Manganese	(2.5–5.0)	mg	1	mg	24
Copper	(2.0–3.0)	mg	0.83	mg	27

AMOUNT PER SERVING		CALORIES PER SERVING	% OF MEAL
Fat	4 grams	36	10
Proteins	19 grams	75	19
Carbohydrates	69 grams	276	71
Cholesterol	2 mg		
Amino acid (essential)			189–248
Fiber	4 grams		

Key: USRDA = Recommended Dietary Allowance
   IU = International Unit
   mg = milligrams
   μg = micrograms
NOTE: The numbers with arrows exceed 100 percent of required USRDA.

Happy Greens

Ingredients:

1 lb collard greens, stems and center spine removed
1 cup spinach, chopped
1 cup chard, chopped
1 tomato, chopped
2 cloves garlic, finely chopped
1 tsp safflower oil
½ cup of chopped onion
¼ cilantro, chopped
1 Tbs wine vinegar
1 Tbs chervil

Preparation: Steam and saute
Time: 35 minutes
Calories: 76 per serving
Serves: 4

Directions

Steam collards for about 10 minutes or until tender. Chop coarsely. Then steam the spinach and chard for 3 minutes. Drain and chop. Heat the oil in a skillet over medium heat. Add the onion and garlic and saute for about 5 minutes. Add tomato, cilantro, and vinegar. Cover and cook about 4 minutes. Add greens and heat to blend. This dish is high in vitamin A, phosphorus, and potassium.

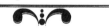

TIP: Tests by the USDA show that cinnamon, apple pie spice, cloves, bay leaves, turmeric, and other common spices may help control diabetes. These spices seem to enhance the ability of insulin to break down glucose, a form of sugar, fivefold, says Richard A. Anderson, lead scientist on the project. The next step is to test this on human beings.

MYTH: Chocolate causes pimples.

FACT: Yale University School of Medicine researchers say that in none of the studies done was there any real evidence of this. They fed chocolate to scores of children, and there was no significant difference in the severity of their acne after the children ate large amounts of chocolate.

Nutrients Contained in: Happy Greens

VITAMINS USRDA			ONE SERVING GIVES YOU APPROXIMATELY		APPROXIMATE PERCENTAGE OF USRDA
A	5,000	IU	7,750	IU	154◄
B$_1$	1.4	mg	0.10	mg	8
B$_2$	1.6	mg	0.20	mg	14
B$_3$	16	mg	0.84	mg	5
B$_5$	10	mg	0.23	mg	2
B$_6$	2.2	mg	0.19	mg	8
B$_{12}$	3	μg	0	μg	0
C	60	mg	41	mg	67
D	400	IU	0	IU	0
E	15	IU	3	IU	19
K	500	μg	48	μg	9
Folic Acid	400	μg	79	μg	19

MINERALS USRDA			ONE SERVING GIVES YOU APPROXIMATELY		APPROXIMATE PERCENTAGE OF USRDA
Sodium	(1,100–3,000)	mg	81	mg	8
Calcium	1,000	mg	184	mg	23
Phosphorus	(800–1,000)	mg	53	mg	6
Potassium	(1,875–5,625)	mg	472	mg	58
Magnesium	400	μg	67	μg	19
Selenium	200	μg	5	μg	2
Iodine	150	mg	0	mg	0
Zinc	15	mg	1	mg	8
Iron	10	mg	3	mg	27
Manganese	(2.5–5.0)	mg	0.94	mg	18
Copper	(2.0–3.0)	mg	0.40	mg	13

AMOUNT PER SERVING		CALORIES PER SERVING	% OF MEAL
Fat	4 grams	34	45
Proteins	3 grams	13	18
Carbohydrates	7 grams	29	38
Cholesterol	0 mg		
Amino acid (essential)			36–44*
Fiber	1 gram		

Key: USRDA = Recommended Dietary Allowance
    IU = International Unit
    mg = milligrams
    μg = micrograms
NOTE: The numbers with arrows exceed 100 percent of required USRDA.

*Complementary food—1 cup of green peas raises EAA to 107–155%.

Sweet Potatoes and Onions

Ingredients:

2 cups sweet potatoes, sliced thin
2 cups onions, sliced very thin
1 ½ cup apple juice
1 tsp brown sugar
1 Tbs margarine

Preparation: Bake and saute

Time: 1 ½ hours

Calories: 288 per serving

Serves: 4

Directions

Preheat oven to 350° F. Use a large round baking dish and place the onions and sweet potato slices in layers. Put the apple juice, brown sugar, and a little cinnamon in a saucepan and stir over medium heat until the sugar dissolves. Put this hot mixture over the onions and sweet potatoes and sprinkle with fresh herbs. Place pieces of margarine over the top and cover the dish with foil. Bake for about 1 hour and then remove foil and bake for another 30 minutes or until the potatoes are tender.

TIP: An article in the *Journal of the American Medical Association* reports that men who exercise vigorously several times a week can reduce by nearly half their chances of getting adult-onset diabetes. This is the most common form of diabetes. Jogging, swimming, cycling, and walking briskly are recommended.

MYTH: Nonfat frozen yogurt, cream cheese, and mozzarella are good foods for diabetics.

FACT: Not if they aren't sugar free. Most of the new fat-free desserts on the shelves are not sugar free. Other fat-free products, like cheeses, may be high in sodium. Foods sweetened with no-cal aspartame or saccharine are suggested as well as low-sodium or reduced-sodium products.

Nutrients Contained in:
Sweet Potatoes and Onions

VITAMINS USRDA			ONE SERVING GIVES YOU APPROXIMATELY		APPROXIMATE PERCENTAGE OF USRDA
A	5,000	IU	2,8117	IU	562◄
B_1	1.4	mg	0.15	mg	12
B_2	1.6	mg	0.26	mg	18
B_3	16	mg	1	mg	7
B_5	10	mg	0.98	mg	9
B_6	2.2	mg	0.55	mg	25
B_{12}	3	μg	0	μg	0
C	60	mg	36	mg	59
D	400	IU	0	IU	0
E	15	IU	3	IU	21
K	500	μg	0	μg	0
Folic Acid	400	μg	34	μg	8

MINERALS USRDA			ONE SERVING GIVES YOU APPROXIMATELY		APPROXIMATE PERCENTAGE OF USRDA
Sodium	(1,100–3,000)	mg	60	mg	5
Calcium	1,000	mg	65	mg	8
Phosphorus	(800–1,000)	mg	76	mg	9
Potassium	(1,875–5,625)	mg	545	mg	68
Magnesium	400	μg	29	μg	8
Selenium	200	μg	2	μg	0
Iodine	150	mg	0	mg	0
Zinc	15	mg	0.60	mg	4
Iron	10	mg	2	mg	16
Manganese	(2.5–5.0)	mg	0.76	mg	15
Copper	(2.0–3.0)	mg	0.32	mg	10

AMOUNT PER SERVING		CALORIES PER SERVING	% OF MEAL
Fat	4 grams	33	11
Proteins	4 grams	15	6
Carbohydrates	60 grams	240	83
Cholesterol	20 mg		
Amino acid (essential)			5-6*
Fiber	2 grams		

Key: USRDA = Recommended Dietary Allowance

IU = International Unit

mg = milligrams

μg = micrograms

NOTE: The numbers with arrows exceed 100 percent of required USRDA.

*Very low EAA.

Linking with Kale

Ingredients:

2 cups kale
2 cups linguine
5 cloves garlic, minced
1 tomato
8 shiitake mushrooms, fresh
¼ cup tomato paste, add ½ cup water
marjoram, basil, chervil, and cayenne pepper
noncaloric spray

Preparation: Saute and steam

Time: 20 minutes

Calories: 254 per serving

Serves: 4

Directions

Steam kale until soft. Saute the garlic in noncaloric spray in skillet for about 5 minutes. Add the kale and saute a minute or two. Stir in the tomato and tomato paste with water. Heat thoroughly. Season to taste with chervil and other spices. Cook about 5 minutes or more. Cook pasta according to package directions. Toss with the other ingredients. This dish is very high in recommended carbohydrates.

TIP: The Mayo Clinic *Health Letter* reports suggest that you choose whole-grain varieties of breads, cereals, and pasta. Eat fresh fruits, vegetables, and legumes. They say these foods contain more fiber and slow the release of glucose into your blood after a meal.

MYTH: The best toothpaste is baking soda.

FACT: Dental associations say that baking soda lacks fluoride and is no better or worse than any other toothpaste. You can always buy the baking soda pastes with fluoride if you want the benefits of cleaning agents in baking soda.

Nutrients Contained in: Linking with Kale

VITAMINS USRDA			ONE SERVING GIVES YOU APPROXIMATELY		APPROXIMATE PERCENTAGE OF USRDA
A	5,000	IU	3,839	IU	76
B₁	1.4	mg	0.23	mg	19
B₂	1.6	mg	0.19	mg	13
B₃	16	mg	5	mg	31
B₅	10	mg	0.11	mg	1
B₆	2.2	mg	0.13	mg	5
B₁₂	3	μg	0.08	μg	2
C	60	mg	53	mg	89
D	400	IU	0	IU	0
E	15	IU	4	IU	27
K	500	μg	3	μg	0
Folic Acid	400	μg	44	μg	10

MINERALS USRDA			ONE SERVING GIVES YOU APPROXIMATELY		APPROXIMATE PERCENTAGE OF USRDA
Sodium	(1,100–3,000)	mg	225	mg	22
Calcium	1,000	mg	67	mg	8
Phosphorus	(800–1,000)	mg	93	mg	11
Potassium	(1,875–5,625)	mg	653	mg	81
Magnesium	400	μg	51	μg	14
Selenium	200	μg	20	μg	10
Iodine	150	mg	0	mg	0
Zinc	15	mg	2	mg	15
Iron	10	mg	2	mg	22
Manganese	(2.5–5.0)	mg	0.30	mg	5
Copper	(2.0–3.0)	mg	0.13	mg	4

AMOUNT PER SERVING		CALORIES PER SERVING	% OF MEAL
Fat	1 gram	10	4
Proteins	9 grams	37	15
Carbohydrates	52 grams	207	81
Cholesterol	0 mg		
Amino acid (essential)			48–78*
Fiber	1 gram		

Key: USRDA = Recommended Dietary Allowance
     IU = International Unit
     mg = milligrams
     μg = micrograms
NOTE: The numbers with arrows exceed 100 percent of required USRDA.

*Complementary food—1/2 cup Brazil nuts raises EAA 182–464%.

Apple of Your Eye

Ingredients:

2 medium apples, cored and coarsely chopped
½ cup pitted prunes
2 stalks celery, coarsely chopped
1 Tbs wheat germ
½ cup chick peas
½ tsp cinnamon
3 Tbs apricot nectar

Preparation: No cooking required

Time: 15 minutes

Calories: 208 per serving

Serves: 4

Directions

Combine all ingredients and chill. Add apricot nectar over salad and season with cinnamon.

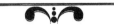

TIP: The ADA recommends that a type II diabetes diet should include about 50 percent of carbohydrates. Each gram of carbohydrate equals 4 calories. Seventy-one percent of the calories in this dish are in carbohydrates. See chart.

MYTH: Smoking just a few cigarettes a day won't hurt you.

FACT: National Cancer Institute studies indicate that the smoke from even one or two cigarettes a day can be harmful and is a greater risk than anything else you're likely to be exposed to on a daily basis.

Nutrients Contained in: Apple of Your Eye

VITAMINS USRDA			ONE SERVING GIVES YOU APPROXIMATELY		APPROXIMATE PERCENTAGE OF USRDA
A	5,000	IU	166	IU	3
B$_1$	1.4	mg	0.23	mg	19
B$_2$	1.6	mg	0.20	mg	14
B$_3$	16	mg	1	mg	7
B$_5$	10	mg	0.68	mg	6
B$_6$	2.2	mg	0.30	mg	13
B$_{12}$	3	μg	0.16	μg	5
C	60	mg	6	mg	9
D	400	IU	13	IU	3
E	15	IU	0.63	IU	4
K	500	μg	0	μg	0
Folic Acid	400	μg	31	μg	7

MINERALS USRDA			ONE SERVING GIVES YOU APPROXIMATELY		APPROXIMATE PERCENTAGE OF USRDA
Sodium	(1,100–3,000)	mg	45	mg	4
Calcium	1,000	mg	109	mg	13
Phosphorus	(800–1,000)	mg	222	mg	27
Potassium	(1,875–5,625)	mg	538	mg	67
Magnesium	400	μg	75	μg	21
Selenium	200	μg	0.34	μg	0
Iodine	150	mg	13	mg	8
Zinc	15	mg	2	mg	14
Iron	10	mg	3	mg	28
Manganese	(2.5–5.0)	mg	2	mg	36
Copper	(2.0–3.0)	mg	0.32	mg	10

AMOUNT PER SERVING		CALORIES PER SERVING	% OF MEAL
Fat	3 grams	24	11
Proteins	9 grams	37	18
Carbohydrates	37 grams	147	71
Cholesterol	2 mg		
Amino acid (essential)			9–16*
Fiber	2 grams		

Key: USRDA = Recommended Dietary Allowance
    IU = International Unit
    mg = milligrams
    μg = micrograms
NOTE: The numbers with arrows exceed 100 percent of required USRDA.

*Complementary food—1 cup sesame seeds raises EAA to 65–100%.

A Stirring Dish

Ingredients:

7	oz halibut, in pieces
3	chicken livers
1	cup zucchini, sliced
1	cup beet greens, cut
2	carrots, sliced in ¼-inch pieces
1	green pepper, seeded and sliced in strips
¼	cup parsley, chopped
2	cloves of garlic, chopped
	Adobo (Goya brand) seasoning
	noncaloric spray
	black pepper
	juice of one lemon

Preparation: Stir-fry

Time: 20 minutes

Calories: 107 per serving

Serves: 4

Directions

Coat large skillet with noncaloric spray and heat on medium high flame. Stir-fry zucchini, beet greens, and carrots and cook about 5 minutes or more. If pan sticks, pour a little water or a little vegetable broth in the pan. Add peppers, garlic, and halibut pieces and cook until done. In a separate pan, use noncaloric spray and cook chicken livers for about 6 minutes until done through. When done, combine with stir-fry mixture adding all the spices. Season with black pepper and lemon juice and sprinkle parsley over all.

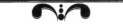

TIP: The ADA suggests that you gradually reach 40 grams of dietary fiber a day. Natural fiber in the diet has been found to have beneficial effects for everyone. Whole wheat products, barley, oats, legumes, and vegetables as well as fruits are the best sources of fiber and other important nutrients. Your chart will show you that this meal gives you 19 grams of fiber.

MYTH: Vitamin B_6 or magnesium will prevent kidney stones.

FACT: A report in the *Wellness Letter* of the University of California at Berkeley says no dietary supplement prevents kidney stones. And there is no evidence that B_6 or magnesium is effective in prevention or treatment.

Nutrients Contained in: A Stirring Dish

VITAMINS USRDA			ONE SERVING GIVES YOU APPROXIMATELY		APPROXIMATE PERCENTAGE OF USRDA
A	5,000	IU	15,906	IU	318◄
B$_1$	1.4	mg	0.14	mg	11
B$_2$	1.6	mg	0.57	mg	40
B$_3$	16	mg	7	mg	43
B$_5$	10	mg	2	mg	17
B$_6$	2.2	mg	0.51	mg	23
B$_{12}$	3	µg	6	µg	200◄
C	60	mg	37	mg	62
D	400	IU	26	IU	6
E	15	IU	2	IU	11
K	500	µg	71	µg	14
Folic Acid	400	µg	199	µg	49

MINERALS USRDA			ONE SERVING GIVES YOU APPROXIMATELY		APPROXIMATE PERCENTAGE OF USRDA
Sodium	(1,100–3,000)	mg	79	mg	7
Calcium	1,000	mg	37	mg	4
Phosphorus	(800–1,000)	mg	261	mg	32
Potassium	(1,875–5,625)	mg	466	mg	58
Magnesium	400	µg	40	µg	11
Selenium	200	µg	1	µg	0
Iodine	150	mg	0	mg	0
Zinc	15	mg	0.63	mg	4
Iron	10	mg	3	mg	32
Manganese	(2.5–5.0)	mg	0.22	mg	4
Copper	(2.0–3.0)	mg	0.30	mg	9

AMOUNT PER SERVING		CALORIES PER SERVING	% OF MEAL
Fat	2 grams	15	14
Proteins	16 grams	63	59
Carbohydrates	7 grams	29	27
Cholesterol	130 mg		
Amino acid (essential)			127–290
Fiber	19 grams		

Key: USRDA = Recommended Dietary Allowance
　　　IU = International Unit
　　　mg = milligrams
　　　µg = micrograms
NOTE: The numbers with arrows exceed 100 percent of required USRDA.

Orient Bean Express

Ingredients:

1 lb green beans
8 shiitake mushrooms, fresh
1 tsp olive oil
chervil
juice of one lemon
basil

Preparation: Steam and saute

Time: 20 minutes

Calories: 148 per serving

Serves: 4

Directions

Steam beans until crisp, about 5 to 7 minutes. Leave beans in steamer with heat off. Heal oil and saute mushrooms until just tender. Combine with beans and sprinkle with chervil and lemon juice. Add a little basil before serving.

TIP: The American Diabetes Association recommends limiting protein intake. Only 12 to 20 percent of daily calorie intake for diabetics should constitute proteins. This means easing up on foods like meat and milk. Each gram of protein equals 4 calories. The protein in this meal is only 9 percent of the calories.

MYTH: You can get salmonella poisoning from frozen raw egg products like Egg Beaters.

FACT: Not so. The USRDA requires all food manufacturers to pasteurize eggs used as an ingredient. The pasteurization process kills microorganisms such as salmonella.

Nutrients Contained in: Orient Bean Express

VITAMINS USRDA			ONE SERVING GIVES YOU APPROXIMATELY		APPROXIMATE PERCENTAGE OF USRDA
A	5,000	IU	417	IU	8
B$_1$	1.4	mg	0.05	mg	3
B$_2$	1.6	mg	0.08	mg	5
B$_3$	16	mg	3	mg	16
B$_5$	10	mg	0.05	mg	0
B$_6$	2.2	mg	0.06	mg	2
B$_{12}$	3	μg	0	μg	0
C	60	mg	6	mg	10
D	400	IU	0	IU	0
E	15	IU	0.44	IU	2
K	500	μg	163	μg	32
Folic Acid	400	μg	51	μg	12

MINERALS USRDA			ONE SERVING GIVES YOU APPROXIMATELY		APPROXIMATE PERCENTAGE OF USRDA
Sodium	(1,100–3,000)	mg	8	mg	0
Calcium	1,000	mg	33	mg	4
Phosphorus	(800–1,000)	mg	24	mg	3
Potassium	(1,875–5,625)	mg	357	mg	44
Magnesium	400	μg	36	μg	10
Selenium	200	μg	0.30	μg	0
Iodine	150	mg	0	mg	0
Zinc	15	mg	2	mg	14
Iron	10	mg	0.86	mg	8
Manganese	(2.5–5.0)	mg	0.19	mg	3
Copper	(2.0–3.0)	mg	0.07	mg	2

AMOUNT PER SERVING		CALORIES PER SERVING	% OF MEAL
Fat	4 grams	32	22
Proteins	3 grams	14	9
Carbohydrates	26 grams	102	69
Cholesterol	0 mg		
Amino acid (essential)			35–39*
Fiber	1 gram		

Key: USRDA = Recommended Dietary Allowance

    IU = International Unit

    mg = milligrams

    μg = micrograms

NOTE: The numbers with arrows exceed 100 percent of required USRDA.

*Complementary food—1 ounce of blue cheese raises EAA to 91–132%.

Lemon Flounder

Ingredients:

1	lb flounder, in 4 pieces	**Preparation:**	Broil
1	Tbs horseradish	**Time:**	25 minutes
¼	cup wheat germ		
1	tsp dill	**Calories:**	104 per serving
	juice of one lime	**Serves:**	4
½	cup Dijon mustard		
	black pepper		

Directions

Preheat broiler. Stir mustard, lime juice, horseradish, wheat germ, and dill until well blended. Place fish on broiler pan. Brush with half the mixture. Grill or broil for about 5 to 7 minutes; turn and brush with remaining mustard mixture. Continue broiling another 6 minutes, or until fish is done.

TIP: The American Diabetes Association recommends that you cut a lot of fat out of your diet. Its members say that calories from fat should account for no more than 30 percent of your total diet. This recipe derives only 11 percent of its calories from fat.

MYTH: All children should have their cholesterol measured.

FACT: Not according to the National Cholesterol Education Program guidelines. According to the guidelines, only children who have a family history of very high cholesterol levels should have their levels measured. High blood cholesterol levels during childhood do not necessarily predict high levels later in life.

Nutrients Contained in: Lemon Flounder

VITAMINS USRDA			ONE SERVING GIVES YOU APPROXIMATELY		APPROXIMATE PERCENTAGE OF USRDA
A	5,000	IU	2	mg	0
B_1	1.4	mg	0.18	mg	15
B_2	1.6	mg	0.11	mg	7
B_3	16	mg	2	mg	13
B_5	10	mg	0.44	mg	4
B_6	2.2	mg	0.07	mg	3
B_{12}	3	μg	0.80	μg	26
C	60	mg	5	mg	9
D	400	IU	0	IU	0
E	15	IU	0	IU	0
K	500	μg	0	μg	0
Folic Acid	400	μg	37	μg	9

MINERALS USRDA			ONE SERVING GIVES YOU APPROXIMATELY		APPROXIMATE PERCENTAGE OF USRDA
Sodium	(1,100–3,000)	mg	60	mg	6
Calcium	1,000	mg	72	mg	8
Phosphorus	(800–1,000)	mg	280	mg	35
Potassium	(1,875–5,625)	mg	461	mg	57
Magnesium	400	μg	54	μg	15
Selenium	200	μg	24	μg	12
Iodine	150	mg	0	mg	0
Zinc	15	mg	1	mg	9
Iron	10	mg	2	mg	15
Manganese	(2.5–5.0)	mg	1	mg	28
Copper	(2.0–3.0)	mg	0.07	mg	2

AMOUNT PER SERVING		CALORIES PER SERVING	% OF MEAL
Fat	1 gram	12	11
Proteins	17 grams	69	67
Carbohydrates	6 grams	23	22
Cholesterol	0 mg		
Amino acid (essential)			111–326
Fiber	0 grams		

Key: USRDA = Recommended Dietary Allowance
     IU = International Unit
     mg = milligrams
     μg = micrograms
NOTE: The numbers with arrows exceed 100 percent of required USRDA.

Green and Orange Special

Ingredients: 4 to 5 carrots, cut in 1-inch pieces

1 ½ cups broccoli, stems peeled and cut in pieces

1 onion, thinly sliced

½ cup low-sodium chicken broth

1 tsp canola oil

juice of one lemon

½ tsp chili powder

½ tsp turmeric

½ tsp cayenne pepper

Preparation: Steam and saute

Time: 20 minutes

Calories: 79 calories per serving

Serves: 4

Directions

Steam carrots and broccoli for about 8 to 10 minutes, letting carrots get a 4-minute headstart. Heat oil in a large skillet. Stir in onions and saute for a few minutes. Add broth, chili, turmeric, and cayenne pepper and blend with heat up for 2 minutes. Add carrots and broccoli and simmer until all ingredients are well blended and the spices have been absorbed. Sprinkle lemon juice over each serving. Note high levels of vitamins A and K and potassium and low calories.

TIP: Founded in 1940, the American Diabetes Association is the nation's leading voluntary health organization supporting diabetes research, education, and patient programs. It has an affiliate office in every state and provides services in more than 800 communities nationwide.

MYTH: All stress is to be avoided to stay healthy.

FACT: Stress experts say that some stress can help people deal with the everyday problems and unexpected events that come up in life. Stress can stimulate us to manage life's problems and adapt to the daily play of life.

Nutrients Contained in: Green and Orange Special

VITAMINS USRDA			ONE SERVING GIVES YOU APPROXIMATELY		APPROXIMATE PERCENTAGE OF USRDA
A	5,000	IU	25,513	IU	510◄
B$_1$	1.4	mg	0.14	mg	11
B$_2$	1.6	mg	0.11	mg	7
B$_3$	16	mg	2	mg	9
B$_5$	10	mg	0.43	mg	4
B$_6$	2.2	mg	0.26	mg	11
B$_{12}$	3	μg	0.04	μg	1
C	60	mg	50	mg	83
D	400	IU	0	IU	0
E	15	IU	11	IU	9
K	500	μg	238	μg	47
Folic Acid	400	μg	46	μg	11

MINERALS USRDA			ONE SERVING GIVES YOU APPROXIMATELY		APPROXIMATE PERCENTAGE OF USRDA
Sodium	(1,100–3,000)	mg	139	mg	13
Calcium	1,000	mg	54	mg	6
Phosphorus	(800–1,000)	mg	76	mg	9
Potassium	(1,875–5,625)	mg	507	mg	63
Magnesium	400	μg	33	μg	9
Selenium	200	μg	7	μg	3
Iodine	150	mg	0	mg	0
Zinc	15	mg	0.42	mg	2
Iron	10	mg	1	mg	10
Manganese	(2.5–5.0)	mg	0.25	mg	5
Copper	(2.0–3.0)	mg	0.08	mg	2

AMOUNT PER SERVING		CALORIES PER SERVING	% OF MEAL
Fat	1 gram	6	7
Proteins	3 grams	12	15
Carbohydrates	15 grams	61	77
Cholesterol	0 mg		
Amino acid (essential)			16–28*
Fiber	2 grams		

Key: USRDA = Recommended Dietary Allowance
IU = International Unit
mg = milligrams
μg = micrograms
NOTE: The numbers with arrows exceed 100 percent of required USRDA.
*Complementary food—1 head of endive raises EAA to 55–94%.

VEGETABLES RANKED IN THE HIGHEST ORDER FOR DIETARY FIBER
PERCENTAGES GIVEN EQUAL ½ CUP

	DIETARY FIBER (GRAMS)	PERCENTAGE OF USRDA
Beans, kidney, canned	10.0	35.7
Beans, pinto, cooked	9.4	33.6
Beans, lima, cooked	7.4	26.4
Beans, lima, frozen	7.4	26.4
Beans, baked, pork/sauce	6.0	21.4
Beans, fava, canned	6.0	21.4
Peas, blackeye, canned	5.7	20.4
Peas, blackeye, cooked	5.7	20.4
Peas, cooked	5.7	20.4
Beans, baked, plain	5.0	17.9
Parsnips, cooked	4.9	17.5
Corn, cooked	4.7	16.8
Potato, baked, with skin	4.4	15.7
Corn on the cob, cooked	3.9	13.9
Broccoli, cooked	3.8	13.6
Broccoli, frozen	3.8	13.6
Potato, sweet	3.7	13.2
Corn, canned	3.3	11.8
Corn, canned, low sodium	3.3	11.8
Brussels sprouts, frozen	3.2	11.4
Spinach, frozen	3.1	11.1
Beans, mung, cooked	3.0	10.7
Vegetables, mixed, low sodium	3.0	10.7

CHAPTER SIX

Healing and Preventive Recipes for Osteoporosis

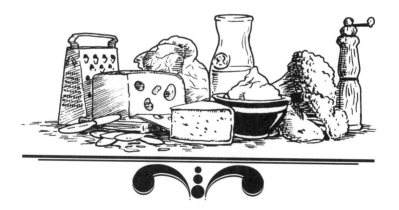

When an idea is wanting, a word can
always be found to take its place.
—Johan von Goethe

Since calcium is an important nutrient that protects against aging bones, you will find recipes in this chapter that emphasize calcium and vitamin D. Researchers have found kale, collards, and broccoli, low-fat and nonfat milk, yogurt, and cheeses to be effective foods for building strong bones. Canned sardines and salmon are equally high on the list.

As stated in the *New England Journal of Medicine*, women who get 1,000 milligrams a day of calcium before menopause and 1,200 to 1,500 milligrams daily after menopause, and who exercise on a regular basis are less apt to get osteoporosis. Getting calcium and vitamin D in your daily meals is good insurance for keeping bones healthy whether you are young or old.

You will also find in this chapter tips on the latest research about the function of calcium and how your body steals calcium from your bones if you don't get enough in your diet.

Each recipe contains ample amounts of these nutrients and others to guide you to the best food sources. The delicious Shrimp Bok Choy gives you a good start; the Salmon with Broccoli, Wheat Germ, and Cheese gives you over 100 percent of your daily vitamin D and 74 percent of your calcium requirements. No single meal, of course, is able to give you the total amount of your calcium and vitamin D that will meet USRDAs, but use the charts to select a variety of healthy and tasty choices. You will know just how much of the USRDAs you are meeting for each important nutrient.

RECOMMENDED DIETARY ALLOWANCES FOR CALCIUM

GROUP/AGE	CALCIUM (MILLIGRAMS)
Infants 0–6 months	360
Infants 6–12 months	540
Children 1–10 years	800
Males 11–18 years	1,200
Males 19+ years	800
Females 11–18 years	1,200
Females 19+ years	800
Pregnant or nursing	
Women 18 years or less	1,600
Women 19+ years	1,200

Shrimp and Bok Choy

Ingredients:

1 lb medium-sized
   shrimp, shelled
1 Tbs corn oil
1 cup sunflower seeds
1 lb Bok choy, chopped
   in medium pieces
1 cup onion, diced
4 garlic cloves, cut in
   fine pieces
   juice of one lime

Preparation: Simmer, sauté

Time: 35 minutes

Calories: 428 per serving

Serves: 4

Directions

Brown seeds in oil in a heavy iron skillet at medium heat. Add garlic and onions and sauté for 5 minutes. To this add the bok choy, juice from lime, and garlic. Cover and cook at medium heat for about 5 minutes. Add shrimp that has been deveined. Mix well and simmer for 8 to 10 minutes. Look at the chart and you will see loads of vitamins A and D, calcium, potassium, and an overflow of natural EAA.

TIP: In addition to vitamin D, there is another benefit you get from cheese. It safeguards your teeth from decay. By stimulating saliva, increasing plaque pH, inhibiting tooth demineralization, and helping tooth remineralization, cheese helps prevent cavities.

MYTH: Some foods are addictive.

FACT: No one has come up with a food that is addictive in the way that drugs, nicotine, and alcohol are addictive. No one seems to develop a physical dependency on sugar or chocolate or experience symptoms associated with truly addictive substances.

Nutrients Contained in: Shrimp and Bok Choy

VITAMINS USRDA			ONE SERVING GIVES YOU APPROXIMATELY		APPROXIMATE PERCENTAGE OF USRDA
A	5,000	IU	2,202	IU	44
B_1	1.4	mg	0.82	mg	67
B_2	1.6	mg	0.18	mg	12
B_3	16	mg	6	mg	39
B_5	10	mg	0.94	mg	9
B_6	2.2	mg	0.64	mg	29
B_{12}	3	μg	1	μg	37
C	60	mg	33	mg	54
D	400	IU	125	IU	31
E	15	IU	37	IU	245◀
K	500	μg	0	μg	0
Folic Acid	400	μg	9	μg	5

MINERALS USRDA			ONE SERVING GIVES YOU APPROXIMATELY		APPROXIMATE PERCENTAGE OF USRDA
Sodium	(1,100–3,000)	mg	207	mg	20
Calcium	1,000	mg	218	mg	27
Phosphorus	(800–1,000)	mg	556	mg	69
Potassium	(1,875–5,625)	mg	1,019	mg	127◀
Magnesium	400	μg	81	μg	23
Selenium	200	μg	40	μg	19
Iodine	150	mg	45	mg	30
Zinc	15	mg	4	mg	25
Iron	10	mg	6	mg	56
Manganese	(2.5–5.0)	mg	0.82	mg	16
Copper	(2.0–3.0)	mg	0.98	mg	32

AMOUNT PER SERVING		CALORIES PER SERVING	% OF MEAL
Fat	25 grams	226	53
Proteins	34 grams	137	32
Carbohydrates	16 grams	65	15
Cholesterol	188 mg		
Amino acid (essential)			257–569*
Fiber	2 grams		

Key: USRDA = Recommended Dietary Allowance
   IU = International Unit
   mg = milligrams
   μg = micrograms
NOTE: The numbers with arrows exceed 100 percent of required USRDA.

*A bonanza.

Salmon with Broccoli, Wheat Germ, and Cheese

Ingredients:

1   16-oz can salmon
2   cups broccoli
1   Tbs margarine
2   cups skim milk
½   cup wheat germ
½   cup half and half cream
¼   cup Parmesan cheese
1   lime

Preparation: Boil and bake

Time: 60 minutes

Calories: 305 per serving

Serves: 6

Directions

Preheat oven to 375° F. Cut broccoli in medium-sized pieces and steam for a few minutes. Melt margarine in a pan and stir in wheat germ. When mixture is smooth, add cream and milk, stirring frequently. Then add cheese, lime juice, broccoli, and salmon. Put into a baking dish and bake covered for about 20 minutes or less. Remove cover and bake an additional 10 minutes. Levels of vitamin D and phosphorus are very good, and notice the bonus amount of essential amino acids.

TIP: The highest bone mass that a person will have is called the peak bone mass, and it is not developed before the mid-20s or early 30s. Researchers such as Dr. Charles Chesnut, director of the Osteoporosis Research Center at the Washington University, St. Louis, says calcium intake is very important during this time to assure that the bone is properly mineralized. Consuming enough nutrients to support the development of peak bone mass when we are young can help.

MYTH: Sweet potatoes are higher in calories than white potatoes.

FACT: You might think so, but a 4 ounce serving of cooked sweet potato contains only about 120 to 140 calories, the same number as a white potato. The sweet potato does, however, have more vitamin C and beta-carotene.

Nutrients Contained in: Salmon with Broccoli, Wheat Germ, and Cheese

VITAMINS USRDA		ONE SERVING GIVES YOU APPROXIMATELY		APPROXIMATE PERCENTAGE OF USRDA
A	5,000 IU	975	IU	19
B$_1$	1.4 mg	0.35	mg	29
B$_2$	1.6 mg	0.34	mg	24
B$_3$	16 mg	9	mg	56
B$_5$	10 mg	2	mg	17
B$_6$	2.2 mg	0.78	mg	35
B$_{12}$	3 μg	4	μg	124◀
C	60 mg	39	mg	64
D	400 IU	575	IU	143◀
E	15 IU	2	IU	13
K	500 μg	100	μg	20
Folic Acid	400 μg	3	μg	0

MINERALS USRDA		ONE SERVING GIVES YOU APPROXIMATELY		APPROXIMATE PERCENTAGE OF USRDA
Sodium	(1,100–3,000) mg	329	mg	32
Calcium	1,000 mg	599	mg	74
Phosphorus	(800–1,000) mg	454	mg	56
Potassium	(1,875–5,625) mg	731	mg	91
Magnesium	400 μg	79	μg	22
Selenium	200 μg	1	μg	0
Iodine	150 mg	4	mg	2
Zinc	15 mg	3	mg	20
Iron	10 mg	2	mg	22
Manganese	(2.5–5.0) mg	2	mg	80
Copper	(2.0–3.0) mg	0.31	mg	10

AMOUNT PER SERVING		CALORIES PER SERVING	% OF MEAL
Fat	14 grams	127	42
Proteins	33 grams	131	43
Carbohydrates	12 grams	47	15
Cholesterol	68 mg		
Amino acid (essential)			280–625*
Fiber	0 grams		

Key: USRDA = Recommended Dietary Allowance
　　　IU = International Unit
　　　mg = milligrams
　　　μg = micrograms

NOTE: The numbers with arrows exceed 100 percent of required USRDA.

*A bonanza.

Halibut Swimming in Chard

Ingredients:
1 ¼ lb halibut
1 lb Swiss chard
1 onion diced
4 cloves, chopped fine
2 tsp safflower oil
3 Tbs dry red wine

Preparation: Saute

Time: 25 minutes

Calories: 372 per serving

Serves: 4

Directions

Heat oil and saute garlic and onions until golden. Add chard and cook at medium heat for a minute or two. Cut fish in 1-inch squares and mix with chard mixture. Add wine, cover, and simmer for about 15 minutes over medium heat until liquid is reduced by half. Note high content of vitamin D needed for calcium synthesis. Also observe high numbers for vitamin K, phosphorus, potassium, and vitamin A.

TIP: Nondairy foods such as fruits, nuts, and fish also supply calcium. But remember that vitamin D is necessary for calcium to be absorbed. Food sources for D include canned sardines, canned salmon, tuna, shrimp, sunflower seeds, nuts, herring, chicken livers, and, of course, milk and cheese.

MYTH: Women need extra calcium during menopause.

FACT: Dr. Robert P. Heaney, professor of medicine at Creighton University in Omaha, says that a woman is getting so much calcium during menopause from the bone she is losing that she doesn't need extra. When menopause is over, however, he says women should have the full 1,500 mg, since the ovaries are no longer producing estrogen.

Nutrients Contained in: Halibut Swimming in Chard

VITAMINS USRDA			ONE SERVING GIVES YOU APPROXIMATELY		APPROXIMATE PERCENTAGE OF USRDA
A	5,000	IU	1,665	IU	33
B₁	1.4	mg	0.26	mg	21
B₂	1.6	mg	0.24	mg	17
B₃	16	mg	28	mg	173◄
B₅	10	mg	0.98	mg	9
B₆	2.2	mg	1	mg	67
B₁₂	3	μg	3	μg	111◄
C	60	mg	4	mg	6
D	400	IU	147	IU	36
E	15	IU	6	IU	38
K	500	μg	0	μg	0
Folic Acid	400	μg	55	μg	13

MINERALS USRDA			ONE SERVING GIVES YOU APPROXIMATELY		APPROXIMATE PERCENTAGE OF USRDA
Sodium	(1,100–3,000)	mg	194	mg	9
Calcium	1,000	mg	54	mg	6
Phosphorus	(800–1,000)	mg	1,050	mg	131◄
Potassium	(1,875–5,625)	mg	783	mg	67
Magnesium	400	μg	85	μg	14
Selenium	200	μg	0.53	μg	0
Iodine	150	mg	0	mg	0
Zinc	15	mg	2	mg	16
Iron	10	mg	3	mg	25
Manganese	(2.5–5.0)	mg	0.14	mg	2
Copper	(2.0–3.0)	mg	0.81	mg	27

AMOUNT PER SERVING		CALORIES PER SERVING	% OF MEAL
Fat	9 grams	77	21
Proteins	71 grams	282	76
Carbohydrates	3 grams	13	4
Cholesterol	167 mg		
Amino acid (essential)			412–999*
Fiber	0 grams		

Key: USRDA = Recommended Dietary Allowance
    IU = International Unit
    mg = milligrams
    μg = micrograms
NOTE: The numbers with arrows exceed 100 percent of required USRDA.

*Batting a thousand.

Lovely Avocado Sprouts

Ingredients:

- 2 ripe avocados
- ½ cup finely chopped almonds, toasted
- ⅓ cup yogurt
- 2 cloves garlic, crushed juice of one lemon
- ¼ cup minced cilantro
- 6 scallions, chopped fine
- 1 cup mung beansprouts

Preparation: Raw

Time: 15 minutes

Calories: 280 per serving

Serves: 4

Directions

Mash avocados until they are a smooth mixture. Add the lemon juice first. Then add remaining ingredients and mix well. Serve on lettuce leaves. Notice high amounts of calcium, phosphorus, and potassium.

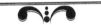

TIP: The Agricultural Research Service of the USDA reports that extra calcium in the diet may help cut down on water retention, menstrual cramps, and moodiness. Consuming more calcium, says psychologist James Penland of the USDA, doesn't have to mean eating a lot of fat. A couple of extra servings of skim milk (302 milligrams of calcium per cup) easily does the trick.

MYTH: Eating "lean meat" means eating chicken or turkey.

FACT: Not so. There are cuts of beef, pork, and even lamb that are lower in fat than dark meat poultry. Recommended portions of meat are 3 to 4 ounces after cooking.

Nutrients Contained in: Lovely Avocado Sprouts

VITAMINS USRDA			ONE SERVING GIVES YOU APPROXIMATELY		APPROXIMATE PERCENTAGE OF USRDA
A	5,000	IU	972	IU	19
B_1	1.4	mg	0.18	mg	14
B_2	1.6	mg	0.34	mg	24
B_3	16	mg	0.82	mg	5
B_5	10	mg	1	mg	14
B_6	2.2	mg	0.43	mg	19
B_{12}	3	μg	0.24	μg	8
C	60	mg	26	mg	43
D	400	IU	19	IU	4
E	15	IU	3	IU	22
K	500	μg	6	μg	1
Folic Acid	400	μg	84	μg	21

MINERALS USRDA			ONE SERVING GIVES YOU APPROXIMATELY		APPROXIMATE PERCENTAGE OF USRDA
Sodium	(1,100–3,000)	mg	51	mg	5
Calcium	1,000	mg	129	mg	16
Phosphorus	(800–1,000)	mg	169	mg	21
Potassium	(1,875–5,625)	mg	877	mg	109◄
Magnesium	400	μg	88	μg	25
Selenium	200	μg	3	μg	1
Iodine	150	mg	20	mg	13
Zinc	15	mg	1	mg	8
Iron	10	mg	2	mg	20
Manganese	(2.5–5.0)	mg	0.48	mg	9
Copper	(2.0–3.0)	mg	0.41	mg	13

AMOUNT PER SERVING		CALORIES PER SERVING	% OF MEAL
Fat	21 grams	188	67
Proteins	7 grams	28	10
Carbohydrates	16 grams	64	23
Cholesterol	3 mg		
Amino acid (essential)			80–92
Fiber	3 grams		

Key: USRDA = Recommended Dietary Allowance
     IU = International Unit
     mg = milligrams
     μg = micrograms
NOTE: The numbers with arrows exceed 100 percent of required USRDA.

Tuna, Cheese, and Pepper Powerhouse

Ingredients:

1 cup of elbow macaroni
1 6 ½-ounce can of tuna
½ cup of chopped onion
¾ cup skimmed milk
2 tsp margarine
1 6-oz. piece Parmesan cheese, crumbled
1 red pepper, seeded and diced
1 tsp dry mustard
¼ cup masa (corn) flower

Preparation: Saute, stir, bake

Time: 50 minutes

Calories: 354 per serving

Serves: 4

Directions

Preheat oven to 375° F. Cook macaroni according to instructions on package. In a skillet, stir together margarine, onions, and pepper and cook over medium heat until the onions and pepper are just tender. Stir in the flour and cook over low heat, stirring all the while until the ingredients are smooth. Remove from heat and stir in the milk. Heat to boiling and boil and stir for 1 minute. Remove from heat, add mustard and cheese. Stir until cheese is melted. Place macaroni in 1 ½-quart baking dish along with the tuna and cheese mixture. Stir cheese sauce into macaroni. Bake uncovered for about 30 minutes. Note very high amounts of calcium and essential amino acids.

TIP: Osteoporosis experts recommend an intake of 1,000 milligrams of calcium a day for men, premenopausal women, and women taking estrogen and 1,500 milligrams for postmenopausal women. One 8-ounce glass of skim milk contains 300 milligrams of calcium.

MYTH: Part-skim cheese is low in fat.

FACT: Nutrition researchers at the University of California at Berkeley say, "Probably not." Most cheeses labeled "slender," "lite," "low-fat," or "part-skim," they say, contain only slightly less fat than regular varieties.

Nutrients Contained in: Tuna, Cheese, and Pepper Powerhouse

VITAMINS USRDA			ONE SERVING GIVES YOU APPROXIMATELY		APPROXIMATE PERCENTAGE OF USRDA
A	5,000	IU	672	IU	13
B_1	1.4	mg	0.13	mg	11
B_2	1.6	mg	0.28	mg	19
B_3	16	mg	6	mg	40
B_5	10	mg	0.41	mg	4
B_6	2.2	mg	0.28	mg	12
B_{12}	3	μg	0.84	μg	27
C	60	mg	22	mg	37
D	400	IU	23	IU	5
E	15	IU	1	IU	8
K	500	μg	0	μg	0
Folic Acid	400	μg	13	μg	3

MINERALS USRDA			ONE SERVING GIVES YOU APPROXIMATELY		APPROXIMATE PERCENTAGE OF USRDA
Sodium	(1,100–3,000)	mg	989	mg	98
Calcium	1,000	mg	575	mg	71
Phosphorus	(800–1,000)	mg	477	mg	59
Potassium	(1,875–5,625)	mg	321	mg	40
Magnesium	400	μg	49	μg	14
Selenium	200	μg	39	μg	19
Iodine	150	mg	2	mg	1
Zinc	15	mg	2	mg	10
Iron	10	mg	2	mg	15
Manganese	(2.5–5.0)	mg	0.07	mg	1
Copper	(2.0–3.0)	mg	0.22	mg	7

AMOUNT PER SERVING		CALORIES PER SERVING	% OF MEAL
Fat	18 grams	161	46
Proteins	31 grams	126	36
Carbohydrates	17 grams	67	19
Cholesterol	86 mg		
Amino acid (essential)			377–615*
Fiber	0 grams		

Key: USRDA = Recommended Dietary Allowance

IU = International Unit

mg = milligrams

μg = micrograms

NOTE: The numbers with arrows exceed 100 percent of required USRDA.

*Well over the top.

Kasha and Pea Pods

Ingredients:

1 cup buckwheat groats
1 cup snap beans, cut
   in small pieces
juice of one lime
1 cup onions, coarsely
   chopped
1 clove garlic, chopped
3 cups water
1 tsp margarine
black pepper

Preparation: Boil, steam, sauté

Time: 25 minutes

Calories: 139 per serving

Serves: 4

Directions

Steam beans for about 7 minutes. While they are cooking, put water on to boil. Sauté onions until light brown. Pour buckwheat into boiling water, lower heat, and cook covered for 5 minutes or so. Just before kasha is done (unroasted buckwheat is quite colorless, but when roasted, it takes on a brown color and the roasted form is known as kasha), stir in the cooked beans and the onions. Add lime juice and black pepper to taste.

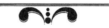

TIP: Cigarette smoking lowers the estrogen level, increasing women's risk of developing osteoporosis. The Osteoporosis Center at the Hospital for Special Surgery in New York also says smokers have been found to have twice as much risk of back fractures as nonsmokers.

MYTH: You can tell by symptoms whether or not you have osteoporosis.

FACT: Not according to the National Osteoporosis Foundation. Its members say that the disease has no symptoms and, up until recently, could not be diagnosed until a fracture occurred. Now there are a number of techniques to measure bone density with accuracy.

Nutrients Contained in: Kasha and Pea Pods

VITAMINS USRDA			ONE SERVING GIVES YOU APPROXIMATELY		APPROXIMATE PERCENTAGE OF USRDA
A	5,000	IU	268	IU	5
B$_1$	1.4	mg	0.20	mg	16
B$_2$	1.6	mg	0.09	mg	5
B$_3$	16	mg	0.98	mg	6
B$_5$	10	mg	0.49	mg	4
B$_6$	2.2	mg	0.23	mg	10
B$_{12}$	3	μg	0	μg	0
C	60	mg	11	mg	18
D	400	IU	0	IU	0
E	15	IU	0.23	IU	1
K	500	μg	81	μg	16
Folic Acid	400	μg	20	μg	4

MINERALS USRDA			ONE SERVING GIVES YOU APPROXIMATELY		APPROXIMATE PERCENTAGE OF USRDA
Sodium	(1,100–3,000)	mg	19	mg	1
Calcium	1,000	mg	39	mg	4
Phosphorus	(800–1,000)	mg	115	mg	14
Potassium	(1,875–5,625)	mg	341	mg	42
Magnesium	400	μg	12	μg	3
Selenium	200	μg	0.95	μg	0
Iodine	150	mg	0	mg	0
Zinc	15	mg	0.21	mg	1
Iron	10	mg	2	mg	18
Manganese	(2.5–5.0)	mg	0.67	mg	13
Copper	(2.0–3.0)	mg	0.24	mg	8

AMOUNT PER SERVING		CALORIES PER SERVING	% OF MEAL
Fat	2 grams	20	15
Proteins	4 grams	17	12
Carbohydrates	25 grams	102	73
Cholesterol	10 mg		
Amino acid (essential)			44–99
Fiber	1 gram		

Key: USRDA = Recommended Dietary Allowance
     IU = International Unit
    mg = milligrams
    μg = micrograms
NOTE: The numbers with arrows exceed 100 percent of required USRDA.

Cauliflower Mushroom Marriage

Ingredients:

4 cups cauliflower, cut in large pieces
2 Tbs mayonnaise
½ cup plain yogurt
2 Tbs Parmesan cheese
prepared mustard

Preparation: Bake

Time: 20 minutes

Calories: 109 per serving

Serves: 4

Directions

Preheat oven to 400°F. Use a medium-sized baking dish or pan and place the cauliflower pieces in the dish. Mix the mayonnaise with the yogurt and spread over the cauliflower; if desired, add a little mustard to the mixture. Sprinkle with cheese and bake for about 10 minutes, making sure that the cheese has melted. Notice large amounts of vitamin K and calcium.

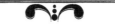

TIP: The USDA indicates that both too little and too much of a nutrient can be harmful. The USRDAs are designed to meet the needs of healthy people, and the allowances have been set high enough so that no improvement in health will be achieved from ingesting higher levels. A varied diet will bring benefits.

MYTH: White spots on your fingernails indicate a vitamin or mineral deficiency.

FACT: A report in the *Wellness Letter* of the University of California at Berkeley says this is not so. The spots are usually the result of minor injury or infections. They are not indicative of nutritional deficiency.

Nutrients Contained in:
Cauliflower Mushroom Marriage

VITAMINS USRDA		ONE SERVING GIVES YOU APPROXIMATELY		APPROXIMATE PERCENTAGE OF USRDA
A	5,000 IU	72	IU	1
B1	1.4 mg	0.09	mg	7
B2	1.6 mg	0.13	mg	9
B3	16 mg	0.68	mg	4
B5	10 mg	0.32	mg	3
B6	2.2 mg	0.25	mg	11
B12	3 μg	16	μg	5
C	60 mg	72	mg	119◄
D	400 IU	13	IU	3
E	15 IU	0.05	IU	0
K	500 μg	3,600	μg	720◄
Folic Acid	400 μg	69	μg	17

MINERALS USRDA		ONE SERVING GIVES YOU APPROXIMATELY		APPROXIMATE PERCENTAGE OF USRDA
Sodium	(1,100–3,000) mg	120	mg	12
Calcium	1,000 mg	115	mg	14
Phosphorus	(800–1,000) mg	109	mg	13
Potassium	(1,875–5,625) mg	427	mg	53
Magnesium	400 μg	21	μg	5
Selenium	200 μg	0.60	μg	0
Iodine	150 mg	13	mg	8
Zinc	15 mg	0.54	mg	3
Iron	10 mg	0.70	mg	6
Manganese	(2.5–5.0) mg	0.20	mg	4
Copper	(2.0–3.0) mg	0.06	mg	1

AMOUNT PER SERVING		CALORIES PER SERVING	% OF MEAL
Fat	7 grams	62	57
Proteins	5 grams	18	17
Carbohydrates	7 grams	29	26
Cholesterol	4 mg		
Amino acid (essential)			52–78*
Fiber	1 gram		

Key: USRDA = Recommended Dietary Allowance

   IU = International Unit

   mg = milligrams

   μg = micrograms

NOTE: The numbers with arrows exceed 100 percent of required USRDA.

*Complementary food—1 cup of mushrooms will raise EAA to 95–158%.

Brussels Sprouts and Jack

Ingredients:

20 brussels sprouts
2 carrots, sliced
2 stalks celery, sliced
   in $\frac{1}{2}$-inch pieces
1 tsp basil
$\frac{1}{4}$ cup Jack cheese
juice of one lemon
black pepper
basil
cayenne pepper

Preparation: Steam

Time: 20 minutes

Calories: 127 per serving

Serves: 4

Directions

Put brussels sprouts, carrots, celery, and basil in steamer and let steam for about 10 minutes (longer if sprouts are very firm). After vegetables have cooked, put them into a large bowl and sprinkle juice of lemon and cheese over them. Add pepper to taste; if desired a speck of cayenne pepper adds a tingle.

TIP: If you don't get enough calcium in your diet, your body "steals" calcium from your bones. This sets the condition for osteoporosis, a disease in which the bones lose mass. That's when they become brittle, thin, and subject to easy breaking.

MYTH: It's healthier to drink raw milk than pasteurized milk.

FACT: University of California at Berkeley reports that this is not so. Raw milk can be contaminated with bacteria that can cause disease and even death, especially in the very young, the elderly, and the ill. Pasteurization destroys harmful bacteria, but it does not affect nutrient content.

Nutrients Contained in:
Brussels Sprouts and Jack

VITAMINS USRDA			ONE SERVING GIVES YOU APPROXIMATELY		APPROXIMATE PERCENTAGE OF USRDA
A	5,000	IU	10,987	IU	219◄
B₁	1.4	mg	0.22	mg	18
B₂	1.6	mg	0.11	mg	7
B₃	16	mg	1	mg	6
B₅	10	mg	0.38	mg	3
B₆	2.2	mg	0.27	mg	12
B₁₂	3	μg	0	μg	0
C	60	mg	85	mg	141◄
D	400	IU	0	IU	0
E	15	IU	2	IU	11
K	500	μg	800	μg	160◄
Folic Acid	400	μg	64	μg	15

MINERALS USRDA			ONE SERVING GIVES YOU APPROXIMATELY		APPROXIMATE PERCENTAGE OF USRDA
Sodium	(1,100–3,000)	mg	122	mg	12
Calcium	1,000	mg	159	mg	19
Phosphorus	(800–1,000)	mg	147	mg	18
Potassium	(1,875–5,625)	mg	527	mg	65
Magnesium	400	μg	31	μg	8
Selenium	200	μg	46	μg	23
Iodine	150	mg	0	mg	0
Zinc	15	mg	0.91	mg	6
Iron	10	mg	2	mg	16
Manganese	(2.5–5.0)	mg	0.39	mg	7
Copper	(2.0–3.0)	mg	0.09	mg	3

AMOUNT PER SERVING		CALORIES PER SERVING	% OF MEAL
Fat	5 grams	42	35
Proteins	7 grams	29	23
Carbohydrates	14 grams	56	42
Cholesterol	13 mg		
Amino acid (essential)			74–102
Fiber	2 grams		

Key: USRDA = Recommended Dietary Allowance
      IU = International Unit
      mg = milligrams
      μg = micrograms
NOTE: The numbers with arrows exceed 100 percent of required USRDA.

Nutty Bok Choy

Ingredients: 1 ½ to 2 cups bok choy, chopped
     1 tsp canola oil
     2 Tbs cinnamon
     ¼ cup peanuts, chopped fine
     black pepper

Preparation: Steam and simmer
Time: 20 minutes
Calories: 96 per serving
Serves: 4

Directions

Steam bok choy for about 5 to 7 minutes. Heat oil in a skillet and add the cooked bok choy, cinnamon, and peanuts. Combine ingredients and heat thoroughly. Add pepper and chili pepper to taste.

TIP: Bok choy, along with collard greens, kale, canned sardines, almonds, cheese, broccoli, cooked beans, onions, buckwheat, millet, oats, tofu, soybeans, and lentils are good sources of calcium.

MYTH: Poultry is lower in cholesterol than beef.

FACT: The USDA Meat and Poultry Division says no. All animal products contain cholesterol—about 20 to 25 milligrams per ounce. A 3.5-ounce serving of chicken breast (with or without skin) has about 75 milligrams of cholesterol, only slightly less than a similar serving of beef.

Nutrients Contained in: Nutty Bok Choy

VITAMINS USRDA			ONE SERVING GIVES YOU APPROXIMATELY		APPROXIMATE PERCENTAGE OF USRDA
A	5,000	IU	1,637	IU	32
B₁	1.4	mg	0.05	mg	4
B₂	1.6	mg	0.05	mg	3
B₃	16	mg	2	mg	11
B₅	10	mg	0.19	mg	1
B₆	2.2	mg	0.04	mg	1
B₁₂	3	μg	0	μg	0
C	60	mg	17	mg	27
D	400	IU	0	IU	0
E	15	IU	1	IU	9
K	500	μg	0	μg	0
Folic Acid	400	μg	0	μg	0

MINERALS USRDA			ONE SERVING GIVES YOU APPROXIMATELY		APPROXIMATE PERCENTAGE OF USRDA
Sodium	(1,100–3,000)	mg	22	mg	2
Calcium	1,000	mg	66	mg	8
Phosphorus	(800–1,000)	mg	55	mg	6
Potassium	(1,875–5,625)	mg	299	mg	37
Magnesium	400	μg	23	μg	6
Selenium	200	μg	0.04	μg	0
Iodine	150	mg	0	mg	0
Zinc	15	mg	0.30	mg	1
Iron	10	mg	0.86	mg	8
Manganese	(2.5–5.0)	mg	0.14	mg	2
Copper	(2.0–3.0)	mg	0.04	mg	1

AMOUNT PER SERVING		CALORIES PER SERVING	% OF MEAL
Fat	8 grams	71	74
Proteins	3 grams	13	14
Carbohydrates	3 grams	12	12
Cholesterol	0 mg		
Amino acid (essential)			31-47*
Fiber	1 gram		

Key: USRDA = Recommended Dietary Allowance

IU = International Unit

mg = milligrams

μg = micrograms

NOTE: The numbers with arrows exceed 100 percent of required USRDA.

*Complementary food–1 3.5-ounce portion of beef chuck raises EAA to 237-624%.

Mellow Melon Salad

Ingredients:
- 1 cantaloupe
- ½ cup pineapple, cut into medium pieces
- ½ cup orange juice
- 2 avocados
- ½ cup apricot nectar
- 6 to 8 iceberg lettuce leaves

Preparation: No cooking required

Time: 15 minutes

Calories: 271 per serving

Serves: 4

Directions

Cut cantaloupe into half-inch pieces and place in a large bowl. Combine the pineapple, orange juice, and apricot nectar and pour the juice over the fruit. Peel the avocados and cut them in half. Remove the pits, fill with the cantaloupe mixture, and serve on lettuce leaves. Use a little Lite Italian dressing if desired. Levels of vitamin A and potassium are high.

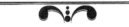

TIP: The Calcium Information Center at the New York Hospital-Cornell Medical Center says one quarter of American women from the age of 20 on never consume even 500 milligrams of calcium a day, and teenagers who drink diet soda instead of milk probably aren't getting enough calcium.

MYTH: Your heart stops when you sneeze.

FACT: Physicians at the Manhattan Ear, Nose, and Throat Hospital says your heart doesn't stop. People do close their eyes by reflex. Blessing one after sneezing came about because people believed that a blessing would ward off infections that sneezes were believed to herald.

Nutrients Contained in: Mellow Melon Salad

VITAMINS USRDA		ONE SERVING GIVES YOU APPROXIMATELY		APPROXIMATE PERCENTAGE OF USRDA
A	5,000 IU	5,449	IU	108◄
B1	1.4 mg	0.20	mg	16
B2	1.6 mg	0.17	mg	12
B3	16 mg	1	mg	7
B5	10 mg	1	mg	12
B6	2.2 mg	0.46	mg	21
B12	3 μg	0	μg	0
C	60 mg	73	mg	122◄
D	400 IU	0	IU	0
E	15 IU	2	IU	14
K	500 μg	71	μg	13
Folic Acid	400 μg	107	μg	26

MINERALS USRDA		ONE SERVING GIVES YOU APPROXIMATELY		APPROXIMATE PERCENTAGE OF USRDA
Sodium	(1,100–3,000) mg	27	mg	2
Calcium	1,000 mg	40	mg	5
Phosphorus	(800–1,000) mg	78	mg	9
Potassium	(1,875–5,625) mg	1,142	mg	142◄
Magnesium	400 μg	61	μg	17
Selenium	200 μg	0.15	μg	0
Iodine	150 mg	0	mg	0
Zinc	15 mg	0.76	mg	5
Iron	10 mg	2	mg	17
Manganese	(2.5–5.0) mg	0.66	mg	13
Copper	(2.0–3.0) mg	0.38	mg	12

AMOUNT PER SERVING		CALORIES PER SERVING	% OF MEAL
Fat	16 grams	144	53
Proteins	4 grams	15	6
Carbohydrates	28 grams	112	41
Cholesterol	1 mg		
Amino acid (essential)			24-31*
Fiber	3 grams		

Key: USRDA = Recommended Dietary Allowance
     IU = International Unit
     mg = milligrams
     μg = micrograms
NOTE: The numbers with arrows exceed 100 percent of required USRDA.

*Complementary food—1 cup of lima beans raises EAA to 173-232%.

Fish and Rice Sitdown

Ingredients:

14 ounce canned salmon
1 cup cooked rice
2 egg whites, hard-boiled
   cut in slices
4 Tbs half and half cream
2 tsp curry
   juice of one lemon
   cayenne pepper

Preparation: Simmer

Time: 20 minutes

Calories: 376 per serving

Serves: 4

Directions

Place salmon in a medium-sized saucepan and stir heating slowly, add the cooked rice and egg whites. The curry should be added to the rice while cooking. Add half and half, lemon juice, and cayenne pepper to taste. Stir together until thoroughly heated. This meal contains very high amounts of needed calcium, vitamin D, and phosphorus and essential amino acids.

TIP: A report from the *Journal of Clinical Endocrinology & Metabolism* says older women with osteoporosis should eat foods high in calcium, take 400 to 800 units of vitamin D each day, and exercise regularly.

MYTH: Chocolate interferes with the body's ability to absorb calcium from milk.

FACT: Research published in the *American Journal of Clinical Nutrition* says there is no cause for concern about this. According to the *Journal*, milk contains a lot of calcium, while the amount of chocolate typically added to milk contains only a little oxalic acid, which is found in chocolate and tends to bind calcium in milk and makes it difficult to absorb.

Nutrients Contained in: Fish and Rice Sitdown

VITAMINS USRDA			ONE SERVING GIVES YOU APPROXIMATELY		APPROXIMATE PERCENTAGE OF USRDA
A	5,000	IU	225	IU	4
B$_1$	1.4	mg	0.34	mg	27
B$_2$	1.6	mg	0.15	mg	10
B$_3$	16	mg	12	mg	75
B$_5$	10	mg	2	mg	19
B$_6$	2.2	mg	0.96	mg	43
B$_{12}$	3	μg	4	μg	135◄
C	60	mg	9	mg	15
D	400	IU	650	IU	162◄
E	15	IU	3	IU	18
K	500	μg	0	μg	0
Folic Acid	400	μg	29	μg	7

MINERALS USRDA			ONE SERVING GIVES YOU APPROXIMATELY		APPROXIMATE PERCENTAGE OF USRDA
Sodium	(1,100–3,000)	mg	151	mg	15
Calcium	1,000	mg	448	mg	55
Phosphorus	(800–1,000)	mg	314	mg	39
Potassium	(1,875–5,625)	mg	590	mg	73
Magnesium	400	μg	75	μg	21
Selenium	200	μg	20	μg	10
Iodine	150	mg	0	mg	0
Zinc	15	mg	2	mg	12
Iron	10	mg	2	mg	20
Manganese	(2.5–5.0)	mg	0.81	mg	16
Copper	(2.0–3.0)	mg	0.31	mg	10

AMOUNT PER SERVING		CALORIES PER SERVING	% OF MEAL
Fat	10 grams	90	24
Proteins	33 grams	131	35
Carbohydrates	39 grams	155	41
Cholesterol	53 mg		
Amino acid (essential)			223–598*
Fiber	0 grams		

Key: USRDA = Recommended Dietary Allowance

IU = International Unit

mg = milligrams

μg = micrograms

NOTE: The numbers with arrows exceed 100 percent of required USRDA.

*Big score.

Rice Under Almonds

Ingredients:

2 cups brown rice
1 cup chopped almonds
1 tsp ground cinnamon
2 whole dried shiitake
  mushrooms
¼ cup safflower oil
1 tsp saffron or turmeric
6 cups water
½ tsp margarine
  juice of one lime
1 Tbs Worcestershire
  sauce

Preparation: Sauté and boil

Time: 45 minutes

Calories: 255 per serving

Serves: 4

Directions

Soak mushrooms until soft. Put Worcestershire sauce and oil in skillet and sauté mushrooms until soft but still firm. Bring the water to boil in a 3-quart saucepan and add turmeric, lime juice, cinnamon, butter, and almonds. Add the rice and mushrooms and cook for about 20 minutes until rice is tender and the water has been absorbed.

TIP: From the nuts and seed family a good source of calcium includes almonds, chia seeds, sesame seeds, Brazil nuts, and filberts.

MYTH: A few weeks of inactivity won't decrease your fitness level if you're physically fit.

FACT: Researchers at the University of Texas at Austin found that even two weeks of inactivity can reduce your fitness level. They studied the fitness of some well-trained athletes who discontinued their workouts for three months and found that their physical fitness declined rapidly in the first 12 days and continued to decline.

Nutrients Contained in: Rice Under Almonds

VITAMINS USRDA			ONE SERVING GIVES YOU APPROXIMATELY		APPROXIMATE PERCENTAGE OF USRDA
A	5,000	IU	0	IU	0
B₁	1.4	mg	0.19	mg	15
B₂	1.6	mg	0.11	mg	7
B₃	16	mg	3	mg	19
B₅	10	mg	0.57	mg	5
B₆	2.2	mg	0.34	mg	15
B₁₂	3	μg	0	μg	0
C	60	mg	0	mg	0
D	400	IU	0	IU	0
E	15	IU	2	IU	13
K	500	μg	0	μg	0
Folic Acid	400	μg	8	μg	1

MINERALS USRDA			ONE SERVING GIVES YOU APPROXIMATELY		APPROXIMATE PERCENTAGE OF USRDA
Sodium	(1,100–3,000)	mg	6	mg	0
Calcium	1,000	mg	38	mg	4
Phosphorus	(800–1,000)	mg	153	mg	19
Potassium	(1,875–5,625)	mg	215	mg	26
Magnesium	400	μg	72	μg	20
Selenium	200	μg	19	μg	9
Iodine	150	mg	0	mg	0
Zinc	15	mg	2	mg	11
Iron	10	mg	1	mg	12
Manganese	(2.5–5.0)	mg	0.97	mg	19
Copper	(2.0–3.0)	mg	0.18	mg	5

AMOUNT PER SERVING		CALORIES PER SERVING	% OF MEAL
Fat	6 grams	51	20
Proteins	6 grams	24	9
Carbohydrates	45 grams	180	71
Cholesterol	0 mg		
Amino acid (essential)			56–85
Fiber	1 gram		

Key: USRDA = Recommended Dietary Allowance
     IU = International Unit
     mg = milligrams
     μg = micrograms
NOTE: The numbers with arrows exceed 100 percent of required USRDA.

Brussels Sprouts Parmesan

Ingredients:

20 Brussels sprouts
 2 carrots
 1 cup onions, sliced
 1 tomato, diced
¼ cup safflower oil
    juice of one lemon
 3 cloves garlic, mashed
 6 Tbs grated Parmesan
      cheese
    juice of one lime
    black pepper
    chervil
    chili pepper

Preparation: Steam

Time: 20 minutes

Calories: 148 per serving

Serves: 6

Directions

Steam brussels sprouts until soft. Then combine onions, carrots cut into thin circles, and tomatoes in large salad bowl. Toss with the oil, juice of lemon and lime, black pepper and chervil, and chili pepper to taste. Sprinkle garlic and cheese over the ingredients and serve in salad bowls. Amounts of vitamins A and K, calcium, and potassium are very high.

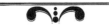

TIP: A 1 ounce serving of cheese, containing approximately 200 grams of calcium, makes an important addition to meeting calcium needs, a need that is reported to provide some protection against osteoporosis.

MYTH: Yellow-skinned chickens are more nutritious than white.

FACT: The poultry industry says the color depends upon what chickens are fed, and the color has no benefit over the white-skinned chickens. The color is a result of breeders trying to meet consumer preferences for color.

Nutrients Contained in: Brussels Sprouts Parmesan

VITAMINS USRDA			ONE SERVING GIVES YOU APPROXIMATELY		APPROXIMATE PERCENTAGE OF USRDA
A	5,000	IU	7,497	IU	149◄
B_1	1.4	mg	0.15	mg	12
B_2	1.6	mg	0.10	mg	7
B_3	16	mg	0.87	mg	5
B_5	10	mg	0.37	mg	3
B_6	2.2	mg	0.24	mg	10
B_{12}	3	μg	0	μg	0
C	60	mg	67	mg	112◄
D	400	IU	0	IU	0
E	15	IU	4	IU	25
K	500	μg	535	μg	107◄
Folic Acid	400	μg	50	μg	12

MINERALS USRDA			ONE SERVING GIVES YOU APPROXIMATELY		APPROXIMATE PERCENTAGE OF USRDA
Sodium	(1,100–3,000)	mg	121	mg	12
Calcium	1,000	mg	113	mg	14
Phosphorus	(800–1,000)	mg	111	mg	13
Potassium	(1,875–5,625)	mg	434	mg	54
Magnesium	400	μg	30	μg	8
Selenium	200	μg	33	μg	16
Iodine	150	mg	0	mg	0
Zinc	15	mg	0.57	mg	3
Iron	10	mg	1	mg	13
Manganese	(2.5–5.0)	mg	0.31	mg	6
Copper	(2.0–3.0)	mg	0.11	mg	3

AMOUNT PER SERVING		CALORIES PER SERVING	% OF MEAL
Fat	9 grams	78	53
Proteins	5 grams	20	14
Carbohydrates	12 grams	50	34
Cholesterol	4 mg		
Amino acid (essential)			52–73*
Fiber	1 gram		

Key: USRDA = Recommended Dietary Allowance
    IU = International Unit
    mg = milligrams
    μg = micrograms
NOTE: The numbers with arrows exceed 100 percent of required USRDA.

*Complementary food—1 egg, large white raises the EAA to 102–148%.

Vegetable Haymaker

Ingredients:

½ cup onions, chopped
½ cup scallions, cut in
    medium pieces
1 tsp canola oil
2 cups cauliflower, cut
    into medium pieces
2 cups broccoli, cut
    into pieces
2 tomatoes, cut into chunks
2 potatoes, cut into
    ¼-inch slices
1 cup red cabbage, shredded
½ tsp ginger, ground
    cayenne pepper
    juice of one lemon
    black pepper

Preparation: Sauté and simmer

Time: 45 minutes

Calories: 153 per serving

Serves: 6

Directions

Sauté onions in a large skillet until soft. Add the cauliflower, broccoli, and about 3 cups of water. Add ginger and cayenne pepper and cook for 10 minutes covered. Add potatoes and tomatoes and cook for about 10 to 15 minutes. Add the red cabbage and cook until vegetables are tender. Sprinkle with black pepper and lemon juice and serve. Notice the large amounts of vitamin K and folic acid; both nutrients are especially good for body growth.

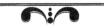

TIP: The National Research Council recommended daily allowance of calcium be increased for young women to 1,200 milligrams daily from 800, on the grounds that the skeletal reserve established during her teens helps to determine bone strength throughout a woman's life.

MYTH: It's not safe to handle chicken with your bare hands because bacteria might penetrate a cut.

FACT: Food experts say it's not dangerous. Salmonella and other bacteria found in chicken have to be eaten to make you sick. It's always a good rule, however, to wash your hands after handling raw chicken because bacteria could be spread to other foods that won't be cooked.

Nutrients Contained in: Vegetable Haymaker

VITAMINS USRDA			ONE SERVING GIVES YOU APPROXIMATELY		APPROXIMATE PERCENTAGE OF USRDA
A	5,000	IU	1,345	IU	26
B$_1$	1.4	mg	0.16	mg	13
B$_2$	1.6	mg	0.12	mg	8
B$_3$	16	mg	2	mg	11
B$_5$	10	mg	0.72	mg	7
B$_6$	2.2	mg	0.40	mg	18
B$_{12}$	3	μg	0	μg	0
C	60	mg	81	mg	134◄
D	400	IU	0	IU	0
E	15	IU	3	IU	17
K	500	μg	1,304	μg	260◄
Folic Acid	400	μg	65	μg	16

MINERALS USRDA			ONE SERVING GIVES YOU APPROXIMATELY		APPROXIMATE PERCENTAGE OF USRDA
Sodium	(1,100–3,000)	mg	26	mg	2
Calcium	1,000	mg	45	mg	5
Phosphorus	(800–1,000)	mg	91	mg	11
Potassium	(1,875–5,625)	mg	646	mg	80
Magnesium	400	μg	39	μg	11
Selenium	200	μg	0.95	μg	0
Iodine	150	mg	0	mg	0
Zinc	15	mg	0.50	mg	3
Iron	10	mg	2	mg	18
Manganese	(2.5–5.0)	mg	0.35	mg	7
Copper	(2.0–3.0)	mg	0.28	mg	9

AMOUNT PER SERVING		CALORIES PER SERVING	% OF MEAL
Fat	5 grams	44	29
Proteins	4 grams	15	10
Carbohydrates	24 grams	94	61
Cholesterol	0 mg		
Amino acid (essential)			34–52*
Fiber	1 gram		

Key: USRDA = Recommended Dietary Allowance

IU = International Unit

mg = milligrams

μg = micrograms

NOTE: The numbers with arrows exceed 100 percent of required USRDA.

*Complementary food—1 head of endive will raise EAA to 79–143%.

Mustards and Collards

Ingredients:
- 3 cups collard greens
- 6 oz ground lean beef
- 1 large onion
- 3 cups mustard greens
- 1 tsp olive oil
- 1 tsp crushed red pepper
- 1 quart water
- black pepper

Preparation: Simmer

Time: 55 minutes

Calories: 125 per serving

Serves: 6

Directions

Cut collards and mustard greens in small pieces. In a large saucepan, place the collards, large onion slices, crushed pepper, and ground beef; season with black pepper for taste. Simmer for 30 minutes. Add the mustard greens and olive oil and cook for 15 minutes or longer until vegetables are tender and water has been absorbed. The chart shows plenty nutritional benefits from vitamins A and C, calcium, and potassium.

TIP: Barbara Levine of the New York Hospital-Cornell Medical Center says she cannot emphasize enough the importance of calcium in our diets. She says teenagers and young adults (up to age 25) need 1,200 milligrams of calcium a day. That equals four 8-ounce glasses of milk. After age 25, the minimum should be 800 milligrams.

MYTH: Fasting is a good way to cleanse your system and should be done occasionally.

FACT: The report from the School of Public Health at the University of California at Berkeley says there's no evidence that a fast can "cleanse" your body. They also say there is no evidence that your body needs this type of cleansing.

Nutrients Contained in: Mustards and Collards

VITAMINS USRDA			ONE SERVING GIVES YOU APPROXIMATELY		APPROXIMATE PERCENTAGE OF USRDA
A	5,000	IU	8,900	IU	178◄
B$_1$	1.4	mg	0.18	mg	15
B$_2$	1.6	mg	0.24	mg	17
B$_3$	16	mg	3	mg	17
B$_5$	10	mg	0.43	mg	4
B$_6$	2.2	mg	0.22	mg	10
B$_{12}$	3	μg	0.50	μg	16
C	60	mg	72	mg	119◄
D	400	IU	0	IU	0
E	15	IU	4	IU	23
K	500	μg	2	μg	0
Folic Acid	400	μg	16	μg	4

MINERALS USRDA			ONE SERVING GIVES YOU APPROXIMATELY		APPROXIMATE PERCENTAGE OF USRDA
Sodium	(1,100–3,000)	mg	58	mg	5
Calcium	1,000	mg	258	mg	32
Phosphorus	(800–1,000)	mg	132	mg	16
Potassium	(1,875–5,625)	mg	559	mg	69
Magnesium	400	μg	53	μg	15
Selenium	200	μg	9	μg	4
Iodine	150	mg	0	mg	0
Zinc	15	mg	2	mg	12
Iron	10	mg	4	mg	37
Manganese	(2.5–5.0)	mg	0.38	mg	7
Copper	(2.0–3.0)	mg	0.27	mg	8

AMOUNT PER SERVING		CALORIES PER SERVING	% OF MEAL
Fat	4 grams	36	30
Proteins	13 grams	51	40
Carbohydrates	9 grams	38	30
Cholesterol	25 mg		
Amino acid (essential)			84–214
Fiber	2 grams		

Key: USRDA = Recommended Dietary Allowance
    IU = International Unit
    mg = milligrams
    μg = micrograms
NOTE: The numbers with arrows exceed 100 percent of required USRDA.

Garlic Tofu Soup

Ingredients:

20	cloves garlic
4 to 6	cups boiling water
1	tsp margarine
¼	cup Italian parsley, chopped
½	cup pea pods
	black pepper
2	5x2 inch tofu squares cut in small cubes

Preparation: Sauté and simmer

Time: 20 minutes

Calories: 80 per serving

Serves: 4

Directions

Sauté whole garlic cloves in a skillet in the margarine until they are light brown. Add tofu cubes, water, parsley, pea pods, and pepper to taste, and simmer for 10 minutes. On a cold day, this is a hot dish.

TIP: A report in the *New England Journal of Medicine* indicated that women who get enough calcium (1,000 milligrams a day before menopause, and 1,200 to 1,500 milligrams daily after menopause), exercise regularly, and might be on hormone-replacement therapy following menopause will probably never get osteoporosis.

MYTH: Women primarily are the ones who suffer from osteoporosis.

FACT: That's what people used to think until researchers found that men from age 30 on lose about 1 percent per year of bone mass in the wrists and hands. The rate of bone loss in the hands and wrists, according to the *Annals of Internal Medicine*, worsens as men get older.

Nutrients Contained in: Garlic Tofu Soup

VITAMINS USRDA			ONE SERVING GIVES YOU APPROXIMATELY		APPROXIMATE PERCENTAGE OF USRDA
A	5,000	IU	427	IU	8
B_1	1.4	mg	0.11	mg	9
B_2	1.6	mg	0.06	mg	4
B_3	16	mg	0.28	mg	1
B_5	10	mg	0.27	mg	2
B_6	2.2	mg	0.02	mg	1
B_{12}	3	μg	0	μg	0
C	60	mg	14	mg	23
D	400	IU	0	IU	0
E	15	IU	0.09	IU	0
K	500	μg	3	μg	0
Folic Acid	400	μg	0.03	μg	8

MINERALS USRDA			ONE SERVING GIVES YOU APPROXIMATELY		APPROXIMATE PERCENTAGE OF USRDA
Sodium	(1,100–3,000)	mg	29	mg	2
Calcium	1,000	mg	106	mg	13
Phosphorus	(800–1,000)	mg	128	mg	16
Potassium	(1,875–5,625)	mg	200	mg	25
Magnesium	400	μg	81	μg	23
Selenium	200	μg	0	μg	0
Iodine	150	mg	0	mg	0
Zinc	15	mg	0.36	mg	2
Iron	10	mg	2	mg	21
Manganese	(2.5–5.0)	mg	0.04	mg	0
Copper	(2.0–3.0)	mg	0.06	mg	1

AMOUNT PER SERVING		CALORIES PER SERVING	% OF MEAL
Fat	4 grams	37	47
Proteins	2 grams	9	11
Carbohydrates	8 grams	34	42
Cholesterol	10 mg		
Amino acid (essential)			58–95
Fiber	1 gram		

Key: USRDA = Recommended Dietary Allowance
     IU = International Unit
     mg = milligrams
     μg = micrograms
NOTE: The numbers with arrows 100 percent of required USRDA.

VEGETABLES RANKED IN THE HIGHEST ORDER FOR CALCIUM
PERCENTAGES GIVEN EQUAL ½ CUP

	CALCIUM (MILLIGRAMS)	PERCENTAGE OF USRDA
Potato, au gratin	146.0	18.3
Spinach, frozen	139.0	17.4
Tofu	130.0	16.3
Spinach, cooked	122.0	15.2
Beans, fava, canned	121.0	15.1
Cauliflower, with cheese	100.0	12.5
Spinach, canned	100.0	12.5
Broccoli, cooked	89.0	11.1
Spinach, cream frozen	80.0	10.0
Beans, baked, pork/sauce	74.0	9.3
Potato, scalloped	70.0	8.8
Beans, baked, plain	64.0	8.0
Beans, navy, cooked	64.0	8.0
Broccoli, with cheese sauce	60.0	7.5
Okra, cooked	50.0	6.3
Peas, frozen	48.0	6.0
Broccoli, frozen	47.0	5.9
Artichoke, cooked	47.0	5.9
Beans, pinto, cooked	43.0	5.4
Beans, kidney, canned	40.0	5.0
Garbanzos, canned	39.0	4.9
Sauerkraut, canned	36.0	4.5
Pumpkin, canned	32.0	4.0
Beans, green, frozen	31.0	3.9
Peas, snow, cooked	29.0	3.6

CHAPTER SEVEN

Healing and Preventive Recipes for Rheumatoid Arthritis

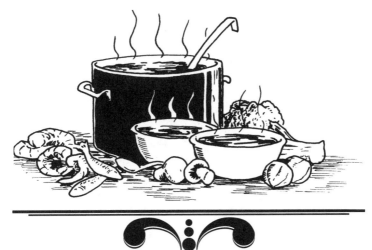

There are lies, damn lies, and statistics.
—Benjamin Disraeli

Rheumatoid arthritis (RA) is an autoimmune disease involving, among other things, a stiffening of joints.

The idea that RA can be eased or protected by nutritional safeguards is controversial. There have been promising results, however, from many studies regarding the inclusion of fish oils in the diet. British researchers reported that people who received fish oil in a test felt less tenderness or pain in their joints than had those in the test who did not receive fish oil. Fish that are high in oils such as omega-3 fatty acids are salmon, sardines, mackerel, and trout.

In studies done in Italy, broccoli soup was found to give significant relief from arthritis pain and stiffness after a month of eating the soup. Some research has indicated in a general way that copper, zinc, and vitamin B may also have a positive effect. Of course, a type of arthritis known as gout has a definite connection to diet. Foods such as anchovies, organ meat, and mushrooms that are a source of purine are known to aggravate arthritis.

Throughout the chapter, you will find many interesting reports on studies that have shown positive results for arthritics. And, of course, all the recipes have been designed to take advantage of whatever ingredients have shown promise in the way of nutrition. Fish and Chicks is an imaginative blend of tuna and chick peas, and Spicy Onion Salmon is excellent for everybody.

Fish and Chicks

Ingredients:

2 6.5-ounce cans tuna packed in water or vegetable oil
1 ½ cups canned chick peas
4 cloves garlic
4 Tbs red wine
1 Tbs Italian parsley
½ tsp black pepper
¼ tsp chili powder
juice of one lime

Preparation: Simmer

Time: 15 minutes

Calories: 416 per serving

Serves: 4

Directions

Put chick peas with their liquid in a large skillet with chopped garlic. Simmer for 5 minutes. Add wine, parsley, pepper, and juice of lime. Cook for another minute. Break tuna into small chunks and add to skillet. Cover and simmer for 5 minutes. If tuna is canned in water, calories will be considerably lesser than given. Amounts of phosphorus, potassium, and magnesium are beneficial. For a surprise, look at EAA percentages on the chart.

TIP: Dr. Norman Childers at Rutgers University in New Jersey made a study of 3,000 arthritis sufferers who avoided so-called nightshade family foods such as eggplant, peppers, potatoes, and tomatoes. Avoiding these foods helped relieve aches, pains, and some disfigurement according to Childers and his researchers.

MYTH: Germs spread more readily in airplanes.

FACT: The U.S. Department of Transportation says there are fewer bacteria and fungi in airplane cabin air than in other indoor environments. They announced this finding after the results of a study undertaken for the DOT were evaluated. According to the DOT, you can catch a cold in an airplane the same as anywhere else.

Nutrients Contained in: Fish and Chicks

VITAMINS USRDA			ONE SERVING GIVES YOU APPROXIMATELY		APPROXIMATE PERCENTAGE OF USRDA
A	5,000	IU	396	IU	7
B$_1$	1.4	mg	0.29	mg	23
B$_2$	1.6	mg	0.17	mg	12
B$_3$	16	mg	13	mg	81
B$_5$	10	mg	1	mg	10
B$_6$	2.2	mg	0.73	mg	32
B$_{12}$	3	µg	1	µg	43
C	60	mg	12	mg	19
D	400	IU	8	IU	1
E	15	IU	2	IU	13
K	500	µg	0	µg	0
Folic Acid	400	µg	5	µg	1

MINERALS USRDA			ONE SERVING GIVES YOU APPROXIMATELY		APPROXIMATE PERCENTAGE OF USRDA
Sodium	(1,100–3,000)	mg	455	mg	45
Calcium	1,000	mg	132	mg	16
Phosphorus	(800–1,000)	mg	463	mg	57
Potassium	(1,875–5,625)	mg	916	mg	114◄
Magnesium	400	µg	143	µg	40
Selenium	200	µg	58	µg	28
Iodine	150	mg	0	mg	0
Zinc	15	mg	3	mg	17
Iron	10	mg	7	mg	66
Manganese	(2.5–5.0)	mg	1	mg	21
Copper	(2.0–3.0)	mg	0.70	mg	23

AMOUNT PER SERVING		CALORIES PER SERVING	% OF MEAL
Fat	5 grams	49	12
Proteins	41 grams	165	40
Carbohydrates	51 grams	202	48
Cholesterol	32 mg		
Amino acid (essential)			353–749
Fiber	4 grams		

Key: USRDA = Recommended Dietary Allowance
   IU = International Unit
   mg = milligrams
   µg = micrograms
NOTE: The numbers with arrows exceed 100 percent of required USRDA.

Spicy Onion Salmon

Ingredients:

4 3.5-ounce salmon steaks
2 cloves garlic, chopped finely
1 Tbs vegetable oil
1 onion, chopped
1 cup scallions, chopped
¼ cup apple cider
2 Tbs marjoram
¼ tsp tarragon
2 cups water or plain broth
1 tsp mint leaves
½ tsp thyme
juice of one lemon
black pepper

Preparation: Sauté

Time: 55 minutes

Calories: 239 per serving

Serves: 4

Directions

In a large iron skillet, sauté garlic in oil. Add chopped onions and scallions and cook until transparent. Add cider, 2 cups of water or plain broth, tarragon, and marjoram. Simmer for 15 minutes. Add thyme, pepper, juice of the lemon, and mint leaves. Cook at low heat for about 15 minutes. Add salmon steaks to this pan and cook covered for about 6 minutes on one side, then turn and cook 6 minutes on the other side. Fish experts measure cooking time by inches, a method that stands up very well. Fish is cooked 10 minutes for every inch at its thickest point. Serve immediately. Observe the high percentages of vitamins A, D, and B_{12}, calcium, phosphorus, and potassium and a whopping amount of EAA.

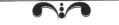

TIP: Researchers at the Academy of Applied Nutrition in Milan, Italy, studied 200 people with arthritis who were given broccoli soup three times a week for 26 weeks. Study director Dr. Aldo Pallucci said 83 percent of the patients reported significant relief from arthritis pain and stiffness after a month of eating the soup as prescribed.

MYTH: Sugar can make you fat.

FACT: A report in the Mayo Clinic Health Letter says sugar is not usually the cause of gaining weight. Fat is more likely the cause. Fat contains twice as many calories as sugar, and the body stores calories from fat more readily than it does from protein or carbohydrates.

Nutrients Contained in: Spicy Onion Salmon

VITAMINS USRDA			ONE SERVING GIVES YOU APPROXIMATELY		APPROXIMATE PERCENTAGE OF USRDA
A	5,000	IU	1,410	IU	28
B$_1$	1.4	mg	0.21	mg	17
B$_2$	1.6	mg	0.10	mg	7
B$_3$	16	mg	10	mg	61
B$_5$	10	mg	1	mg	13
B$_6$	2.2	mg	0.77	mg	34
B$_{12}$	3	μg	4	μg	133◄
C	60	mg	24	mg	39
D	400	IU	650	IU	162◄
E	15	IU	3	IU	16
K	500	μg	0	μg	0
Folic Acid	400	μg	38	μg	9

MINERALS USRDA			ONE SERVING GIVES YOU APPROXIMATELY		APPROXIMATE PERCENTAGE OF USRDA
Sodium	(1,100–3,000)	mg	119	mg	11
Calcium	1,000	mg	441	mg	55
Phosphorus	(800–1,000)	mg	217	mg	27
Potassium	(1,875–5,625)	mg	604	mg	75
Magnesium	400	μg	40	μg	11
Selenium	200	μg	0.80	μg	0
Iodine	150	mg	0	mg	0
Zinc	15	mg	1	mg	7
Iron	10	mg	2	mg	18
Manganese	(2.5–5.0)	mg	0.07	mg	1
Copper	(2.0–3.0)	mg	0.24	mg	8

AMOUNT PER SERVING		CALORIES PER SERVING	% OF MEAL
Fat	11 grams	99	41
Proteins	28 grams	112	47
Carbohydrates	7 grams	28	12
Cholesterol	47 mg		
Amino acid (essential)			166–543
Fiber	0 grams		

Key: USRDA = Recommended Dietary Allowance
     IU = International Unit
     mg = milligrams
     μg = micrograms
NOTE: The numbers with arrows exceed 100 percent of required USRDA.

Nuts to Apples

Ingredients: 4   large apples   **Preparation:** Bake
2   tsp margarine
1   cup brown sugar   **Time:** 50 minutes
1   cup peanuts, chopped
juice of one lemon   **Calories:** 989 per serving
$\frac{1}{2}$ cup water   **Serves:** 4

Directions

Preheat oven to 450° F. Core the apples and spread $\frac{1}{2}$ tsp of the margarine over them. In a large bowl, mix $\frac{1}{4}$ cup of the sugar with peanuts. Roll the apples in the mixture. Set them in a baking dish. Mix $\frac{1}{2}$ cup of the sugar with the remaining peanut-sugar mixture and use this to put into the core of the apples. Heat the water and mix with the juice of the lemon and the final $\frac{1}{4}$ cup sugar and pour around the apples. Use the remaining margarine to sprinkle around the apples and in the core. Bake for 20 minutes covered. Use the pan juices to cover apples as they bake. Cover and bake another 10 minutes or until apples are tender or slightly brown. This meal has very high percentages of magnesium, potassium, phosphorus, and EAA.

TIP: Just as some foods can aggravate arthritis, it is thought some foods or nutrients may help if added to the diet. Dr. Richard Panush, professor and chairman of the Department of Medicine at St. Barnabas Medical Center in Livingston, New Jersey, says copper, zinc, vitamin B, and fish oil and a number of other substances may have some positive affect.

MYTH: Yeast infections come from eating sugar and starches.

FACT: Dietitians registered with the American Dietetic Association indicate that sugars and starches are unrelated to yeast infection in the body. They have no evidence that sugar you eat is the cause of yeast infections or that it affects the immune system.

Nutrients Contained in: Nuts to Apples

VITAMINS USRDA			ONE SERVING GIVES YOU APPROXIMATELY		APPROXIMATE PERCENTAGE OF USRDA
A	5,000	IU	196	IU	3
B₁	1.4	mg	0.14	mg	11
B₂	1.6	mg	0.07	mg	5
B₃	16	mg	6	mg	39
B₅	10	mg	0.86	mg	8
B₆	2.2	mg	0.22	mg	10
B₁₂	3	µg	0	µg	0
C	60	mg	16	mg	25
D	400	IU	0	IU	0
E	15	IU	4	IU	24
K	500	µg	3	µg	0
Folic Acid	400	µg	5	µg	1

MINERALS USRDA			ONE SERVING GIVES YOU APPROXIMATELY		APPROXIMATE PERCENTAGE OF USRDA
Sodium	(1,100–3,000)	mg	72	mg	7
Calcium	1,000	mg	173	mg	21
Phosphorus	(800–1,000)	mg	220	mg	27
Potassium	(1,875–5,625)	mg	817	mg	102◀
Magnesium	400	µg	184	µg	52
Selenium	200	µg	4	µg	1
Iodine	150	mg	0	mg	0
Zinc	15	mg	1	mg	8
Iron	10	mg	6	mg	59
Manganese	(2.5–5.0)	mg	0.60	mg	12
Copper	(2.0–3.0)	mg	0.22	mg	7

AMOUNT PER SERVING		CALORIES PER SERVING	% OF MEAL
Fat	21 grams	188	19
Proteins	10 grams	39	4
Carbohydrates	191 grams	762	77
Cholesterol	0 mg		
Amino acid (essential)			67–126
Fiber	2 grams		

Key: USRDA = Recommended Dietary Allowance
     IU = International Unit
     mg = milligrams
     µg = micrograms
NOTE: The numbers with arrows exceed 100 percent of required USRDA.

Green and Yellow Vibrancy

Ingredients:

2 cups kale
2 cups yellow turnips, peeled and sliced
1 tsp vegetable oil
4 cloves garlic, minced
1 cup onions, chopped
½ cup green peppers, diced
½ cup low-sodium chicken or vegetable broth
1 tsp allspice
½ tsp chervil
black pepper

Preparation: Sauté and boil
Time: 45 minutes
Calories: 96 per serving
Serves: 4

Directions

Bring a pot of water to boil, add turnips, turn down heat, and let simmer for about 20 minutes. Sauté garlic in oil; add onions, broth, and allspice; and bring to a boil. Add kale, lower heat, and cook for about 7 minutes, covered. After 5 minutes add the green pepper and turnips. Remove kale from pan and cut it into coarse pieces. Add chervil and black pepper. Vitamin C, vitamin A, and potassium are very high.

TIP: Of the more than 100 types of arthritis recorded, only gout has a definite connection to diet. Foods high in purines can cause problems and aggravate arthritis. Purines are found in anchovies, organ meat, and mushrooms, among others says Dr. Richard S. Panush, professor and chairman of the Department of Medicine at St. Barnabas Medical Center in New Jersey.

MYTH: Eggs microwaved with their shells on are not as dangerous as those microwaved without them.

FACT: Egg distributors report that with their shells on eggs can present some danger of exploding. The suggestion is to remove eggs from their shells before microwaving and pierce the yolks.

Nutrients Contained in: Green and Yellow Vibrancy

VITAMINS USRDA			ONE SERVING GIVES YOU APPROXIMATELY		APPROXIMATE PERCENTAGE OF USRDA
A	5,000	IU	3,021	IU	60
B₁	1.4	mg	0.11	mg	9
B₂	1.6	mg	0.08	mg	5
B₃	16	mg	1	mg	7
B₅	10	mg	0.22	mg	2
B₆	2.2	mg	0.24	mg	10
B₁₂	3	μg	0.04	μg	1
C	60	mg	77	mg	128◄
D	400	IU	0	IU	0
E	15	IU	5	IU	31
K	500	μg	0	μg	0
Folic Acid	400	μg	30	μg	7

MINERALS USRDA			ONE SERVING GIVES YOU APPROXIMATELY		APPROXIMATE PERCENTAGE OF USRDA
Sodium	(1,100–3,000)	mg	158	mg	15
Calcium	1,000	mg	77	mg	9
Phosphorus	(800–1,000)	mg	57	mg	7
Potassium	(1,875–5,625)	mg	402	mg	50
Magnesium	400	μg	26	μg	7
Selenium	200	μg	1	μg	0
Iodine	150	mg	0	mg	0
Zinc	15	mg	0.31	mg	2
Iron	10	mg	1	mg	11
Manganese	(2.5–5.0)	mg	0.33	mg	6
Copper	(2.0–3.0)	mg	0.13	mg	4

AMOUNT PER SERVING		CALORIES PER SERVING	% OF MEAL
Fat	4 grams	36	37
Proteins	3 grams	12	13
Carbohydrates	12 grams	48	50
Cholesterol	0 mg		
Amino acid (essential)			20–30*
Fiber	1 gram		

Key: USRDA = Recommended Dietary Allowance

IU = International Unit

mg = milligrams

μg = micrograms

NOTE: The numbers with arrows exceed 100 percent of required USRDA.

*Complementary food–1 cup wheat germ raises EAA to 352–598%.

Corn the Great

Ingredients:

- 1 cup corn
- 1 red pepper, seeded and sliced into strips
- 1 cup scallion, chopped
- 1 cup frozen peas, thawed
- 1 cup black fungus mushrooms
- 1 tsp Italian parsley
- 2 tsp lime juice
- $\frac{1}{2}$ tsp chervil
- 1 tsp chili powder
- black pepper
- $\frac{1}{4}$ cup water

Preparation: Simmer

Time: 30 minutes

Calories: 249 calories per serving

Serves: 4

Directions

Stir together corn, red pepper, scallions, and peas in a nonstick pan and add water. Cover and simmer over low heat until green pepper and peas are tender but not mushy, about 15 minutes or so. Soak mushrooms in water for about 15 minutes. Stir in mushrooms, chervil, chili powder, and pepper and simmer for a few minutes. Sprinkle lime juice and parsley over preparation.

TIP: A report of a study in the British medical publication *The Lancet* said that in the last 13 years three studies have shown that fasting produces objective improvement in symptoms for people with rheumatoid arthritis. The downside is the pain, stiffness, tenderness, and swelling returns once fasting ends, say University of Oslo researchers.

MYTH: Fasting will shrink your stomach.

FACT: Health researchers report there is no evidence to support this idea.

Nutrients Contained in: Corn the Great

VITAMINS USRDA			ONE SERVING GIVES YOU APPROXIMATELY		APPROXIMATE PERCENTAGE OF USRDA
A	5,000	IU	1,592	IU	31
B1	1.4	mg	0.13	mg	10
B2	1.6	mg	0.17	mg	12
B3	16	mg	4	mg	23
B5	10	mg	0.10	mg	1
B6	2.2	mg	0.18	mg	8
B12	3	μg	0	μg	0
C	60	mg	40	mg	67
D	400	IU	0	IU	0
E	15	IU	6	IU	39
K	500	μg	110	μg	22
Folic Acid	400	μg	87	μg	21

MINERALS USRDA			ONE SERVING GIVES YOU APPROXIMATELY		APPROXIMATE PERCENTAGE OF USRDA
Sodium	(1,100–3,000)	mg	186	mg	18
Calcium	1,000	mg	56	mg	6
Phosphorus	(800–1,000)	mg	58	mg	7
Potassium	(1,875–5,625)	mg	464	mg	57
Magnesium	400	μg	54	μg	15
Selenium	200	μg	0.25	μg	0
Iodine	150	mg	0	mg	0
Zinc	15	mg	3	mg	18
Iron	10	mg	2	mg	15
Manganese	(2.5–5.0)	mg	0.23	mg	4
Copper	(2.0–3.0)	mg	0.10	mg	3

AMOUNT PER SERVING		CALORIES PER SERVING	% OF MEAL
Fat	7 grams	67	27
Proteins	6 grams	24	10
Carbohydrates	39 grams	158	63
Cholesterol	0 mg		
Amino acid (essential)			23-35*
Fiber	3 grams		

Key: USRDA = Recommended Dietary Allowance
     IU = International Unit
    mg = milligrams
    μg = micrograms
NOTE: The numbers with arrows exceed 100 percent of required USRDA.

*Complementary food—1 oz Gouda cheese raises EAA to 121-457%.

Baked Winter Comfort

Ingredients:

1 large winter squash, peeled and cut into cubes
1 tsp allspice
¼ cup honey
¼ tsp cinnamon
1 tsp margarine
2 tsp fresh lime juice
dash paprika and cayenne

Preparation: Bake

Time: 60 minutes

Calories: 178 per serving

Serves: 4

Directions

Preheat oven to 375° F. Put squash cubes in a baking dish and sprinkle with cinnamon, honey, and spices. Sprinkle margarine and lime juice on top and bake for about 40 minutes or until tender.

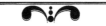

TIP: Because ancient South American Indians ate corn exclusively and their bones show no evidence of rheumatic arthritis, some modern researchers feel that arthritis sufferers might benefit from eating rice, oatmeal, and corn bread as an alternative to wheat bread.

MYTH: Eating some specific food or nutrient will give you a healthy, beautiful skin.

FACT: There is no evidence that any one nutrient or food will give you beautiful skin. The best approach with food is to have a balanced diet according to nutritionists.

Nutrients Contained in: Baked Winter Comfort

VITAMINS USRDA			ONE SERVING GIVES YOU APPROXIMATELY		APPROXIMATE PERCENTAGE OF USRDA
A	5,000	IU	3,806	IU	76
B₁	1.4	mg	0.14	mg	11
B₂	1.6	mg	0.07	mg	5
B₃	16	mg	0.93	mg	5
B₅	10	mg	0.69	mg	6
B₆	2.2	mg	0.21	mg	9
B₁₂	3	µg	0	µg	0
C	60	mg	20	mg	33
D	400	IU	0	IU	0
E	15	IU	0.68	IU	4
K	500	µg	2	µg	0
Folic Acid	400	µg	54	µg	13

MINERALS USRDA			ONE SERVING GIVES YOU APPROXIMATELY		APPROXIMATE PERCENTAGE OF USRDA
Sodium	(1,100–3,000)	mg	6	mg	0
Calcium	1,000	mg	33	mg	4
Phosphorus	(800–1,000)	mg	46	mg	5
Potassium	(1,875–5,625)	mg	687	mg	85
Magnesium	400	µg	23	µg	6
Selenium	200	µg	0.80	µg	0
Iodine	150	mg	0	mg	0
Zinc	15	mg	0.46	mg	3
Iron	10	mg	0.94	mg	9
Manganese	(2.5–5.0)	mg	0.33	mg	6
Copper	(2.0–3.0)	mg	0.19	mg	6

AMOUNT PER SERVING		CALORIES PER SERVING	% OF MEAL
Fat	5 grams	42	23
Proteins	2 grams	8	5
Carbohydrates	32 grams	128	72
Cholesterol	0 mg		
Amino acid (essential)			19–28*
Fiber	2 grams		

Key: USRDA = Recommended Dietary Allowance
    IU = International Unit
    mg = milligrams
    µg = micrograms
NOTE: The numbers with arrows exceed 100 percent of required USRDA.

*Complementary food—1 cup buttermilk raises EAA to 120–172%.

Peachy Sweet Potatoes

Ingredients:

4	sweet potatoes
1	tsp margarine
2	Tbs syrup
½	cup water
1	cup peach nectar
	dash of white pepper

Preparation: Bake

Time: 60 minutes

Calories: 280 per serving

Serves: 4

Directions

Preheat oven to 400° F. Slice sweet potatoes in half and place in baking pan. Mix all remaining ingredients and pour over the potatoes. Bake for about 35 to 40 minutes. The chart shows that you will exceed USRDA percentages for vitamin A and that you will do pretty well with fiber and potassium.

TIP: Word from scientists at the Albany Medical College in Albany, New York, is that reducing saturated fats in the diet can reduce arthritic pain. They found that saturated fats from meat and dairy products promote morning stiffness, joint pain, swelling, and tenderness. Fatty acids, however, found in fish and polyunsaturated oils relieve pain by suppressing the production of pain-promoting prostaglandin according to the researchers.

MYTH: Honey is better for your health than sugar.

FACT: According to the American Dietetic Association, honey has a few B vitamins and trace minerals, but to derive any benefits from it, you would have to eat a whole jar of honey. Table sugar has no B vitamins and trace minerals.

Nutrients Contained in: Peachy Sweet Potatoes

VITAMINS USRDA			ONE SERVING GIVES YOU APPROXIMATELY		APPROXIMATE PERCENTAGE OF USRDA
A	5,000	IU	13,007	IU	260◄
B$_1$	1.4	mg	0.11	mg	9
B$_2$	1.6	mg	0.18	mg	12
B$_3$	16	mg	0.83	mg	5
B$_5$	10	mg	2	mg	22
B$_6$	2.2	mg	0.37	mg	16
B$_{12}$	3	μg	0	μg	0
C	60	mg	30	mg	50
D	400	IU	0	IU	0
E	15	IU	6	IU	39
K	500	μg	2	μg	0
Folic Acid	400	μg	41	μg	10

MINERALS USRDA			ONE SERVING GIVES YOU APPROXIMATELY		APPROXIMATE PERCENTAGE OF USRDA
Sodium	(1,100–3,000)	mg	17	mg	1
Calcium	1,000	mg	54	mg	6
Phosphorus	(800–1,000)	mg	87	mg	10
Potassium	(1,875–5,625)	mg	596	mg	74
Magnesium	400	μg	36	μg	10
Selenium	200	μg	0.65	μg	0
Iodine	150	mg	0	mg	0
Zinc	15	mg	0.43	mg	2
Iron	10	mg	0.98	mg	9
Manganese	(2.5–5.0)	mg	1	mg	21
Copper	(2.0–3.0)	mg	0.51	mg	16

AMOUNT PER SERVING		CALORIES PER SERVING	% OF MEAL
Fat	4 grams	36	13
Proteins	21 grams	82	29
Carbohydrates	40 grams	162	58
Cholesterol	0 mg		
Amino acid (essential)			65–89
Fiber	4 grams		

Key: USRDA = Recommended Dietary Allowance
     IU = International Unit
     mg = milligrams
     μg = micrograms

NOTE: The numbers with arrows exceed 100 percent of required USRDA.

Little Sprouts

Ingredients:

- 1 cup cauliflower, cut into pieces
- 2 cups mung bean sprouts
- 1 cup zucchini, sliced
- 1 tsp vegetable oil
- 3 stalks celery, sliced
- 1 onion, chopped
- 8 shiitake mushrooms, fresh
- 1 tsp chervil
- black pepper
- 1 tsp Adobo (Goya product) seasoning

Preparation: Sauté

Time: 20 minutes

Calories: 180 per serving

Serves: 4

Directions

Sauté bean sprouts in vegetable oil until tender, about 5 minutes. Add cauliflower, zucchini, celery, onion, mushrooms, and spices. Heat through and serve. If desired, sprinkle lemon juice over servings for taste. Check your chart for large vitamin K and potassium percentages.

TIP: While some foods are good, some are particularly negative for arthritis sufferers. Items such as cake and other foods that are made from wheat flour, which contains the protein gluten, and are high in sugar, cholesterol, and fat, could be a big mistake if eaten. Dr. Raympiid Shatin of the Alfred Hospital in Melbourne, Florida, says that areas of the planet where gluten-high cereals are eaten correspond to areas where rheumatoid arthritis is most found.

MYTH: Canola oil is unsafe because it contains erucic acid, thought to be harmful to the liver and heart.

FACT: Researchers at the University of California at Berkeley *Wellness Letter* report that canola oil is safe and a good choice for salads and cooking and is widely used in the United States and Canada.

Nutrients Contained in: Little Sprouts

VITAMINS USRDA			ONE SERVING GIVES YOU APPROXIMATELY		APPROXIMATE PERCENTAGE OF USRDA
A	5,000	IU	161	IU	3
B$_1$	1.4	mg	0.12	mg	9
B$_2$	1.6	mg	0.14	mg	9
B$_3$	16	mg	3	mg	20
B$_5$	10	mg	0.40	mg	4
B$_6$	2.2	mg	0.24	mg	10
B$_{12}$	3	μg	0	μg	0
C	60	mg	32	mg	53
D	400	IU	0	IU	0
E	15	IU	2	IU	11
K	500	μg	900	μg	180◀
Folic Acid	400	μg	97	μg	24

MINERALS USRDA			ONE SERVING GIVES YOU APPROXIMATELY		APPROXIMATE PERCENTAGE OF USRDA
Sodium	(1,100–3,000)	mg	298	mg	29
Calcium	1,000	mg	45	mg	5
Phosphorus	(800–1,000)	mg	86	mg	10
Potassium	(1,875–5,625)	mg	614	mg	76
Magnesium	400	μg	54	μg	15
Selenium	200	μg	1	μg	0
Iodine	150	mg	0	mg	0
Zinc	15	mg	2	mg	16
Iron	10	mg	1	mg	12
Manganese	(2.5–5.0)	mg	0.32	mg	6
Copper	(2.0–3.0)	mg	0.16	mg	5

AMOUNT PER SERVING		CALORIES PER SERVING	% OF MEAL
Fat	4 grams	34	19
Proteins	6 grams	22	12
Carbohydrates	31 grams	124	69
Cholesterol	0 mg		
Amino acid (essential)			28-40*
Fiber	1 gram		

Key: USRDA = Recommended Dietary Allowance

IU = International Unit

mg = milligrams

μg = micrograms

NOTE: The numbers with arrows exceed 100 percent of required USRDA.

*Complementary food—1 cup peas raises EAA to 103–138%.

Bow Ties and Black Hats

Ingredients:

8	ounces bow ties pasta
¼	cup scallions, chopped
2	cloves garlic
12	shiitake mushrooms
5	tomatoes
¼	lemon, juiced
½	tsp chervil
1	Tbs canola oil
2	Tbs Parmesan cheese
½	tsp marjoram
½	tsp chili powder
	black pepper

Preparation: Boil

Time: 30 minutes

Calories: 277 per serving

Serves: 4

Directions

Cut tomatoes into small chunks and put tomatoes, scallions, lemon juice, half of the oil, and seasonings into a blender. Blend all ingredients until a thick sauce develops. Set aside for about 1 hour, longer if you want a stronger flavor. Cook bow ties according to package instructions, al dente. Sprinkle on cheese and add sauce.

TIP: According to the Department of Health, Education and Welfare, the cause of arthritis is not exactly known, and there are no 100 percent-certain cures or methods of prevention. Diet, however, they say is believed by many to be a part of the cause of this disorder, as well as a key to its relief.

MYTH: You should not be concerned about the lead used in printed designs and writing on plastic bags used to wrap breads sold at supermarkets.

FACT: Maybe you should be. Based on a study at the Environmental and Occupational Health Sciences Institute in Piscataway, New Jersey, it found that lead can flake off onto food if you turn the bags inside out and reuse them to store food or pack lunches for children.

Nutrients Contained in: Bow Ties and Black Hats

VITAMINS USRDA			ONE SERVING GIVES YOU APPROXIMATELY		APPROXIMATE PERCENTAGE OF USRDA
A	5,000	IU	2,077	IU	41
B$_1$	1.4	mg	0.17	mg	14
B$_2$	1.6	mg	0.17	mg	11
B$_3$	16	mg	5	mg	29
B$_5$	10	mg	0.43	mg	4
B$_6$	2.2	mg	0.12	mg	5
B$_{12}$	3	μg	0	μg	0
C	60	mg	38	mg	62
D	400	IU	0	IU	0
E	15	IU	2	IU	16
K	500	μg	13	μg	2
Folic Acid	400	μg	62	μg	15

MINERALS USRDA			ONE SERVING GIVES YOU APPROXIMATELY		APPROXIMATE PERCENTAGE OF USRDA
Sodium	(1,100–3,000)	mg	69	mg	6
Calcium	1,000	mg	63	mg	7
Phosphorus	(800–1,000)	mg	87	mg	10
Potassium	(1,875–5,625)	mg	648	mg	80
Magnesium	400	μg	65	μg	18
Selenium	200	μg	14	μg	6
Iodine	150	mg	0	mg	0
Zinc	15	mg	3	mg	21
Iron	10	mg	1	mg	14
Manganese	(2.5–5.0)	mg	0.19	mg	3
Copper	(2.0–3.0)	mg	0.14	mg	4

AMOUNT PER SERVING		CALORIES PER SERVING	% OF MEAL
Fat	5 grams	43	15
Proteins	8 grams	31	11
Carbohydrates	51 grams	203	73
Cholesterol	2 mg		
Amino acid (essential)			42–52*
Fiber	1 gram		

Key: USRDA = Recommended Dietary Allowance

  IU = International Unit

  mg = milligrams

  μg = micrograms

NOTE: The numbers with arrows exceed 100 percent of required USRDA.

*Complementary food—1 ounce pine nuts raises EAA to 107–154%.

A Touch of Walnuts

Ingredients:

1 lb Brussels sprouts
1 cup low-sodium
   chicken or clear broth
2 tsp lime juice
1 tsp basil
1 cup black fungus
   mushrooms, sliced
1 tsp basil
1 Tbs horseradish
1 cup summer squash,
   sliced
¼ cup walnuts, chopped
1 tsp Adobo (Goya
   product) seasoning
dash of cayenne pepper

Preparation: Steam and boil

Time: 30 minutes

Calories: 132 per serving

Serves: 4

Directions

After cutting brussels sprouts in half, steam them until tender, about 8 minutes or so. Use a large pan and bring the broth to a boil. Reduce heat to medium and stir in lime juice, basil, and horseradish. Add the mushrooms and squash and boil until the squash is done and broth is reduced, about 5 minutes. Add the brussels sprouts. High percentages of vitamin C, vitamin K, and potassium are shown on the chart.

TIP: The advice from Dr. Barbara Klein of the University of Illinois is that the most nutritious methods for cooking frozen vegetables are microwaving and boiling. Steaming doesn't enhance the taste of frozen vegetables. To boil, use just enough water to prevent scorching. Bring the water to a boil before you add the vegetables. Then cover the pot, return to a boil, and reduce the heat. Bet you knew that already.

MYTH: Copper bracelets, mussel extracts, and snake venom are remedies for arthritis sufferers.

FACT: According to the Food and Drug Administration, remedies such as those mentioned above are among the top 10 unproven health frauds in the United States.

Nutrients Contained in: A Touch of Walnuts

VITAMINS USRDA			ONE SERVING GIVES YOU APPROXIMATELY		APPROXIMATE PERCENTAGE OF USRDA
A	5,000	IU	975	IU	19
B_1	1.4	mg	0.21	mg	17
B_2	1.6	mg	0.25	mg	17
B_3	16	mg	4	mg	22
B_5	10	mg	1	mg	12
B_6	2.2	mg	0.34	mg	15
B_{12}	3	μg	0.08	μg	2
C	60	mg	93	mg	154◀
D	400	IU	0	IU	0
E	15	IU	2	IU	10
K	500	μg	754	μg	150◀
Folic Acid	400	μg	77	μg	19

MINERALS USRDA			ONE SERVING GIVES YOU APPROXIMATELY		APPROXIMATE PERCENTAGE OF USRDA
Sodium	(1,100–3,000)	mg	221	mg	22
Calcium	1,000	mg	66	mg	8
Phosphorus	(800–1,000)	mg	142	mg	17
Potassium	(1,875–5,625)	mg	696	mg	86
Magnesium	400	μg	52	μg	14
Selenium	200	μg	57	μg	28
Iodine	150	mg	0	mg	0
Zinc	15	mg	1	mg	7
Iron	10	mg	3	mg	25
Manganese	(2.5–5.0)	mg	0.57	mg	11
Copper	(2.0–3.0)	mg	0.40	mg	13

AMOUNT PER SERVING		CALORIES PER SERVING	% OF MEAL
Fat	5 grams	45	35
Proteins	7 grams	27	20
Carbohydrates	15 grams	60	45
Cholesterol	0 mg		
Amino acid (essential)			37–77*
Fiber	2 grams		

Key: USRDA = Recommended Dietary Allowance
    IU = International Unit
    mg = milligrams
    μg = micrograms
NOTE: The numbers with arrows exceed 100 percent of required USRDA.

*Complementary food—one head of endive raises EAA to 104–162%.

Cabbage and Wild Friends

Ingredients:

½ cup wild rice
4 cups cabbage
12 shiitake mushrooms, sliced
4 cloves garlic, chopped
1 Tbs olive oil
1 cup low-sodium chicken broth
1 onion, diced
1 cup corn
¼ cup sesame seed
2 tomatoes, diced
black pepper

Preparation: Sauté, boil

Time: 55 minutes

Calories: 297 per serving

Serves: 6

Directions

Cook rice according to package instructions. Once done, set aside. Sauté mushroom and garlic in ½ tsp of the oil in a large iron skillet until mushrooms are tender. Add a little broth or water if more moisture is needed. Add the broth and corn and heat. In another pan, sauté onion in remaining oil for a few minutes. Add the onions, cabbage, sesame seeds, and black pepper to the mushrooms. Sauté for 5 minutes. Add the tomatoes and simmer for 10 minutes. Place rice and cabbage mixture on a large serving plate. This meal is high in potassium, vitamin C, and folic acid.

TIP: Dr. David T. Felson of Boston University says that people with arthritis should avoid being overweight. He says keeping weight down can be especially helpful if there's a family history of arthritis and if you are in the early stages of arthritis. He adds that one should get more calcium from dairy products, sardines, and leafy green vegetables and avoid alcohol.

MYTH: Taking an annual flu shot will give you a case of the flu.

FACT: The National Institutes of Health report that studies do not support this concern. People over age 65 should not be hesitant about getting flu shots.

Nutrients Contained in:
Cabbage and Wild Friends

VITAMINS USRDA			ONE SERVING GIVES YOU APPROXIMATELY		APPROXIMATE PERCENTAGE OF USRDA
A	5,000	IU	695	IU	13
B$_1$	1.4	mg	0.26	mg	21
B$_2$	1.6	mg	0.13	mg	9
B$_3$	16	mg	5	mg	31
B$_5$	10	mg	0.85	mg	8
B$_6$	2.2	mg	0.31	mg	13
B$_{12}$	3	μg	0.05	μg	1
C	60	mg	66	mg	109◄
D	400	IU	0	IU	0
E	15	IU	2	IU	14
K	500	μg	54	μg	10
Folic Acid	400	μg	122	μg	30

MINERALS USRDA			ONE SERVING GIVES YOU APPROXIMATELY		APPROXIMATE PERCENTAGE OF USRDA
Sodium	(1,100–3,000)	mg	171	mg	17
Calcium	1,000	mg	82	mg	10
Phosphorus	(800–1,000)	mg	160	mg	20
Potassium	(1,875–5,625)	mg	777	mg	97
Magnesium	400	μg	83	μg	23
Selenium	200	μg	9	μg	4
Iodine	150	mg	0	mg	0
Zinc	15	mg	3	mg	23
Iron	10	mg	2	mg	17
Manganese	(2.5–5.0)	mg	0.61	mg	12
Copper	(2.0–3.0)	mg	0.23	mg	7

AMOUNT PER SERVING		CALORIES PER SERVING	% OF MEAL
Fat	5 grams	43	14
Proteins	9 grams	35	12
Carbohydrates	55 grams	219	74
Cholesterol	0 mg		
Amino acid (essential)			57–85
Fiber	2 grams		

Key: USRDA = Recommended Dietary Allowance
     IU = International Unit
     mg = milligrams
     μg = micrograms
NOTE: The numbers with arrows exceed 100 percent of required USRDA.

Salmon Potassium King

Ingredients: 1 ½ lb salmon steaks
3 Tbs Dijon mustard
1 8-oz. can tomatoes
4 Tbs finely chopped shallots
1 green pepper, diced
1 tsp dill weed
1 tsp paprika
½ tsp chili powder
2 cloves garlic, minced
dash cayenne pepper

Preparation: Bake

Time: 40 minutes

Calories: 329 per serving

Serves: 4

Directions

Preheat oven to 450° F. Prepare salmon by sprinkling garlic on the salmon surface, season with pepper and mustard. Place in a baking dish. Mix the tomatoes, shallots, green pepper, and seasonings, pour over salmon and bake in oven for half hour or less; check every 10 minutes to see if salmon is flaky. Look at chart for the high percentage of vitamins B_3, B_{12}, and D, calcium, phosphorus, and potassium, quite a nutritional bonanza.

TIP: Dr. Arthur I. Grayzel, senior vice president of medical affairs for the Arthritis Foundation, and other researchers say eating oily fish three to five times a week is safer than taking fish oil capsules. Best fish for omega-3 intake are salmon, tuna, halibut, and sardines. Pure fish oil contains lots of vitamins A and D, which can be toxic in high doses.

MYTH: You are better off sweetening your foods when called for with fruit juice rather than sugar.

FACT: The American Dietetic Association says there's no nutritional advantage in using fruit juice. Sugar is sugar, regardless of its source.

Nutrients Contained in: Salmon Potassium King

VITAMINS USRDA			ONE SERVING GIVES YOU APPROXIMATELY		APPROXIMATE PERCENTAGE OF USRDA
A	5,000	IU	843	IU	16
B_1	1.4	mg	0.33	mg	27
B_2	1.6	mg	0.14	mg	9
B_3	16	mg	18	mg	110◄
B_5	10	mg	2	mg	22
B_6	2.2	mg	1	mg	58
B_{12}	3	μg	7	μg	233◄
C	60	mg	48	mg	79
D	400	IU	1,138	IU	284◄
E	15	IU	4	IU	26
K	500	μg	0	μg	0
Folic Acid	400	μg	48	μg	12

MINERALS USRDA			ONE SERVING GIVES YOU APPROXIMATELY		APPROXIMATE PERCENTAGE OF USRDA
Sodium	(1,100–3,000)	mg	315	mg	31
Calcium	1,000	mg	746	mg	93
Phosphorus	(800–1,000)	mg	342	mg	42
Potassium	(1,875–5,625)	mg	959	mg	119◄
Magnesium	400	μg	62	μg	17
Selenium	200	μg	0.18	μg	0
Iodine	150	mg	0	mg	0
Zinc	15	mg	2	mg	21
Iron	10	mg	3	mg	27
Manganese	(2.5–5.0)	mg	0.02	mg	0
Copper	(2.0–3.0)	mg	0.37	mg	12

AMOUNT PER SERVING		CALORIES PER SERVING	% OF MEAL
Fat	13 grams	119	36
Proteins	48 grams	193	59
Carbohydrates	4 grams	17	5
Cholesterol	82 mg		
Amino acid (essential)			279–935
Fiber	5 grams		

Key: USRDA = Recommended Dietary Allowance
IU = International Unit
mg = milligrams
μg = micrograms
NOTE: The numbers with arrows exceed 100 percent of required USRDA.

Easy Sardines

Ingredients:
2 cans sardines
3 Tbs prepared mustard
1 Tbs horseradish
¼ cup wheat germ
juice of one lime

Preparation: Broil

Time: 10 minutes

Calories: 153 per serving

Serves: 4

Directions

Preheat broiler. Mix the oil from the two cans of sardines with the mustard and horseradish. Place this mixture on top of the sardines and roll them in the wheat germ. Place under broiler until they brown. Sprinkle lime juice on each and serve. Exceeds the USRDA for vitamin B_{12} and rather high percentages of magnesium and vitamin D.

TIP: Researchers at Harvard Medical School and in Australia report that fish oil, a polyunsaturated fat, might help reduce inflammation because it contains omega-3 fatty acids instead of omega-6, which is found in other polyunsaturated fats. The body turns omega-6 fatty acids into inflammatory chemicals, whereas the effects of omega-3 fatty acids are much less inflammatory.

MYTH: In order to keep warm in the cold, one should take hot drinks.

FACT: The U.S. Army Research Institute of Environmental Medicine at Natick, Massachusetts, says hot liquids can dilate blood vessels in the skin and this may make you feel warmer, but actually causes a small amount of heat loss. According to their research the important idea is to keep your fluid intake up when you're out in the cold with hot or cold fluids, but don't expect to raise body temperature.

Nutrients Contained in: Easy Sardines

VITAMINS USRDA			ONE SERVING GIVES YOU APPROXIMATELY		APPROXIMATE PERCENTAGE OF USRDA
A	5,000	IU	147	IU	2
B₁	1.4	mg	0.28	mg	23
B₂	1.6	mg	0.22	mg	15
B₃	16	mg	3	mg	19
B₅	10	mg	0.23	mg	2
B₆	2.2	mg	0.21	mg	9
B₁₂	3	μg	4	μg	126◄
C	60	mg	6	mg	9
D	400	IU	128	IU	31
E	15	IU	0.15	IU	1
K	500	μg	0	μg	0
Folic Acid	400	μg	56	μg	14

MINERALS USRDA			ONE SERVING GIVES YOU APPROXIMATELY		APPROXIMATE PERCENTAGE OF USRDA
Sodium	(1,100–3,000)	mg	219	mg	21
Calcium	1,000	mg	176	mg	22
Phosphorus	(800–1,000)	mg	166	mg	20
Potassium	(1,875–5,625)	mg	330	mg	41
Magnesium	400	μg	63	μg	18
Selenium	200	μg	0	μg	0
Iodine	150	mg	0	mg	0
Zinc	15	mg	3	mg	19
Iron	10	mg	3	mg	26
Manganese	(2.5–5.0)	mg	3	mg	56
Copper	(2.0–3.0)	mg	0.10	mg	3

AMOUNT PER SERVING		CALORIES PER SERVING	% OF MEAL
Fat	6 grams	57	38
Proteins	15 grams	59	39
Carbohydrates	9 grams	37	24
Cholesterol	61 mg		
Amino acid (essential)			44–72
Fiber	0 grams		

Key: USRDA = Recommended Dietary Allowance
     IU = International Unit
     mg = milligrams
     μg = micrograms
NOTE: The numbers with arrows exceed 100 percent of required USRDA.

Blues Are Not Bad

Ingredients:

2 lb bluefish, boned and scaled
1 tsp garlic salt
$\frac{1}{2}$ tsp black pepper
1 tsp margarine
1 onion, sliced
dash of cayenne pepper
juice of one lemon
$\frac{1}{2}$ cup low-sodium chicken broth
4 Tbs horseradish
2 egg whites
1 cup half and half cream

Preparation: Bake

Time: 45 minutes

Calories: 413 per serving

Serves: 5

Directions

Preheat oven to 450° F. Season fish inside and out with pepper and a little salt. Place fish into a baking dish with the chicken broth. Cover with onion slices and bake in oven for about 20 minutes or less, depending on thickness of the fish. While fish is baking, mix together the horseradish, salt, and pepper. Beat egg whites until stiff; then beat half and half cream (or heavy cream if thicker mix is desired) until stiff and blend the two. Add the horseradish mixture and the lemon juice. Mix and chill. Pour over fish when ready to serve. Chart shows a very high vitamin B_{12} percentage.

TIP: Dr. Joel Kremer, professor of medicine at Albany Medical College, New York, has made numerous studies on the effects of fish oil. In his fourth study, he compared two different doses of fish oil to olive oil in 49 people with rheumatoid arthritis. He found signs of inflammation pain, morning stiffness, and fatigue improved much more in those who received the omega-3 fatty acid from fish oil than in those who received olive oil.

MYTH: A prenatal multivitamin/mineral supplement is a necessary routine for all pregnant women.

FACT: Medical experts have different opinions about prenatal nutrition, especially concerning the kinds of supplements a pregnant woman should take. The American College of Obstetricians and Gynecologists advises at least 400 micrograms of supplemental folic acid a day for most pregnant women. The consensus seems to be that prenatal vitamin/mineral supplements are unnecessary if a woman eats a well-balanced diet.

Nutrients Contained in: Blues Are Not Bad

VITAMINS USRDA			ONE SERVING GIVES YOU APPROXIMATELY		APPROXIMATE PERCENTAGE OF USRDA
A	5,000	IU	511	IU	10
B$_1$	1.4	mg	0.21	mg	17
B$_2$	1.6	mg	0.36	mg	26
B$_3$	16	mg	6	mg	34
B$_5$	10	mg	0.39	mg	3
B$_6$	2.2	mg	0.53	mg	24
B$_{12}$	3	µg	7	µg	230◄
C	60	mg	20	mg	33
D	400	IU	5	IU	1
E	15	IU	0.42	IU	2
K	500	µg	0	µg	0
Folic Acid	400	µg	49	µg	12

MINERALS USRDA			ONE SERVING GIVES YOU APPROXIMATELY		APPROXIMATE PERCENTAGE OF USRDA
Sodium	(1,100–3,000)	mg	336	mg	33
Calcium	1,000	mg	133	mg	16
Phosphorus	(800–1,000)	mg	81	mg	10
Potassium	(1,875–5,625)	mg	211	mg	26
Magnesium	400	µg	91	µg	26
Selenium	200	µg	4	µg	1
Iodine	150	mg	0	mg	0
Zinc	15	mg	2	mg	13
Iron	10	mg	2	mg	18
Manganese	(2.5–5.0)	mg	0.05	mg	0
Copper	(2.0–3.0)	mg	0.05	mg	1

AMOUNT PER SERVING		CALORIES PER SERVING	% OF MEAL
Fat	19 grams	170	41
Proteins	53 grams	210	51
Carbohydrates	8 grams	33	8
Cholesterol	225 mg		
Amino acid (essential)			Very high
Fiber	0 grams		

Key: USRDA = Recommended Dietary Allowance
     IU = International Unit
    mg = milligrams
    µg = micrograms
NOTE: The numbers with arrows exceed 100 percent of required USRDA.

Mackerel and Mushrooms

Ingredients:

2 lb king mackerel, dressed
1 tsp margarine
2 cloves garlic, crushed
12 shiitake mushrooms (fresh if available)
1 tsp chili powder
2 tsp lemon juice
   chopped fresh parsley
1 tsp pepper
   noncaloric spray

Preparation: Broil and sauté

Time: 20 minutes

Calories: 444 per serving

Serves: 4

Directions

Preheat broiler. Broil the mackerel in a large skillet with noncaloric spray. Broil about 3 to 4 minutes on each side. Set aside on a platter. Using the same skillet, heat the margarine and add the garlic, chili powder, mushrooms, and lemon juice; sauté for about 3 minutes. Pour this mixture over the mackerel and sprinkle with chopped fresh parsley. Check your chart to see the tremendous percentages of B_{12}, vitamin D, and potassium.

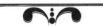

TIP: The National Fisheries Institute says when baking fish, cook it at 450° F allowing about 10 minutes for every inch of thickness. The important point to note is that the fish should not be heated at 325 to 350° F for 30 minutes or more.

MYTH: The way to avoid a hangover is to take an aspirin before you drink.

FACT: From information published in the *Journal of the American Medical Association*, men who took two aspirin an hour before drinking ended up with blood alcohol concentration 30 percent higher than when they didn't take aspirin before drinking. The best remedy is to drink in moderation.

Nutrients Contained in: Mackerel and Mushrooms

VITAMINS USRDA			ONE SERVING GIVES YOU APPROXIMATELY		APPROXIMATE PERCENTAGE OF USRDA
A	5,000	IU	611	IU	12
B$_1$	1.4	mg	0.18	mg	15
B$_2$	1.6	mg	0.54	mg	38
B$_3$	16	mg	11	mg	66
B$_5$	10	mg	0.04	mg	0
B$_6$	2.2	mg	0.55	mg	24
B$_{12}$	3	μg	20	μg	666◄
C	60	mg	15	mg	24
D	400	IU	744	IU	185◄
E	15	IU	4	IU	24
K	500	μg	0	μg	0
Folic Acid	400	μg	64	μg	16

MINERALS USRDA			ONE SERVING GIVES YOU APPROXIMATELY		APPROXIMATE PERCENTAGE OF USRDA
Sodium	(1,100–3,000)	mg	100	mg	9
Calcium	1,000	mg	34	mg	4
Phosphorus	(800–1,000)	mg	5	mg	0
Potassium	(1,875–5,625)	mg	729	mg	91
Magnesium	400	μg	142	μg	40
Selenium	200	μg	3	μg	1
Iodine	150	mg	0	mg	0
Zinc	15	mg	4	mg	26
Iron	10	mg	2	mg	20
Manganese	(2.5–5.0)	mg	0.04	mg	0
Copper	(2.0–3.0)	mg	0.02	mg	0

AMOUNT PER SERVING		CALORIES PER SERVING	% OF MEAL
Fat	22 grams	200	45
Proteins	29 grams	114	26
Carbohydrates	33 grams	130	29
Cholesterol	80 mg		
Amino acid (essential)			High level
Fiber	0 grams		

Key: USRDA = Recommended Dietary Allowance
　　　IU = International Unit
　　　mg = milligrams
　　　μg = micrograms
NOTE: The numbers with arrows exceed 100 percent of required USRDA.

CHAPTER EIGHT

Healing and Preventive Recipes for Gallbladder

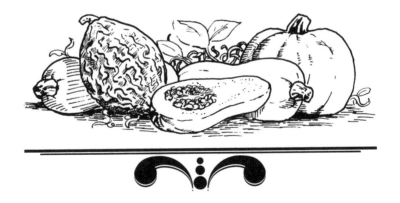

The less people know about how sausages and laws
are made, the better they'll sleep at night.
—Bismarck

Gallstones are the most common reason gallbladders become inflamed. And doctors say that gallstones form when there's too much cholesterol and too little bile acid. This concentrated cholesterol clumps together and interferes with the flow of bile.

The recipes in this chapter have been designed to follow the recommendation by doctors on what works best nutritionally to help the digestive system function properly. They advise a diet that maintains a moderate cholesterol level; appropriate body weight; a low-fat, high-fiber diet; and the eating of frequent small meals.

With these ideas in mind, you won't find fatty meats, butter, or high-fat cheeses in these recipes. But you will enjoy such fare as Baked Acorn Squash with zero cholesterol; Yellow Jewels, an appetizing way of eating millet and getting some fiber; and a beef fillet with minimum fat and maximum fiber. You will also find recipes that include the foods thought to be best for gallbladder problems such as fish, poultry, grains, vegetables, dried beans, and tubers.

Even if you don't have gallbladder concerns, this is not a bad way to eat to avoid other problems such as overweight and heart problems. And with your handy nutritional chart, you will always know the USRDA percentages met in each meal.

Red Baked Acorn Squash

Ingredients: 2   medium acorn squash   **Preparation:** Bake
1   banana, mashed
¼   cup cranberry juice   **Time:** 1 hour, 15 minutes
¼   cup water   **Calories:** 158 per serving

                                                   Serves: 4

Directions

Preheat oven to 425° F. Cut squash in half and clean out seeds and fibers. Place cut sides down in baking pan large enough to hold the four pieces; pierce shell with fork to release steam. Pour ¼ cup cranberry juice and ¼ cup water into pan. Bake for 25 minutes. Turn squash, brush with mashed banana, and pour remaining cranberry juice into the open halves. Bake, basting frequently with the juice for about 30 minutes or until tender. This table queen is at least 2,000 years old. Very high percentages of vitamin A and potassium are recorded on the chart.

TIP: Boston or Bibb lettuce has twice as much vitamin C and three times as much vitamin A by weight as iceberg lettuce. Romaine has even six times as much C and eight times as much A as iceberg.

MYTH: A sure sign of low risk for a heart attack is a blood cholesterol reading of 185.

FACT: The National Institutes of Health report that specific measurement is not enough. You need to have your physician determine how much of your total cholesterol consists of "good" HDL cholesterol. An HDL cholesterol reading below 35 indicates a "very high risk" of heart disease even with cholesterol readings at less than 200.

Nutrients Contained in: Red Baked Acorn Squash

VITAMINS USRDA			ONE SERVING GIVES YOU APPROXIMATELY		APPROXIMATE PERCENTAGE OF USRDA
A	5,000	IU	7,324	IU	146◄
B₁	1.4	mg	0.19	mg	15
B₂	1.6	mg	0.09	mg	6
B₃	16	mg	2	mg	10
B₅	10	mg	0.79	mg	7
B₆	2.2	mg	0.31	mg	14
B₁₂	3	μg	0	μg	0
C	60	mg	37	mg	62
D	400	IU	0	IU	0
E	15	IU	0.51	IU	3
K	500	μg	0.55	μg	0
Folic Acid	400	μg	63	μg	15

MINERALS USRDA			ONE SERVING GIVES YOU APPROXIMATELY		APPROXIMATE PERCENTAGE OF USRDA
Sodium	(1,100–3,000)	mg	6	mg	0
Calcium	1,000	mg	50	mg	6
Phosphorus	(800–1,000)	mg	1,023	mg	127◄
Potassium	(1,875–5,625)	mg	44	mg	12
Magnesium	400	μg	0.38	μg	0
Selenium	200	μg	0.55	μg	0
Iodine	150	mg	0	mg	0
Zinc	15	mg	0.61	mg	4
Iron	10	mg	0.86	mg	8
Manganese	(2.5–5.0)	mg	0.48	mg	9
Copper	(2.0–3.0)	mg	0.22	mg	7

AMOUNT PER SERVING		CALORIES PER SERVING	% OF MEAL
Fat	1 gram	13	8
Proteins	2 grams	8	6
Carbohydrates	34 grams	137	86
Cholesterol	0 mg		
Amino acid (essential)			21–32*
Fiber	2 grams		

Key: USRDA = Recommended Dietary Allowance

IU = International Unit

mg = milligrams

μg = micrograms

NOTE: The numbers with arrows exceed 100 percent of required USRDA.

*Complementary food—1 broiled lamp chop raises EAA to 155–249%.

Yellow Jewels

Ingredients:
- 1 cup millet
- 1 quart low-sodium chicken broth
- 1 tsp salt
- 1 large apple, cored and sliced
- dash of cayenne

Preparation: Boil

Time: 55 minutes

Calories: 262 per serving

Serves: 4

Directions

Follow directions on the package for cooking the millet. It's a good idea to sauté the millet in a pan for 5 minutes or so until it's roasted a bit. Then add to the boiling broth with salt and simmer for about 45 minutes. During the last 5 minutes add apple slices. Serve hot.

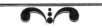

TIP: Millet is a yellow grain that can serve you well when it comes to putting carbohydrates, fiber, and vegetable protein in your diet. It's also a pretty good source of iron compared to other grains such as barley, rice, and pasta.

MYTH: Age spots or so-called liver spots lead to cancers.

FACT: Dermatologists say that these spots are almost always harmless. They can be removed, and you can avoid developing them by staying out of the sun.

Nutrients Contained in: Yellow Jewels

VITAMINS USRDA			ONE SERVING GIVES YOU APPROXIMATELY		APPROXIMATE PERCENTAGE OF USRDA
A	5,000	IU	19	IU	0
B1	1.4	mg	0.43	mg	35
B2	1.6	mg	0.29	mg	20
B3	16	mg	5	mg	29
B5	10	mg	0.02	mg	0
B6	2.2	mg	0.04	mg	1
B12	3	μg	0.30	μg	10
C	60	mg	2	mg	3
D	400	IU	0	IU	0
E	15	IU	1	IU	8
K	500	μg	0	μg	0
Folic Acid	400	μg	6	μg	1

MINERALS USRDA			ONE SERVING GIVES YOU APPROXIMATELY		APPROXIMATE PERCENTAGE OF USRDA
Sodium	(1,100–3,000)	mg	776	mg	77
Calcium	1,000	mg	23	mg	2
Phosphorus	(800–1,000)	mg	180	mg	22
Potassium	(1,875–5,625)	mg	495	mg	61
Magnesium	400	μg	96	μg	27
Selenium	200	μg	0.18	μg	0
Iodine	150	mg	0	mg	0
Zinc	15	mg	0.26	mg	1
Iron	10	mg	4	mg	44
Manganese	(2.5–5.0)	mg	0.02	mg	0
Copper	(2.0–3.0)	mg	0.01	mg	0

AMOUNT PER SERVING		CALORIES PER SERVING	% OF MEAL
Fat	3 grams	29	11
Proteins	11 grams	42	16
Carbohydrates	48 grams	191	73
Cholesterol	1 mg		
Amino acid (essential)			44–145
Fiber	2 grams		

Key: USRDA = Recommended Dietary Allowance

IU = International Unit

mg = milligrams

μg = micrograms

NOTE: The numbers with arrows exceed 100 percent of required USRDA.

No Small Matter Shrimp

Ingredients: 1 ½ lb shrimp, peeled
                4 Tbs lemon juice
                ¼ tsp Tabasco
                4 tsp chervil
                ¼ tsp salt
                1 Tbs olive oil
                1 tsp garlic powder

Preparation: Boil

Time: 40 minutes

Calories: 229 per serving

Serves: 4

Directions

Put a quart of water in a large kettle, bring to boil, put shrimp in the water, return to boil, and turn off the flame. Cover and let stand for 1 minute. Remove to cold water bath. Devein and chill. While shrimp chills, prepare sauce. In a small bowl, combine 4 Tbs lemon juice, olive oil, salt, garlic powder, and chervil. Serve shrimp with this sauce and lemon wedges. Note the high vitamin D and EAA levels on the chart.

TIP: Research at the Harvard Medical School indicates that women may have more risk for gallbladder disease because of hormones. The hormone estrogen is known to increase the rate of fat buildup, which interferes with gallbladder movement. Birth control pills also increase the cholesterol content of bile as they contain estrogen. For this reason, it is reported that there is a risk of gallbladder disease in women under 29 who have taken birth control pills for less than 5 years.

MYTH: Beef labeled "good" is inferior to "choice" or "prime."

FACT: The U.S. Department of Agriculture says "good" beef is actually leaner, although it may be a little tougher. They say it is more nutritious per calorie than either choice or prime beef.

Nutrients Contained in: No Small Matter Shrimp

VITAMINS USRDA			ONE SERVING GIVES YOU APPROXIMATELY		APPROXIMATE PERCENTAGE OF USRDA
A	5,000	IU	4	IU	0
B$_1$	1.4	mg	0.04	mg	2
B$_2$	1.6	mg	0.05	mg	3
B$_3$	16	mg	5	mg	30
B$_5$	10	mg	0.45	mg	4
B$_6$	2.2	mg	0.16	mg	7
B$_{12}$	3	μg	1	μg	44
C	60	mg	11	mg	17
D	400	IU	150	IU	37
E	15	IU	2	IU	13
K	500	μg	0	μg	0
Folic Acid	400	μg	18	μg	4

MINERALS USRDA			ONE SERVING GIVES YOU APPROXIMATELY		APPROXIMATE PERCENTAGE OF USRDA
Sodium	(1,100–3,000)	mg	335	mg	33
Calcium	1,000	mg	98	mg	12
Phosphorus	(800–1,000)	mg	251	mg	31
Potassium	(1,875–5,625)	mg	350	mg	43
Magnesium	400	μg	70	μg	20
Selenium	200	μg	50	μg	24
Iodine	150	mg	79	mg	52
Zinc	15	mg	2	mg	15
Iron	10	mg	2	mg	24
Manganese	(2.5–5.0)	mg	0.05	mg	0
Copper	(2.0–3.0)	mg	0.37	mg	12

AMOUNT PER SERVING		CALORIES PER SERVING	% OF MEAL
Fat	8 grams	74	32
Proteins	33 grams	133	58
Carbohydrates	6 grams	22	10
Cholesterol	263 mg		
Amino acid (essential)			166–563
Fiber	0 grams		

Key: USRDA = Recommended Dietary Allowance
     IU = International Unit
     mg = milligrams
     μg = micrograms
NOTE: The numbers with arrows exceed 100 percent of required USRDA.

On the Half Shell

Ingredients:

24 oysters (Bluepoints if possible)
4 cloves garlic, minced
2 Tbs margarine
4 Tbs parsley, chopped
½ cup apple cider
½ tsp salt
1 tsp black pepper
¼ tsp cayenne pepper
lemons or limes

Preparation: Bake

Time: 20 minutes

Calories: 79 per serving

Serves: 4

Directions

Preheat oven to 350° F. Keep oysters in place on the half shell. Melt the margarine and then combine with the garlic, parsley, salt, pepper, and apple cider and spoon half of the sauce on each one, about 1 tsp per oyster. Bake for 6 minutes; spoon the remaining sauce over the oysters. Serve immediately with lemon or lime quarters.

TIP: Dr. Harris of the University of Massachusetts School of Public Health in Amherst compared the diets of 84 female and 16 male gallbladder patients to patients admitted to a hospital (for other than gallbladder problems). He concluded that there is some risk of gallbladder disease in women who frequently consume starchy foods such as breads, pasta, rice, and potatoes. A small protective effect was reported among women who consume high amounts of vegetables of all kinds.

MYTH: Sustained low blood pressure can cause weakness, headaches, or chronic fatigue.

FACT: The National Institutes of Health report that many people have low blood pressure for a lifetime with no problems. According to the NIH, low blood pressure (90/60) seems to go with long life and health.

Nutrients Contained in: On the Half Shell

VITAMINS USRDA			ONE SERVING GIVES YOU APPROXIMATELY		APPROXIMATE PERCENTAGE OF USRDA
A	5,000	IU	789	IU	15
B₁	1.4	mg	0.15	mg	12
B₂	1.6	mg	0.20	mg	13
B₃	16	mg	1	mg	7
B₅	10	mg	0.01	mg	0
B₆	2.2	mg	0.02	mg	0
B₁₂	3	μg	15	μg	500◄
C	60	mg	47	mg	77
D	400	IU	50	IU	12
E	15	IU	0.89	IU	5
K	500	μg	0	μg	0
Folic Acid	400	μg	9	μg	2

MINERALS USRDA			ONE SERVING GIVES YOU APPROXIMATELY		APPROXIMATE PERCENTAGE OF USRDA
Sodium	(1,100–3,000)	mg	98	mg	9
Calcium	1,000	mg	49	mg	6
Phosphorus	(800–1,000)	mg	11	mg	1
Potassium	(1,875–5,625)	mg	272	mg	34
Magnesium	400	μg	50	μg	14
Selenium	200	μg	0	μg	0
Iodine	150	mg	0	mg	0
Zinc	15	mg	76	mg	507◄
Iron	10	mg	6	mg	59
Manganese	(2.5–5.0)	mg	0.07	mg	1
Copper	(2.0–3.0)	mg	0.03	mg	1

AMOUNT PER SERVING		CALORIES PER SERVING	% OF MEAL
Fat	2 grams	19	24
Proteins	7 grams	29	37
Carbohydrates	8 grams	31	39
Cholesterol	46 mg		
Amino acid (essential)			1–2*
Fiber	0 grams		

Key: USRDA = Recommended Dietary Allowance

IU = International Unit

mg = milligrams

μg = micrograms

NOTE: The numbers with arrows exceed 100 percent of required USRDA.

*Complementary food—1 cup grape nuts raises EAA to 93–254%.

Back to Your Roots

Ingredients:

2 parsnips, peeled and sliced
1 cup green beans, chopped
3 white potatoes, peeled and sliced
1 onion, chopped
2 cloves garlic, minced
1 tsp vegetable oil
1 tsp dried marjoram
¼ cup water
   juice of one lemon
¼ tsp chervil

Preparation: Sauté

Time: 40 minutes

Calories: 167 per serving

Serves: 4

Direction

Sauté garlic and onion in oil until tender. Add parsnips, green beans, and potatoes. Sauté, stirring occasionally, another 6 minutes. Add water and marjoram; stir gently. Cook for another 15 to 20 minutes or until desired tenderness. Season with lemon juice and chervil.

TIP: The U.S. Department of Agriculture in Beltsville, Maryland says you should be alert to the type of margarine you select. They report that trans fatty acids, produced when vegetable oils are converted to margarine or other solid shortenings can raise cholesterol levels and create a possible heart-disease risk. The suggestion is to use diet soft margarine, which has fewer trans fatty acids.

MYTH: Special insoles will prevent sports injuries.

FACT: Experts say it is unlikely. One study from the University of Calgary in Alberta says they don't think such insoles significantly increase the shock-absorbing ability of good athletic shoes. They suggest selecting shoes that provide appropriate cushioning by themselves. When the shoes wear out replace them, do not add insoles they caution.

Nutrients Contained in: Back to Your Roots

VITAMINS USRDA			ONE SERVING GIVES YOU APPROXIMATELY		APPROXIMATE PERCENTAGE OF USRDA
A	5,000	IU	209	IU	4
B$_1$	1.4	mg	0.16	mg	13
B$_2$	1.6	mg	0.05	mg	3
B$_3$	16	mg	2	mg	9
B$_5$	10	mg	0.59	mg	5
B$_6$	2.2	mg	0.36	mg	16
B$_{12}$	3	μg	0	μg	0
C	60	mg	20	mg	33
D	400	IU	0	IU	0
E	15	IU	2	IU	14
K	500	μg	81	μg	16
Folic Acid	400	μg	50	μg	12

MINERALS USRDA			ONE SERVING GIVES YOU APPROXIMATELY		APPROXIMATE PERCENTAGE OF USRDA
Sodium	(1,100–3,000)	mg	13	mg	1
Calcium	1,000	mg	48	mg	5
Phosphorus	(800–1,000)	mg	67	mg	8
Potassium	(1,875–5,625)	mg	643	mg	80
Magnesium	400	μg	44	μg	12
Selenium	200	μg	0.95	μg	0
Iodine	150	mg	0	mg	0
Zinc	15	mg	0.49	mg	3
Iron	10	mg	0.89	mg	8
Manganese	(2.5–5.0)	mg	0.29	mg	5
Copper	(2.0–3.0)	mg	0.22	mg	7

AMOUNT PER SERVING		CALORIES PER SERVING	% OF MEAL
Fat	2 grams	18	11
Proteins	3 grams	14	8
Carbohydrates	34 grams	135	81
Cholesterol	0 mg		
Amino acid (essential)			26–42*
Fiber	2 grams		

Key: USRDA = Recommended Dietary Allowance

    IU = International Unit

    mg = milligrams

    μg = micrograms

NOTE: The numbers with arrows exceed 100 percent of required USRDA.

*Complementary food—1 cup peas raises EAA to 105–149%.

Savory Beef Fillet

Ingredients:

- 1 lb beef fillet, cubed
- 1 cup onion, chopped
- ½ tsp sage
- 1 cup chick peas
- 1 cup carrots, sliced
- ½ tsp paprika
- 2 tomatoes, quartered
- 1 red pepper, seeded and cut into strips
- ½ tsp vegetable oil
- 1 ½ cups boiling water
- black pepper

Preparation: Bake and sauté

Time: 50 minutes

Calories: 529 per serving

Serves: 4

Directions

Preheat oven to 325°F. While oven is heating, heat oil in a large skillet. Cook the meat and onion until the beef is brown. Season with the sage and paprika and use black pepper to taste. Pour this mixture into a medium size casserole dish, cover with the water. Bake with a cover until meat is tender, about 55 minutes. Then mix in the chick peas, carrots, tomatoes, and red pepper and bake 30 minutes more. Check your chart for large percentages of vitamin A, potassium, magnesium, calcium, and phosphorus and a whopping amount of EAA.

TIP: Researchers at the Harvard School of Public Health make the point that since the gallbladder is part of the digestive system, its condition depends in large measure on one's diet. They observed after studying thousands of women that even moderate overweight can raise the risk of gallbladder problems leading to stones and the very obese probably faces a sixfold higher risk.

MYTH: Since the prostate gland contains zinc, one should increase the amount of zinc beyond what one receives in a balanced diet.

FACT: The Recommended Dietary Allowance of zinc is 12 milligrams for women and 15 milligrams for men, but taking more does not do more good. Researchers at the University of Wyoming showed that megadoses of zinc may reduce levels of "good" HDL cholesterol. Other studies have shown that even 50 to 75 milligrams of zinc a day can cause HDL levels to drop.

Nutrients Contained in: Savory Beef Fillet

VITAMINS USRDA			ONE SERVING GIVES YOU APPROXIMATELY		APPROXIMATE PERCENTAGE OF USRDA
A	5,000	IU	10,444	IU	208◄
B_1	1.4	mg	0.38	mg	31
B_2	1.6	mg	0.72	mg	51
B_3	16	mg	0.06	mg	37
B_5	10	mg	0.02	mg	15
B_6	2.2	mg	0.01	mg	45
B_{12}	3	μg	0.02	μg	80
C	60	mg	0.32	mg	53
D	400	IU	0.00	IU	0
E	15	IU	0.03	IU	22
K	500	μg	0.63	μg	12
Folic Acid	400	μg	0.18	μg	4

MINERALS USRDA			ONE SERVING GIVES YOU APPROXIMATELY		APPROXIMATE PERCENTAGE OF USRDA
Sodium	(1,100–3,000)	mg	90	mg	8
Calcium	1,000	mg	117	mg	14
Phosphorus	(800–1,000)	mg	477	mg	59
Potassium	(1,875–5,625)	mg	1,240	mg	155◄
Magnesium	400	μg	119	μg	33
Selenium	200	μg	32	μg	16
Iodine	150	mg	0	mg	0
Zinc	15	mg	6	mg	36
Iron	10	mg	9	mg	92
Manganese	(2.5–5.0)	mg	83	mg	16
Copper	(2.0–3.0)	mg	0.51	mg	16

AMOUNT PER SERVING		CALORIES PER SERVING	% OF MEAL
Fat	21 grams	188	35
Proteins	46 grams	184	35
Carbohydrates	39 grams	157	30
Cholesterol	70 mg		
Amino acid (essential)			373–859
Fiber	3 grams		

Key: USRDA=Recommended Dietary Allowance
     IU = International Unit
     mg = milligrams
     μg = micrograms
NOTE: The numbers with arrows exceed 100 percent of required USRDA.

Pleasant Crabs

Ingredients: 24   live hard-shell crabs   **Preparation:** Boil
               juice of one lemon   **Time:** 25 minutes
            2   Tbs horseradish   **Calories:** 364 per serving

                                              Serves: 6

Directions

In a large kettle add water to just cover the bottom of the kettle. Cover and heat to boiling. Place the crabs in the kettle and reduce heat. Simmer for about 15 to 20 minutes. When done, break off large claws. Pull off top shell and break off the legs. Remove digestive tract and organs located in the center part of the body. These members of the shellfish family should show signs of life when you purchase them, for example, a little movement of claws or general movement. Do not buy them if they are dead. Add lemon juice and horseradish and serve. The chart shows a bonanza of vitamin A, calcium, phosphorus, potassium, magnesium, and selenium.

TIP: The National Cancer Institute suggests daily intake of 2,030 grams of fiber, recommending that you eat the fiber in the skin and membranes of fruits and vegetables such as apples, peaches, tomatoes, and carrots. Instead of mashed potatoes, eat baked potatoes with the skins. NCI reminds you that, as you gradually increase the amount of dietary fiber you eat, you should remember to drink more water.

MYTH: Frozen desserts made from skim milk or nonfat solids do not contain more calcium than ice cream.

FACT: According to analyses of these desserts, they may actually contain more calcium than ice creams. The lack of fat leaves more room for other important ingredients.

Nutrients Contained in: Pleasant Crabs

VITAMINS USRDA			ONE SERVING GIVES YOU APPROXIMATELY		APPROXIMATE PERCENTAGE OF USRDA
A	5,000	IU	8,686	IU	173◄
B₁	1.4	mg	0.65	mg	53
B₂	1.6	mg	0.32	mg	23
B₃	16	mg	11	mg	70
B₅	10	mg	2	mg	24
B₆	2.2	mg	1	mg	55
B₁₂	3	μg	40	μg	1,333◄
C	60	mg	18	mg	30
D	400	IU	0	IU	0
E	15	IU	0.40	IU	2
K	500	μg	3	μg	0
Folic Acid	400	μg	62	μg	15

MINERALS USRDA			ONE SERVING GIVES YOU APPROXIMATELY		APPROXIMATE PERCENTAGE OF USRDA
Sodium	(1,100–3,000)	mg	5	mg	0
Calcium	1,000	mg	180	mg	22
Phosphorus	(800–1,000)	mg	705	mg	88
Potassium	(1,875–5,625)	mg	761	mg	95
Magnesium	40	μg	147	μg	42
Selenium	200	μg	4	μg	2
Iodine	150	mg	0	mg	0
Zinc	15	mg	14	mg	96
Iron	10	mg	3	mg	33
Manganese	(2.5–5.0)	mg	0.08	mg	1
Copper	(2.0–3.0)	mg	1	mg	36

AMOUNT PER SERVING		CALORIES PER SERVING	% OF MEAL
Fat	8 grams	69	19
Proteins	69 grams	278	76
Carbohydrates	4 grams	17	5
Cholesterol	400 mg		
Amino acid (essential)			526–999
Fiber	0 grams		

Key: USRDA=Recommended Dietary Allowance

IU = International Unit

mg = milligrams

μg = micrograms

NOTE: The numbers with arrows exceed 100 percent of required USRDA.

Greens L'Italia

Ingredients:

2	lbs kale and turnip greens
2	cloves garlic, chopped
1	tsp vegetable oil
½	tsp marjoram
	juice of one lemon
¼	tsp basil leaves
	juice of one lime
	dash of cayenne

Preparation: Steam and sauté

Time: 20 minutes

Calories: 48 per serving

Serves: 6

Directions

Cut off and discard any heavy stems or roots on the kale. Cut both greens into small pieces (reduces cooking time). Wash leaves to be sure they are clean of sand and grit. Place them in a steamer for about 10 minutes. Heat oil in a large pan, sauté garlic, and add the greens. Add all the seasonings except the lime juice and cayenne. Heat through for about 2 minutes. Add the juice of the lime and the cayenne and serve. Kale, a member of the cabbage family and believed to be the earliest cultivated form of cabbage, is very high in vitamin A.

TIP: A note in *The Lancet* reports that any diet that is low in fiber and high in sugar, fat, and calories can put anyone at risk of gallstones and other health problems.

MYTH: Light scanning is just as good as mammography for detection of breast cancer at an early stage.

FACT: According to the National Cancer Institute, the Centers for Disease Control, and other groups, light scanning supplies no useful clinical information and is more prone to error than mammography.

Nutrients Contained in: Greens L'Italia

VITAMINS USRDA			ONE SERVING GIVES YOU APPROXIMATELY		APPROXIMATE PERCENTAGE OF USRDA
A	5,000	IU	5,966	IU	119◄
B₁	1.4	mg	0.09	mg	7
B₂	1.6	mg	0.13	mg	9
B₃	16	mg	0.23	mg	1
B₅	10	mg	0.21	mg	2
B₆	2.2	mg	0.06	mg	2
B₁₂	3	μg	0	μg	0
C	60	mg	60	mg	100◄
D	400	IU	0	IU	0
E	15	IU	5	IU	30
K	500	μg	62	μg	12
Folic Acid	400	μg	23	μg	5

MINERALS USRDA			ONE SERVING GIVES YOU APPROXIMATELY		APPROXIMATE PERCENTAGE OF USRDA
Sodium	(1,100–3,000)	mg	22	mg	2
Calcium	1,000	mg	133	mg	16
Phosphorus	(800–1,000)	mg	40	mg	4
Potassium	(1,875–5,625)	mg	269	mg	33
Magnesium	400	μg	32	μg	9
Selenium	200	μg	2	μg	1
Iodine	150	mg	0	mg	0
Zinc	15	mg	0.13	mg	0
Iron	10	mg	2	mg	17
Manganese	(2.5–5.0)	mg	0.13	mg	2
Copper	(2.0–3.0)	mg	0.08	mg	2

AMOUNT PER SERVING		CALORIES PER SERVING	% OF MEAL
Fat	2 grams	14	28
Proteins	2 grams	9	20
Carbohydrates	6 grams	25	52
Cholesterol	0 mg		
Amino acid (essential)			13–34*
Fiber	1 gram		

Key: USRDA = Recommended Dietary Allowance

IU = International Unit

mg = milligrams

μg = micrograms

NOTE: The numbers with arrows exceed 100 percent of required USRDA.

*Complementary food—1 cup peas raises EAA to 94–139%.

Green and Brown Beans

Ingredients:

- 1 lb green beans, cut crosswise in thirds
- ½ cup chick peas
- ½ cup green peppers, seeded and chopped
- ½ cup onion, chopped
- ¼ tsp thyme
- 1 tsp turmeric
- 1 tsp ground savory
- black pepper
- juice of one lemon

Preparation: Boil and simmer

Time: 15 minutes

Calories: 134 per serving

Serves: 4

Directions

Place beans in a little water to cover and heat to boiling. Cook for about 5 minutes. Add green peppers and onions and cook another 2 minutes. Add chick peas and cook covered for 2 minutes. Add all seasonings and cook for another minute. Add juice of one lemon and black pepper and serve. High amounts of potassium and vitamin K are recorded.

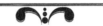

TIP: Gallbladder removal is the most common of all procedures for treatment of gallstones. Gallstones consist mainly of cholesterol, and many treatment options try to dissolve the stones, but only surgical removal of the gallbladder insures no recurrence of stones.

MYTH: You should bundle up to avoid catching a cold.

FACT: Dr. Jack Gwaltney, professor of medicine at the University of Virginia Medical School, says in repeated experiments at the Common Cold Unit in Salisbury, England, people left shivering out in the cold were no more likely to catch cold than were those who stayed warm indoors. He says it all depends on a virus getting to you in the right place; if not, no cold.

Nutrients Contained in: Green and Brown Beans

VITAMINS USRDA			ONE SERVING GIVES YOU APPROXIMATELY		APPROXIMATE PERCENTAGE OF USRDA
A	5,000	IU	469	IU	9
B$_1$	1.4	mg	0.15	mg	12
B$_2$	1.6	mg	0.11	mg	7
B$_3$	16	mg	0.95	mg	5
B$_5$	10	mg	0.43	mg	4
B$_6$	2.2	mg	0.21	mg	9
B$_{12}$	3	μg	0	μg	0
C	60	mg	26	mg	42
D	400	IU	0	IU	0
E	15	IU	0.49	IU	3
K	500	μg	163	μg	32
Folic Acid	400	μg	27	μg	6

MINERALS USRDA			ONE SERVING GIVES YOU APPROXIMATELY		APPROXIMATE PERCENTAGE OF USRDA
Sodium	(1,100–3,000)	mg	10	mg	0
Calcium	1,000	mg	76	mg	9
Phosphorus	(800–1,000)	mg	116	mg	14
Potassium	(1,875–5,625)	mg	449	mg	56
Magnesium	400	μg	63	μg	17
Selenium	200	μg	4	μg	1
Iodine	150	mg	0	mg	0
Zinc	15	mg	0.96	mg	6
Iron	10	mg	3	mg	27
Manganese	(2.5–5.0)	mg	0.55	mg	10
Copper	(2.0–3.0)	mg	0.28	mg	9

AMOUNT PER SERVING		CALORIES PER SERVING	% OF MEAL
Fat	2 grams	14	10
Proteins	7 grams	27	20
Carbohydrates	23 grams	93	70
Cholesterol	0 mg		
Amino acid (essential)			62–99
Fiber	2 grams		

Key: USRDA = Recommended Dietary Allowance
     IU = International Unit
     mg = milligrams
     μg = micrograms
NOTE: The numbers with arrows exceed 100 percent of required USRDA.

Breast Over Broccoli

Ingredients:

- 1 lb chicken breast, boned and sliced into strips
- 1 cup brown rice
- 2 lbs fresh broccoli, chopped
- ½ cup onion, chopped
- 1 tsp vegetable oil
- ½ cup herb-seasoned mix
- ½ cup grape nut flakes
- black pepper

Preparation: Bake

Time: 1 hour, 15 minutes

Calories: 281 per serving

Serves: 4

Directions

Preheat oven to 350° F. Cook the rice as directed on the package. In the meantime, heat the oil in a large skillet, add herb mix and stir; sauté the onions until transparent. Add the chicken strips, cook for a minute then add the chopped broccoli. Continue to cook until the broccoli is almost done. During the last 5 minutes of cooking time for the rice, fold rice, broccoli, and chicken mix in a large casserole dish. Sprinkle the crushed grape nut flakes over the dish and bake for 5 to 10 minutes. Thomas Jefferson, unlike former President George Bush, was fond of broccoli. Good amounts of potassium, vitamin A, and EAA.

TIP: Physicians recommend as a dietary goal that 20 to 35 grams of soluble and insoluble fiber should be eaten daily. Foods such as dried beans, broccoli, carrots, corn, peas, sweet potatoes, cereals, whole wheat, rye, and pumpernickel breads, and whole wheat crackers, as well as fruits such as prunes, pears, apples, and oranges are good sources.

MYTH: Pregnant women have a craving for pickles.

FACT: According to a report in the Tufts University *Diet and Nutrition Letter*, a study by Advance Pregnancy Test found that women who do have unusual food cravings (3 out of 10 do not) tend toward ice cream and fruit, not pickles.

Nutrients Contained in: Breast Over Broccoli

VITAMINS USRDA			ONE SERVING GIVES YOU APPROXIMATELY		APPROXIMATE PERCENTAGE OF USRDA
A	5,000	IU	1,309	IU	26
B$_1$	1.4	mg	0.44	mg	36
B$_2$	1.6	mg	0.30	mg	21
B$_3$	16	mg	7	mg	46
B$_5$	10	mg	1	mg	11
B$_6$	2.2	mg	0.75	mg	34
B$_{12}$	3	μg	0.84	μg	27
C	60	mg	45	mg	74
D	400	IU	0	IU	0
E	15	IU	1	IU	8
K	500	μg	150	μg	30
Folic Acid	400	μg	90	μg	22

MINERALS USRDA			ONE SERVING GIVES YOU APPROXIMATELY		APPROXIMATE PERCENTAGE OF USRDA
Sodium	(1,100–3,000)	mg	131	mg	13
Calcium	1,000	mg	55	mg	6
Phosphorus	(800–1,000)	mg	225	mg	28
Potassium	(1,875–5,625)	mg	410	mg	51
Magnesium	400	μg	74	μg	21
Selenium	200	μg	20	μg	10
Iodine	150	mg	0	mg	0
Zinc	15	mg	2	mg	11
Iron	10	mg	2	mg	21
Manganese	(2.5–5.0)	mg	0.96	mg	19
Copper	(2.0–3.0)	mg	0.19	mg	6

AMOUNT PER SERVING		CALORIES PER SERVING	% OF MEAL
Fat	2 grams	14	5
Proteins	12 grams	48	17
Carbohydrates	55 grams	219	78
Cholesterol	20 mg		
Amino acid (essential)			125–166
Fiber	2 grams		

Key: USRDA = Recommended Dietary Allowance
      IU = International Unit
      mg = milligrams
      μg = micrograms
NOTE: The numbers with arrows exceed 100 percent of required USRDA.

OK Lima Beans

Ingredients:

2 cups dried lima beans
1 green pepper, seeded and chopped
½ cup parsley, chopped
1 cup onion, chopped
½ cup low-sodium chicken broth
2 cups okra
2 fresh tomatoes, cut into pieces
½ tsp chervil
black pepper
½ tsp salt

Preparation: Cook

Time: 20 minutes

Calories: 163 per serving

Serves: 4

Directions

Soak beans 6 to 8 hours and keep the soaking water. Then cook beans according to package instructions. Cook celery, onions, and green pepper in a little chicken broth. Season with chervil. When vegetables are crispy, add the tomatoes and okra. Simmer all together for about 12 minutes. Add parsley, salt, and pepper and serve. If you go to New Orleans, you must order this Creole dish. It has very high potassium levels.

TIP: Health experts from the National Institutes of Health say that there is no sure way to prevent gallstones. What many doctors recommend is that you eat prudently by maintaining a moderate cholesterol level and by eating a low-fat, high-fiber diet. They also advise that you eat several small meals rather than one or two large ones.

MYTH: Fatty meat has more cholesterol than lean meat.

FACT: Fatty meat has about the same amount of cholesterol as lean cuts. This is because cholesterol is found primarily in the lean tissue, not in the fat.

Nutrients Contained in: OK Lima Beans

VITAMINS USRDA		ONE SERVING GIVES YOU APPROXIMATELY		APPROXIMATE PERCENTAGE OF USRDA
A	5,000 IU	1,980	IU	39
B_1	1.4 mg	0.29	mg	24
B_2	1.6 mg	0.18	mg	12
B_3	16 mg	2	mg	14
B_5	10 mg	0.57	mg	5
B_6	2.2 mg	0.37	mg	16
B_{12}	3 μg	0.04	μg	1
C	60 mg	46	mg	76
D	400 IU	0	IU	0
E	15 IU	1	IU	8
K	500 μg	5	μg	1
Folic Acid	400 μg	168	μg	42

MINERALS USRDA		ONE SERVING GIVES YOU APPROXIMATELY		APPROXIMATE PERCENTAGE OF USRDA
Sodium	(1,100–3,000) mg	125	mg	12
Calcium	1,000 mg	98	mg	12
Phosphorus	(800–1,000) mg	173	mg	21
Potassium	(1,875–5,625) mg	905	mg	113◀
Magnesium	400 μg	105	μg	29
Selenium	200 μg	1	μg	0
Iodine	150 mg	0	mg	0
Zinc	15 mg	1	mg	7
Iron	10 mg	3	mg	34
Manganese	(2.5–5.0) mg	2	mg	35
Copper	(2.0–3.0) mg	0.83	mg	27

AMOUNT PER SERVING		CALORIES PER SERVING	% OF MEAL
Fat	1 gram	7	4
Proteins	9 grams	35	21
Carbohydrates	30 grams	121	74
Cholesterol	0 mg		
Amino acid (essential)			78–121
Fiber	3 grams		

Key: USRDA = Recommended Dietary Allowance
    IU = International Unit
    mg = milligrams
    μg = micrograms
NOTE: The numbers with arrows exceed 100 percent of required USRDA.

Carrots' Cousin

Ingredients:

1 lb parsnips, peeled and sliced thin cross-wise
½ cup low-sodium chicken broth
½ tsp thyme
2 stalks celery, diced
juice of one lemon
1 small bunch watercress
1 tsp chervil

Preparation: Boil and steam

Time: 20 minutes

Calories: 47 per serving

Serves: 4

Directions

Pour broth into a large skillet and heat. Add parsnips and celery. Cover, bring to a boil, and steam about 10 minutes or less if parsnips are tender. Add chervil. When ready to serve, add juice of lemon and black pepper. Surround with watercress. Parsnips go back to the early Greeks and Romans and was Europe's contribution to native Americans during colonial times.

TIP: Dr. James Everhart, of the National Institute of Diabetes and Digestive and Kidney Diseases in Bethesda, Maryland, says that most gallstones cause no symptoms at all and are detected only when patients are treated for unrelated ailments or when an attack occurs during vacations or special occasions when we change our eating patterns.

MYTH: Cans or jars of meat will last on a kitchen shelf for only six months or so.

FACT: The U.S. Department of Agriculture says they will keep from two to five years. The reason—they are sterilized at very high temperatures before they are packaged. After opening, of course, they should be used within a week, even when stored under refrigeration.

Nutrients Contained in: Carrots' Cousin

VITAMINS USRDA			ONE SERVING GIVES YOU APPROXIMATELY		APPROXIMATE PERCENTAGE OF USRDA
A	5,000	IU	30	IU	0
B$_1$	1.4	mg	0.02	mg	1
B$_2$	1.6	mg	0	mg	0
B$_3$	16	mg	0.11	mg	0
B$_5$	10	mg	0.06	mg	0
B$_6$	2.2	mg	0.02	mg	1
B$_{12}$	3	μg	0	μg	0
C	60	mg	15	mg	25
D	400	IU	0	IU	0
E	15	IU	4	IU	28
K	500	μg	3	μg	0
Folic Acid	400	μg	31	μg	7

MINERALS USRDA			ONE SERVING GIVES YOU APPROXIMATELY		APPROXIMATE PERCENTAGE OF USRDA
Sodium	(1,100–3,000)	mg	119	mg	11
Calcium	1,000	mg	29	mg	3
Phosphorus	(800–1,000)	mg	7	mg	0
Potassium	(1,875–5,625)	mg	256	mg	32
Magnesium	400	μg	24	μg	6
Selenium	200	μg	3	μg	1
Iodine	150	mg	0	mg	0
Zinc	15	mg	0.06	mg	0
Iron	10	mg	0.21	mg	2
Manganese	(2.5–5.0)	mg	0.03	mg	0
Copper	(2.0–3.0)	mg	0.01	mg	0

AMOUNT PER SERVING		CALORIES PER SERVING	% OF MEAL
Fat	0 grams	2	5
Proteins	1 gram	6	12
Carbohydrates	10 grams	39	83
Cholesterol	0 mg		
Amino acid (essential)			Very low*
Fiber	1 gram		

Key: USRDA = Recommended Dietary Allowance

　　　　IU = International Unit

　　　　mg = milligrams

　　　　μg = micrograms

NOTE: The numbers with arrows exceed 100 percent of required USRDA.

*Complementary food—1 head of endive raises EAA to 29–183%.

Ole for Sole

Ingredients:

4 slices fillet of sole
1 cucumber, sliced
½ tsp paprika
1 tsp prepared mustard
juice of one lemon
lettuce leaves

Preparation: Bake

Time: 20 minutes

Calories: 157 per serving

Serves: 4

Directions

Preheat oven to 450° F. Pour the juice of one lemon over fish. Spread mustard over each slice and sprinkle with paprika. Arrange the cucumber slices around the fish. Wrap slices of fillet in lettuce leaves to retain moisture. Bake for about 10 minutes or less if fillet slices are very thin. High percentages of phosphorus, potassium, and EAA are recorded.

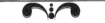

TIP: Physicians at Lenox Hill Hospital in New York City say gallbladder attacks typically occur shortly after eating. Sharp abdominal pains as well as nausea and vomiting may also occur. Once a stone, which can be as small as a dot or the size of an egg, passes back into the gallbladder or into the small intestine, the pain subsides.

MYTH: Beef is the only standard when referring to red meat.

FACT: According to the USDA, there is no official definition of red meat. The term is used for all meat other than poultry. This includes pork, lamb, and game.

Nutrients Contained in: Ole for Sole

VITAMINS USRDA			ONE SERVING GIVES YOU APPROXIMATELY		APPROXIMATE PERCENTAGE OF USRDA
A	5,000	IU	350	IU	6
B1	1.4	mg	0.16	mg	13
B2	1.6	mg	0.13	mg	9
B3	16	mg	4	mg	23
B5	10	mg	0.87	mg	8
B6	2.2	mg	0.04	mg	1
B12	3	μg	2	μg	53
C	60	mg	16	mg	27
D	400	IU	0	IU	0
E	15	IU	0.55	IU	3
K	500	μg	1	μg	0
Folic Acid	400	μg	36	μg	9

MINERALS USRDA			ONE SERVING GIVES YOU APPROXIMATELY		APPROXIMATE PERCENTAGE OF USRDA
Sodium	(1,100–3,000)	mg	114	mg	11
Calcium	1,000	mg	147	mg	18
Phosphorus	(800–1,000)	mg	411	mg	51
Potassium	(1,875–5,625)	mg	894	mg	111◄
Magnesium	400	μg	70	μg	19
Selenium	200	μg	48	μg	24
Iodine	150	mg	0	mg	0
Zinc	15	mg	0.84	mg	5
Iron	10	mg	2	mg	21
Manganese	(2.5–5.0)	mg	0.09	mg	1
Copper	(2.0–3.0)	mg	0.08	mg	2

AMOUNT PER SERVING		CALORIES PER SERVING	% OF MEAL
Fat	1 gram	10	7
Proteins	31 grams	123	78
Carbohydrates	6 grams	24	15
Cholesterol	0 mg		
Amino acid (essential)			179–597
Fiber	1 gram		

Key: USRDA = Recommended Dietary Allowance

IU = International Unit

mg = milligrams

μg = micrograms

NOTE: The numbers with arrows exceed 100 percent of required USRDA.

Soup of Beans

Ingredients:
$\frac{1}{2}$ cup dried navy beans
$\frac{1}{2}$ cup dried kidney beans
$\frac{1}{2}$ cup dried lentils
$\frac{1}{2}$ cup dried pinto beans
1 cup canned tomatoes
$\frac{1}{2}$ cup parsnips, chopped
$\frac{1}{2}$ cup celery, chopped
1 cup large onion, chopped
2 cloves garlic, chopped into fine pieces
$\frac{1}{2}$ tsp each basil, thyme, black pepper, and oregano
1 Tbs Adobo (Goya product) seasoning

Preparation: Boil

Time: 1 $\frac{1}{2}$ hours

Calories: 125 per serving

Serves: 5

Directions

Soaking dried beans replaces water that was lost in the drying process. Use the old-fashioned method and soak the washed beans in a covered pot from 6 to 8 hours. You can save the water and use it as the package instructs for cooking the beans. Combine the beans with all the other ingredients (except the tomatoes, the acid slows down the cooking of the beans) and simmer for about one and a half hours. Check beans to make certain they don't stick and are not overdone; add a little water if necessary. Finally, add the tomatoes and blend thoroughly.

TIP: Members of the American Academy of Family Physicians report that obesity has always been considered a risk factor for cholesterol-induced stone formation. Very obese persons have a higher incidence of gallstones as compared with lean persons. Ethnic background also has a major effect on the prevalence of gallstones which may be due to genetic factors or factors such as diet and environment.

MYTH: We are getting plenty of complex carbohydrates as long as we eat four servings of breads and cereals a day.

FACT: Not if we abide by the federal dietary guidelines for Americans which recommends 6 to 11 daily helpings of carbohydrate-rich grains such as cereal, rice, pasta, or bread.

Nutrients Contained in: Soup of Beans

VITAMINS USRDA			ONE SERVING GIVES YOU APPROXIMATELY		APPROXIMATE PERCENTAGE OF USRDA
A	5,000	IU	8,222	IU	164◄
B$_1$	1.4	mg	0.15	mg	12
B$_2$	1.6	mg	0.09	mg	6
B$_3$	16	mg	1	mg	7
B$_5$	10	mg	0.41	mg	4
B$_6$	2.2	mg	0.21	mg	9
B$_{12}$	3	μg	0	μg	0
C	60	mg	14	mg	23
D	400	IU	0	IU	0
E	15	IU	1	IU	8
K	500	μg	40	μg	8
Folic Acid	400	μg	33	μg	8

MINERALS USRDA			ONE SERVING GIVES YOU APPROXIMATELY		APPROXIMATE PERCENTAGE OF USRDA
Sodium	(1,100–3,000)	mg	116	mg	11
Calcium	1,000	mg	60	mg	7
Phosphorus	(800–1,000)	mg	104	mg	12
Potassium	(1,875–5,625)	mg	555	mg	69
Magnesium	400	μg	31	μg	8
Selenium	200	μg	4	μg	1
Iodine	150	mg	0	mg	0
Zinc	15	mg	0.73	mg	4
Iron	10	mg	2	mg	22
Manganese	(2.5–5.0)	mg	0.10	mg	2
Copper	(2.0–3.0)	mg	0.15	mg	5

AMOUNT PER SERVING		CALORIES PER SERVING	% OF MEAL
Fat	1 gram	6	4
Proteins	7 grams	28	23
Carbohydrates	23 grams	91	73
Cholesterol	0 mg		
Amino acid (essential)			63–227
Fiber	7 grams		

Key: USRDA = Recommended Dietary Allowance
　　　IU = International Unit
　　　mg = milligrams
　　　μg = micrograms
NOTE: The numbers with arrows exceed 100 percent of required USRDA.

Simple Zucchini and Carrots

Ingredients: 1 ½ cups carrots
(about 4 carrots)
2 zucchini, sliced cross-
wise
2 stalks celery, chopped
1 bunch scallions, cut
into large pieces
8 fresh shiitake mushrooms
½ cup vegetable or
low-sodium chicken
broth
½ tsp thyme
juice of one lemon
½ tsp chervil
cayenne pepper

Preparation: Simmer

Time: 25 minutes

Calories: 191 per serving

Serves: 4

Directions

Place carrots, zucchini, celery, mushrooms, onion, and ½ cup of chicken or vegetable broth in large saucepan. Add the thyme and a dash of cayenne pepper. Simmer carrots for about 5 minutes; then add zucchini and simmer for about 10 minutes more. Add chervil and juice of lemon. Mushrooms have been a favorite since ancient Egypt and with Roman soldiers in the belief it gave them strength. While there are many types of mushrooms, most of the recipes in this book favor shiitake and black fungus for reasons given throughout. Notice high percentages of potassium and vitamin A.

TIP: Researchers at King Fahd Hospital in Saudia Arabia found that eating fatty foods can give you gallstones. They noticed that the number of gallbladder operations performed annually was about 10 times higher in 1986 than in 1977. The local population had only a 67 percent growth. The Saudis had changed their eating habits from high-fiber grains to a diet higher in calories and with 197 percent more fat.

MYTH: Poisonous mushrooms turn a silver spoon black.

FACT: There is no evidence to support this old wives' tale, and there is no evidence that nonpoisonous ones do not.

Nutrients Contained in:
Simple Zucchini and Carrots

VITAMINS USRDA			ONE SERVING GIVES YOU APPROXIMATELY		APPROXIMATE PERCENTAGE OF USRDA
A	5,000	IU	21,412	IU	428◄
B$_1$	1.4	mg	0.12	mg	9
B$_2$	1.6	mg	0.13	mg	9
B$_3$	16	mg	4	mg	26
B$_5$	10	mg	0.25	mg	2
B$_6$	2.2	mg	0.19	mg	8
B$_{12}$	3	μg	0	μg	0
C	60	mg	21	mg	35
D	400	IU	0	IU	0
E	15	IU	0.66	IU	4
K	500	μg	100	μg	20
Folic Acid	400	μg	70	μg	17

MINERALS USRDA			ONE SERVING GIVES YOU APPROXIMATELY		APPROXIMATE PERCENTAGE OF USRDA
Sodium	(1,100–3,000)	mg	37	mg	3
Calcium	1,000	mg	49	mg	6
Phosphorus	(800–1,000)	mg	67	mg	8
Potassium	(1,875–5,625)	mg	723	mg	90
Magnesium	400	μg	60	μg	17
Selenium	200	μg	2	μg	1
Iodine	150	mg	0	mg	0
Zinc	15	mg	3	mg	22
Iron	10	mg	1	mg	11
Manganese	(2.5–5.0)	mg	0.22	mg	4
Copper	(2.0–3.0)	mg	0.11	mg	3

AMOUNT PER SERVING		CALORIES PER SERVING	% OF MEAL
Fat	0 grams	2	1
Proteins	5 grams	20	10
Carbohydrates	42 grams	169	89
Cholesterol	0 mg		
Amino acid (essential)			11–18*
Fiber	1 gram		

Key: USRDA = Recommended Dietary Allowance

   IU = International Unit

   mg = milligrams

   μg = micrograms

NOTE: The numbers with arrows exceed 100 percent of required USRDA.

*Complementary food—3-inch square of tofu raises EAA to 111–184%.

Lobster for a Change

Ingredients:

3 live lobsters
   (about 1 ½ lbs each)
4 quarts of water
2 lemons, cut into
   wedges
   garlic salt

Preparation: Boil

Time: 20 minutes

Calories: 205 per serving

Serves: 4

Directions

Lobster serving should approximate about 6 4-inch pieces for each. Boil water in a large kettle. Put lobsters in water and cover. Return to boil, reduce heat, and simmer for about 10 minutes. When done, place lobster on its back. Cut lengthwise in half. Remove the stomach in back of the head and the intestinal vein. You can find this beginning at the stomach to the tip of the tail. The coral roe and green liver are edible. Serve with lemon wedges and garlic salt. See tip about large amount of cholesterol. See chart for percentage of important selenium.

TIP: Shellfish, despite its high cholesterol level, is fine once in a while as it has only minuscule amount of saturated fat. And nutritionists say saturated fat is the bigger concern when it comes to health.

MYTH: Potatoes and onions should be stored at cool room temperatures, preferable under the sink.

FACT: Do not store root vegetables and/or onions under the sink, where most of us store our detergents and cleansers. In addition, drains and other pipes under the sink might contribute heat to the area and make the temperature too warm for storage.

Nutrients Contained in: Lobster for a Change

VITAMINS USRDA			ONE SERVING GIVES YOU APPROXIMATELY		APPROXIMATE PERCENTAGE OF USRDA
A	5,000	IU	0	IU	0
B$_1$	1.4	mg	0.80	mg	66
B$_2$	1.6	mg	0.10	mg	7
B$_3$	16	mg	3	mg	18
B$_5$	10	mg	2	mg	20
B$_6$	2.2	mg	0	mg	0
B$_{12}$	3	µg	0.60	µg	20
C	60	mg	0	mg	0
D	400	IU	0	IU	0
E	15	IU	5	IU	30
K	500	µg	0	µg	0
Folic Acid	400	µg	22	µg	5

MINERALS USRDA			ONE SERVING GIVES YOU APPROXIMATELY		APPROXIMATE PERCENTAGE OF USRDA
Sodium	(1,100–3,000)	mg	0	mg	0
Calcium	1,000	mg	58	mg	7
Phosphorus	(800–1,000)	mg	366	mg	45
Potassium	(1,875–5,625)	mg	300	mg	37
Magnesium	400	µg	44	µg	12
Selenium	200	µg	132	µg	66
Iodine	150	mg	0	mg	0
Zinc	15	mg	3	mg	20
Iron	10	mg	1	mg	12
Manganese	(2.5–5.0)	mg	0.04	mg	0
Copper	(2.0–3.0)	mg	1	mg	33

AMOUNT PER SERVING		CALORIES PER SERVING	% OF MEAL
Fat	7 grams	65	32
Proteins	34 grams	136	66
Carbohydrates	1 gram	4	2
Cholesterol	400 mg		
Amino acid (essential)			252–729
Fiber	0 grams		

Key: USRDA = Recommended Dietary Allowance
IU = International Unit
mg = milligrams
µg = micrograms
NOTE: The numbers with arrows exceed 100 percent of required USRDA.

MEATS RANKED IN THE HIGHEST ORDER FOR CHOLESTEROL MILLIGRAMS GIVEN EQUAL 3 OUNCES IN MOST INSTANCES

	CHOLESTEROL (MILLIGRAMS)
Liver, chicken	536.0
Liver, beef, fried	410.0
Liver, calf	331.0
Kidney, veal	329.0
Liver, calf, fried	280.0
Beef, corned, hash	206.0
Chicken, pot pie, 8 oz	175.0
Beef, meatballs, 1.5 inch dia	169.0
Beef, chili, with beans	133.0
Beef, meatloaf	125.6
Chicken, diced, 1 cup	116.0
Chicken liver pate, 1 oz.	111.0
Veal, cutlets	109.0
Beef, Sloppy Joe	105.0
Pork, spare ribs	103.0
Beef, Philadelphia steak	99.0
Pork, chop, loin	91.0
Beef, tongue	91.0
Chicken, breast, fried	88.0
Veal, breast	84.0
Veal, chop	84.0
Beef, corned, cooked	83.0
Pork, steak, lean	83.0
Chicken, breast, roasted, 3 $\frac{1}{2}$ oz	83.0
Rabbit	82.0
Goose, roasted, without skin	82.0
Beef, ground patty	80.0
Ham, fresh	80.0
Lamb, loin chop	79.0
Pork, tenderloin	79.0
Beef, short ribs, lean	79.0
Beef, brisket, lean/fat	79.0
Turkey, white meat, diced, 1 cup	77.0
Goose, roasted	77.0
Turkey, dark meat	76.0

(*continued*)

MEATS RANKED IN THE HIGHEST ORDER FOR CHOLESTEROL MILLIGRAMS GIVEN EQUAL 3 OUNCES IN MOST INSTANCES (continued)

	CHOLESTEROL (MILLIGRAMS)
Duck, roasted, without skin	76.0
Beef, steak, sirloin lean	76.0
Lamb, gyros	76.0
Beef, ground, 70% lean	76.0
Pork, butt	75.0

CHAPTER NINE

Healing and Preventive Recipes for Constipation

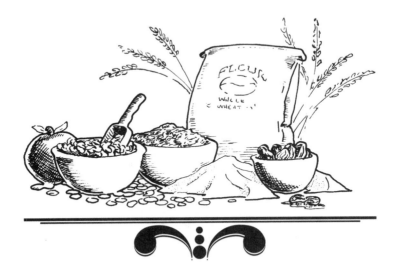

Let food be your medicine and medicine be your food.

Hippocrates

In spite of the strong emphasis on fiber alone as an antidote for constipation, many researchers advocate regular exercise combined with a balanced diet with a reasonable fiber content as the best strategy for preventing constipation.

Throughout the recipes in this chapter, in the "Tip" section you will find up-to-date reports and explanations regarding dietary fiber, constipation, and what the current thinking is on the use of fiber. Everyone seems to agree that both kinds of fiber, soluble and insoluble, are helpful to the diet, although soluble gets second billing.

Such foods as bran, all whole grains, fruit, beans, whole wheat flour, rice, nuts, and of course, prunes are featured in the recipes that have been constructed to alleviate this problem. Another benefit of a diet that includes these ingredients is that bran found in food helps you to lose weight by making you feel full as you eat less. You will find Chicken Con Carne not only full of fiber but full of taste surprises.

Carrot Cabbage

Ingredients:

3 carrots, shredded
1 lb green cabbage
1 quart water
1 Tbs brown sugar
½ tsp salt
1 tsp garlic powder
1 ½ cup skimmed milk
½ cup whole wheat flour
1 tsp dill
¼ tsp oregano
3 Tbs Parmesan cheese

Preparation: Bake and boil

Time: 1 hour, 20 minutes

Calories: 185 per serving

Serves: 4

Directions

Preheat oven to 425° F. Removing the core from cabbage, shred or chop finely, and mix with water, sugar, and salt. Bring to a boil, cover, and cook over a low heat about one hour. Remove cabbage and drain. Steam carrots for about 5 minutes. Combine the milk, flour, and garlic powder. Bring to a boil stirring. Combine with the cabbage. Stir in 1 tablespoon of the cheese and blend. Pour cabbage mixture into a baking pan. Sprinkle dill, oregano, and remaining cheese over all; bake until thoroughly heated and cheese has melted. This meal has very high vitamin A content with good fiber amounts.

TIP: Too many fiber-filled foods could interfere with your body's ability to make use of the calcium, magnesium, zinc, and iron you eat, but only, says Dr. James Anderson, chief of the endocrine metabolism section of The Veterans Administration Medical Center in Lexington, Kentucky, if you overdo it by ingesting large quantities. The advice when switching to high-fiber eating is to go slowly at first.

MYTH: Fat and cholesterol must be monitored in a child's diet as soon as he or she starts eating solid food.

FACT: A low-fat, low-cholesterol diet applies only after the age of 2, according to the American Heart Association. Diets for children age 2 and up are like those for adults.

Nutrients Contained in: Carrot Cabbage

VITAMINS USRDA			ONE SERVING GIVES YOU APPROXIMATELY		APPROXIMATE PERCENTAGE OF USRDA
A	5,000	IU	15,357	IU	307◄
B$_1$	1.4	mg	0.23	mg	18
B$_2$	1.6	mg	0.23	mg	16
B$_3$	16	mg	2	mg	9
B$_5$	10	mg	0.59	mg	5
B$_6$	2.2	mg	0.28	mg	12
B$_{12}$	3	μg	0.36	μg	12
C	60	mg	60	mg	100◄
D	400	IU	38	IU	9
E	15	IU	2	IU	10
K	500	μg	125	μg	25
Folic Acid	400	μg	85	μg	21

MINERALS USRDA			ONE SERVING GIVES YOU APPROXIMATELY		APPROXIMATE PERCENTAGE OF USRDA
Sodium	(1,100–3,000)	mg	158	mg	15
Calcium	1,000	mg	244	mg	30
Phosphorus	(800–1,000)	mg	175	mg	21
Potassium	(1,875–5,625)	mg	681	mg	85
Magnesium	400	μg	59	μg	16
Selenium	200	μg	3	μg	1
Iodine	150	mg	5	mg	3
Zinc	15	mg	1	mg	7
Iron	10	mg	2	mg	18
Manganese	(2.5–5.0)	mg	0.26	mg	5
Copper	(2.0–3.0)	mg	0.10	mg	3

AMOUNT PER SERVING		CALORIES PER SERVING	% OF MEAL
Fat	2 grams	17	9
Proteins	9 grams	34	19
Carbohydrates	33 grams	134	72
Cholesterol	5 mg		
Amino acid (essential)			86–109
Fiber	3 grams		

Key: USRDA = Recommended Dietary Allowance

    IU = International Unit

    mg = milligrams

    μg = micrograms

NOTE: The numbers with arrows exceed 100 percent of required USRDA.

The Big Herb with Beans

Ingredients:

2 cups spinach, shredded
2 Tbs prune juice
3 cloves garlic, chopped
½ cup cooked chick peas
1 cup cooked navy beans
1 tsp vegetable oil
1 tomato
1 cup onion, chopped
   coarsely
2 Tbs horseradish
¼ tsp marjoram
1 tsp chervil
   juice of one lemon
¼ tsp cinnamon

Preparation: No cooking required

Time: 30 minutes

Calories: 231 per serving

Serves: 4

Directions

Mix prune juice, oil, and horseradish in a medium bowl. Add the garlic, oregano, marjoram, chervil, and lemon juice. In a larger bowl, combine the spinach, chick peas, navy beans, tomatoes, and onions; sprinkle cinnamon on top. Pour the dressing and mix together and serve. High vitamin A, folic acid, potassium, and fiber are shown in the chart.

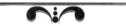

TIP: Physicians say inactivity can also contribute to constipation. Exercises like jogging, aerobics, and brisk walking are recommended to help stimulate the bowel. Any increased activity will be beneficial.

MYTH: Constipation is caused by disease.

FACT: There is no evidence that disease causes constipation. According to Dr. Marvin M. Lipman, medical adviser at Consumers Union, life-style and living habits are more likely the cause. He says the most common problem is too little fiber in the diet.

Nutrients Contained in: The Big Herb with Beans

VITAMINS USRDA			ONE SERVING GIVES YOU APPROXIMATELY		APPROXIMATE PERCENTAGE OF USRDA
A	5,000	IU	7,733	IU	154◄
B₁	1.4	mg	0.28	mg	23
B₂	1.6	mg	0.31	mg	22
B₃	16	mg	2	mg	10
B₅	10	mg	0.58	mg	5
B₆	2.2	mg	0.42	mg	19
B₁₂	3	μg	0	μg	0
C	60	mg	18	mg	30
D	400	IU	0	IU	0
E	15	IU	5	IU	30
K	500	μg	93	μg	18
Folic Acid	400	μg	142	μg	35

MINERALS USRDA			ONE SERVING GIVES YOU APPROXIMATELY		APPROXIMATE PERCENTAGE OF USRDA
Sodium	(1,100–3,000)	mg	85	mg	8
Calcium	1,000	mg	202	mg	25
Phosphorus	(800–1,000)	mg	233	mg	29
Potassium	(1,875–5,625)	mg	1,019	mg	127◄
Magnesium	400	μg	128	μg	36
Selenium	200	μg	13	μg	6
Iodine	150	mg	0	mg	0
Zinc	15	mg	2	mg	13
Iron	10	mg	7	mg	67
Manganese	(2.5–5.0)	mg	1	mg	25
Copper	(2.0–3.0)	mg	0.42	mg	14

AMOUNT PER SERVING		CALORIES PER SERVING	% OF MEAL
Fat	4 grams	32	14
Proteins	13 grams	50	22
Carbohydrates	37 grams	149	64
Cholesterol	0 mg		
Amino acid (essential)			157–307
Fiber	3 grams		

Key: USRDA = Recommended Dietary Allowance
IU = International Unit
mg = milligrams
μg = micrograms
NOTE: The numbers with arrows exceed 100 percent of required USRDA.

Arabian Pockets

Ingredients:

- ½ cup lentils
- 1 cup canned chick peas
- 1 cup low-sodium chicken broth
- ½ cup bulgur
- 4 cloves garlic
- 2 Tbs whole wheat flour
- ½ cup wheat germ
- 1 Tbs lemon juice
- 2 Tbs tomato paste
- 1 egg white
- 1 tsp sunflower seeds
- 1 cup nonfat sour cream
- 1 tsp vegetable oil
- 4 whole wheat pita bread
- 1 cup diced tomatoes
- 1 tsp oregano
- 2 tsp tarragon
- ¼ cup bean sprouts

Preparation: Sauté, boil

Time: 1 hour, 20 minutes

Calories: 512 per serving

Serves: 4

Directions

Place lentils in a saucepan with water to cover. Bring to a boil, reduce heat, and let simmer for about 30 minutes. Drain chick peas from can and puree peas and lentils in a blender. Bring half cup of broth to a boil and add the bulgur, garlic, and sunflower seeds. Cover, remove from heat, and let stand about 30 minutes. Add to the chick peas and lentil mixture. In the same pan blend together the whole wheat flour, tomato paste, and remaining broth. Cook until the mixture becomes thick. Add to the chick peas and lentils. Add wheat germ, oregano, tarragon, and lemon juice. Mix ingredients well, cover, and refrigerate for 40 minutes or longer. Use the mixture to form 14 cakes about ½ inch thick. In a small bowl, beat the egg white adding a little water. Dip the cakes into the mixture and coat with more wheat germ. Use a large skillet and sauté the cakes in the oil until done on both sides. Serve in the pita pockets with the tomatoes, sour cream, and bean sprouts.

TIP: Counting grams can be tedious, but Dr. Peter Greenwald, director of the division of cancer control at the National Cancer Institute, says you don't really need to count fiber grams. The foods that are high in fiber are the complex carbohydrates that nutritionists are already telling you to add to your diet such as dried peas and beans.

Nutrients Contained in: Arabian Pockets

VITAMINS USRDA			ONE SERVING GIVES YOU APPROXIMATELY		APPROXIMATE PERCENTAGE OF USRDA
A	5,000	IU	921	IU	18
B₁	1.4	mg	0.83	mg	70
B₂	1.6	mg	0.98	mg	70
B₃	16	mg	6	mg	38
B₅	10	mg	1	mg	13
B₆	2.2	mg	0.73	mg	32
B₁₂	3	μg	0.05	μg	1
C	60	mg	22	mg	37
D	400	IU	0	IU	0
E	15	IU	2	IU	12
K	500	μg	0	μg	0
Folic Acid	400	μg	112	μg	28

MINERALS USRDA			ONE SERVING GIVES YOU APPROXIMATELY		APPROXIMATE PERCENTAGE OF USRDA
Sodium	(1,100–3,000)	mg	348	mg	35
Calcium	1,000	mg	124	mg	16
Phosphorus	(800–1,000)	mg	404	mg	51
Potassium	(1,875–5,625)	mg	1,071	mg	134◄
Magnesium	400	μg	220	μg	63
Selenium	200	μg	5	μg	2
Iodine	150	mg	0	mg	0
Zinc	15	mg	5	mg	33
Iron	10	mg	8	mg	79
Manganese	(2.5–5.0)	mg	0.6	mg	20
Copper	(2.0–3.0)	mg	0.25	mg	8

AMOUNT PER SERVING		CALORIES PER SERVING	% OF MEAL
Fat	9 grams	78	26
Proteins	27 grams	108	42
Carbohydrates	81 grams	326	32
Cholesterol	0 mg		
Amino acid (essential)			216–326
Fiber	9 grams		

Key: USRDA = Recommended Dietary Allowance

IU = International Unit

mg = milligrams

μg = micrograms

NOTE: The numbers with arrows exceed 100 percent of required USRDA.

Semolina with Color

Ingredients:
- 1 cup couscous
- 1 ½ cups low-sodium chicken broth
- 1 ½ cups carrots, chopped
- 1 cup broccoli, chopped
- 2 cloves garlic, chopped
- 1 tsp paprika
- 1 tsp marjoram
- 2 Tbs dill
- 1 Tbs lemon juice
- ½ tsp oregano
- ½ tsp vegetable oil
- ½ tsp soy sauce

Preparation: Boil and sauté

Time: 30 minutes

Calories: 91 calories per serving

Serves: 4

Directions

Bring the broth to a boil in a large saucepan. Add the couscous. Cover and remove from heat. Let stand about 5 minutes. Heat oil and soy sauce in a skillet. Add the carrots and sauté for about 4 minutes; then add broccoli, garlic, and seasonings. Cook until vegetables are tender. Stir in lemon juice. Add the couscous and combine.

TIP: Gail Levey, R.D., a nutrition consultant in New York City, says insoluble fiber won't break down in water, but it does absorb water in the digestive tract, causing waste to move up and out at the best possible pace. Consequently, a diet high in insoluble fiber can prevent constipation, alleviate irritable bowel syndrome, and help cut down on intestinal disorders.

MYTH: Bananas are fattening.

FACT: Since one banana has only 105 calories, it is not fattening. And nutritionally, a banana is much better for you than fruit packed in syrup. A cup of pineapple in syrup, for example, has about 200 calories.

Nutrients Contained in: Semolina with Color

VITAMINS USRDA			ONE SERVING GIVES YOU APPROXIMATELY		APPROXIMATE PERCENTAGE OF USRDA
A	5,000	IU	5,509	IU	110◄
B$_1$	1.4	mg	0.12	mg	9
B$_2$	1.6	mg	0.11	mg	8
B$_3$	16	mg	2	mg	13
B$_5$	10	mg	0.22	mg	2
B$_6$	2.2	mg	0.09	mg	4
B$_{12}$	3	μg	0.11	μg	3
C	60	mg	33	mg	55
D	400	IU	0	IU	0
E	15	IU	0.43	IU	2
K	500	μg	138	μg	27
Folic Acid	400	μg	28	μg	6

MINERALS USRDA			ONE SERVING GIVES YOU APPROXIMATELY		APPROXIMATE PERCENTAGE OF USRDA
Sodium	(1,100–3,000)	mg	308	mg	30
Calcium	1,000	mg	29	mg	3
Phosphorus	(800–1,000)	mg	58	mg	7
Potassium	(1,875–5,625)	mg	289	mg	36
Magnesium	400	μg	20	μg	5
Selenium	200	μg	11	μg	5
Iodine	150	mg	0	mg	0
Zinc	15	mg	0.29	mg	1
Iron	10	mg	0.98	mg	9
Manganese	(2.5–5.0)	mg	0.10	mg	2
Copper	(2.0–3.0)	mg	0.03	mg	1

AMOUNT PER SERVING		CALORIES PER SERVING	% OF MEAL
Fat	1 gram	8	9
Proteins	5 grams	20	21
Carbohydrates	16 grams	63	70
Cholesterol	0 mg		
Amino acid (essential)			22–37*
Fiber	1 gram		

Key: USRDA = Recommended Dietary Allowance

　　　IU = International Unit

　　　mg = milligrams

　　　μg = micrograms

NOTE: The numbers with arrows exceed 100 percent of required USRDA.

*Complementary food—1 large egg raises EAA to 116–143%.

Grandma's Oats

Ingredients: 3 ½ cups dry oats
6 ½ cups water
⅓ cup rice bran
¼ tsp cinnamon

Preparation: Boil

Time: 30 minutes

Calories: 224 per serving
(about 7 ounces)

Serves: 4

Directions

Bring water to boil and stir in oats. Reduce heat and let the mixture cook slowly. Cook about 15 minutes, stirring occasionally. For a softer result, cover near the end of cooking time. Serve with cinnamon and rice bran sprinkled over top. A hearty meal.

TIP: Dietary fiber is plant material which is largely undigested and unabsorbed by the body. Fiber is not necessarily crucial to your health, says Dr. Marie Cassidy, professor of physiology at George Washington University in Washington, D.C. Unlike vitamins and minerals, fiber has no nutritional value per se, but it does have nutritional impact, says Cassidy.

MYTH: Defrosted food must be used immediately or thrown out.

FACT: If the food is safe to eat, it is safe to refreeze, according to the USDA Nutrition Center. The taste might not be up to par or the vitamins, however.

Nutrients Contained in: Grandma's Oats

VITAMINS USRDA			ONE SERVING GIVES YOU APPROXIMATELY		APPROXIMATE PERCENTAGE OF USRDA
A	5,000	IU	200	IU	3
B$_1$	1.4	mg	0.46	mg	38
B$_2$	1.6	mg	0.13	mg	8
B$_3$	16	mg	3	mg	18
B$_5$	10	mg	0.06	mg	2
B$_6$	2.2	mg	0.44	mg	19
B$_{12}$	3	µg	0	µg	0
C	60	mg	2	mg	2
D	400	IU	0	IU	0
E	15	IU	0	IU	0
K	500	µg	0	µg	0
Folic Acid	400	µg	0	µg	0

MINERALS USRDA			ONE SERVING GIVES YOU APPROXIMATELY		APPROXIMATE PERCENTAGE OF USRDA
Sodium	(1,100–3,000)	mg	0	mg	0
Calcium	1,000	mg	34	mg	4
Phosphorus	(800–1,000)	mg	19	mg	2
Potassium	(1,875–5,625)	mg	400	mg	49
Magnesium	400	µg	115	µg	32
Selenium	200	µg	0	µg	0
Iodine	150	mg	0	mg	0
Zinc	15	mg	2	mg	10
Iron	10	mg	3	mg	33
Manganese	(2.5–5.0)	mg	0.05	mg	1
Copper	(2.0–3.0)	mg	0.10	mg	3

AMOUNT PER SERVING		CALORIES PER SERVING	% OF MEAL
Fat	4 grams	33	15
Proteins	7 grams	28	12
Carbohydrates	41 grams	163	73
Cholesterol	0 mg		
Amino acid (essential)			very low*
Fiber	1 gram		

Key: USRDA = Recommended Dietary Allowance
    IU = International Unit
    mg = milligrams
    µg = micrograms
NOTE: The numbers with arrows exceed 100 percent of required USRDA.
*Complementary food—1 cup lima beans raises EAA to 149–427%.

Bulgur Variations

Ingredients:

1 cup bulgur wheat
1 cup zucchini, chopped fine
1 cup spring onions, chopped fine
½ cup mint, chopped
½ cup lemon juice
2 tomatoes, chopped
2 cloves garlic, minced
romaine lettuce leaves

Preparation: Boil

Time: 4 hours

Calories: 115 per serving

Serves: 4

Directions

Cover bulgur wheat and zucchini with boiling water and let soak for 2 hours. Drain. Add the remaining ingredients and mix thoroughly. Let stand for 2 hours or longer in refrigerator. Serve in a bowl and garnish with romaine lettuce leaves.

TIP: If you forget to increase the amount of fluids you drink while gradually adding bran to your diet, you may develop excessive gas, stomach cramps, and/or diarrhea. And too much bran can prevent absorption of some essential nutrients.

MYTH: You should avoid jelly and jam as they contain loads of calories.

FACT: A tablespoon of jelly on your toast adds only 50 calories; a tablespoon of jam, 55. And they are without saturated fat or cholesterol. The same amount of butter contains about 100 calories and is 100 percent saturated fat.

Nutrients Contained in: Bulgur Variations

VITAMINS USRDA			ONE SERVING GIVES YOU APPROXIMATELY		APPROXIMATE PERCENTAGE OF USRDA
A	5,000	IU	1,834	IU	36
B$_1$	1.4	mg	0.19	mg	16
B$_2$	1.6	mg	0.45	mg	31
B$_3$	16	mg	6	mg	39
B$_5$	10	mg	3	mg	29
B$_6$	2.2	mg	0.23	mg	10
B$_{12}$	3	μg	0.09	μg	2
C	60	mg	37	mg	61
D	400	IU	0	IU	0
E	15	IU	0.89	IU	5
K	500	μg	80	μg	16
Folic Acid	400	μg	63	μg	15

MINERALS USRDA			ONE SERVING GIVES YOU APPROXIMATELY		APPROXIMATE PERCENTAGE OF USRDA
Sodium	(1,100–3,000)	mg	20	mg	2
Calcium	1,000	mg	51	mg	6
Phosphorus	(800–1,000)	mg	182	mg	22
Potassium	(1,875–5,625)	mg	791	mg	98
Magnesium	400	μg	53	μg	15
Selenium	200	μg	15	μg	7
Iodine	150	mg	0	mg	0
Zinc	15	mg	2	mg	10
Iron	10	mg	4	mg	36
Manganese	(2.5–5.0)	mg	0.38	mg	7
Copper	(2.0–3.0)	mg	0.72	mg	23

AMOUNT PER SERVING		CALORIES PER SERVING	% OF MEAL
Fat	1 gram	8	7
Proteins	6 grams	22	19
Carbohydrates	21 grams	85	74
Cholesterol	0 mg		
Amino acid (essential)			47–85[*]
Fiber	2 grams		

Key: USRDA = Recommended Dietary Allowance
   IU = International Unit
   mg = milligrams
   μg = micrograms
NOTE: The numbers with arrows exceed 100 percent of required USRDA.
[*]Complementary food—1 cup grape nut flakes raises EAA to 176–337%.

Bran Oat Wheatloaf

Ingredients:

1 cup wheat bran
1 cup bean sprouts
1 cup cooked brown rice
1 tsp vegetable oil
¼ cup beef broth
⅓ cup rice bran
⅓ cup dry oats
½ cup wheat germ
½ cup spring onions, minced
¼ tsp thyme
1 tsp savory
salt to taste

Preparation: Bake

Time: 35 minutes

Calories: 370 per serving

Serves: 4

Directions

Preheat oven to 400° F. Mix all ingredients together and bake in pan with a little oil for 35 minutes. Serve with a favorite type tomato or spaghetti. Very high EAA, magnesium, potassium, and manganese are recorded.

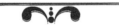

TIP: The National Cancer Institute recommends that everyone eat 20 to 30 grams of fiber a day. Yet the average American is reported to eat only about 11 grams daily. One easy way to increase your fiber intake is to include more bran in your diet. Bran has more dietary fiber than almost any other food.

MYTH: Apple juice is good for children who are thirsty.

FACT: Registered dietitian Mona Sutnick in Philadelphia says apple juice's nutritional benefits are negligible. So-called "100 percent apple juice" holds mostly water and fruit sugar. Apple juice cannot make up for a vitamin-poor diet. And some studies indicate that apple juice may cause chronic diarrhea in some children. Apricot nectar is a good choice.

Nutrients Contained in: Bran Oat Wheatloaf

VITAMINS	USRDA		ONE SERVING GIVES YOU APPROXIMATELY		APPROXIMATE PERCENTAGE OF USRDA
A	5,000	IU	708	IU	14
B₁	1.4	mg	0.80	mg	66
B₂	1.6	mg	0.29	mg	20
B₃	16	mg	6	mg	39
B₅	10	mg	2	mg	16
B₆	2.2	mg	1	mg	50
B₁₂	3	μg	0	μg	0
C	60	mg	18	mg	29
D	400	IU	0	IU	0
E	15	IU	1	IU	7
K	500	μg	95	μg	19
Folic Acid	400	μg	159	μg	39

MINERALS	USRDA		ONE SERVING GIVES YOU APPROXIMATELY		APPROXIMATE PERCENTAGE OF USRDA
Sodium	(1,100–3,000)	mg	8	mg	0
Calcium	1,000	mg	106	mg	13
Phosphorus	(800–1,000)	mg	359	mg	44
Potassium	(1,875–5,625)	mg	707	mg	88
Magnesium	400	μg	291	μg	83
Selenium	200	μg	34	μg	17
Iodine	150	mg	0	mg	0
Zinc	15	mg	5	mg	32
Iron	10	mg	5	mg	52
Manganese	(2.5–5.0)	mg	4	mg	87
Copper	(2.0–3.0)	mg	0.26	mg	8

AMOUNT PER SERVING		CALORIES PER SERVING	% OF MEAL
Fat	7 grams	65	18
Proteins	16 grams	65	18
Carbohydrates	60 grams	240	64
Cholesterol	0 mg		
Amino acid (essential)			157–224
Fiber	2 grams		

Key: USRDA = Recommended Dietary Allowance

IU = International Unit

mg = milligrams

μg = micrograms

NOTE: The numbers with arrows exceed 100 percent of required USRDA.

Chicken Con Carne

Ingredients:

1 lb ground chicken
1 onion, chopped
1 tsp Brewer's yeast
2 cups canned tomatoes
1 tsp chili powder
1 cup Picante sauce
2 cups cooked kidney
   beans
½ tsp garlic powder
¼ tsp oregano
1 tsp vegetable oil

Preparation: Sauté and simmer

Time: 50 minutes

Calories: 202 per serving

Serves: 4

Directions

In a large skillet sauté onions until golden. Add ground chicken, oregano, and garlic and continue to simmer for a few minutes stirring throughout. Add remaining ingredients and simmer for 30 minutes. Add a little water if mixture gets dry. This dish is high in fiber.

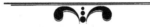

TIP: When choosing bran cereals, choose those containing at least 3 grams of dietary fiber per serving. A good choice will contain no more than 1 or 2 grams of fat per serving and fewer than 5 or 6 grams of sugar.

MYTH: Cottage cheese is a terrific diet food.

FACT: Not unless it is a low-fat cottage cheese. A cup of large-curd cottage cheese that is 4 percent fat has 235 calories, and the fat represents 40 percent of the calories.

Nutrients Contained in: Chicken Con Carne

VITAMINS USRDA			ONE SERVING GIVES YOU APPROXIMATELY		APPROXIMATE PERCENTAGE OF USRDA
A	5,000	IU	191	IU	3
B$_1$	1.4	mg	1	mg	97
B$_2$	1.6	mg	0.35	mg	24
B$_3$	16	mg	6	mg	37
B$_5$	10	mg	0.98	mg	9
B$_6$	2.2	mg	0.38	mg	17
B$_{12}$	3	μg	0.84	μg	27
C	60	mg	13	mg	21
D	400	IU	0	IU	0
E	15	IU	4	IU	26
K	500	μg	0	μg	0
Folic Acid	400	μg	234	μg	58

MINERALS USRDA			ONE SERVING GIVES YOU APPROXIMATELY		APPROXIMATE PERCENTAGE OF USRDA
Sodium	(1,100–3,000)	mg	149	mg	14
Calcium	1,000	mg	81	mg	10
Phosphorus	(800–1,000)	mg	295	mg	36
Potassium	(1,875–5,625)	mg	696	mg	87
Magnesium	400	μg	34	μg	9
Selenium	200	μg	0.80	μg	0
Iodine	150	mg	0	mg	0
Zinc	15	mg	1	mg	7
Iron	10	mg	4	mg	39
Manganese	(2.5–5.0)	mg	0.08	mg	1
Copper	(2.0–3.0)	mg	0.68	mg	22

AMOUNT PER SERVING		CALORIES PER SERVING	% OF MEAL
Fat	3 grams	25	12
Proteins	16 grams	64	32
Carbohydrates	28 grams	113	56
Cholesterol	20 mg		
Amino acid (essential)			240–539
Fiber	7 grams		

Key: USRDA = Recommended Dietary Allowance

IU = International Unit

mg = milligrams

μg = micrograms

NOTE: The numbers with arrows exceed 100 percent of required USRDA.

Really Stuffed Green and Red Pepper

Ingredients:

4 peppers, 2 red and 2 green
½ cup oat bran
½ cup wheat germ
1 cup okra
1 cup tomato paste
1 cup cooked brown rice
1 tsp soy sauce
1 tsp savory
½ cup onion, chopped
1 tsp vegetable oil

Preparation: Bake and sauté

Time: 1 hour, 10 minutes

Calories: 336 per serving

Serves: 4

Directions

Preheat oven to 400° F. Prepare peppers by placing them in a baking pan after they have been washed, cored, and seeded. Add a little hot water to cover the bottom of the dish. Meanwhile sauté chopped onions in oil and soy sauce until soft. Add oat bran, wheat germ, okra, rice, and savory to skillet and heat through. Remove from heat and fill each pepper with mixture. If there is mixture left over, use additional peppers and fill. Bake for about 40 minutes or until peppers are tender. This gives a lot of vitamin C, potassium, iron, and B_1.

TIP: Linda Van Horn, Ph.D., R.D. at Chicago's Northwestern University Medical School, indicates that the number one fiber-rich food is bran, which promotes regularity, fends off diseases of the gastrointestinal tract, and improves blood sugar control in diabetics. Oat bran seems to be the best.

MYTH: You must feel pain to benefit from exercise.

FACT: Sports experts say that actual pain can be a sign of injury and indicates that too much exercise has been done. One could have a sprain, or one could strain muscles. The suggestion is to warm up and exercise slowly, gradually increasing your exercise maximum.

Nutrients Contained in: Really Stuffed Green and Red Pepper

VITAMINS USRDA			ONE SERVING GIVES YOU APPROXIMATELY		APPROXIMATE PERCENTAGE OF USRDA
A	5,000	IU	2,615	IU	52
B$_1$	1.4	mg	0.66	mg	54
B$_2$	1.6	mg	0.26	mg	18
B$_3$	16	mg	6	mg	35
B$_5$	10	mg	0.86	mg	8
B$_6$	2.2	mg	0.52	mg	23
B$_{12}$	3	μg	0	μg	0
C	60	mg	119	mg	198◄
D	400	IU	0	IU	0
E	15	IU	2	IU	12
K	500	μg	0	μg	0
Folic Acid	400	μg	89	μg	20

MINERALS USRDA			ONE SERVING GIVES YOU APPROXIMATELY		APPROXIMATE PERCENTAGE OF USRDA
Sodium	(1,100–3,000)	mg	34	mg	3
Calcium	1,000	mg	66	mg	8
Phosphorus	(800–1,000)	mg	365	mg	45
Potassium	(1,875–5,625)	mg	984	mg	123◄
Magnesium	400	μg	116	μg	33
Selenium	200	μg	20	μg	10
Iodine	150	mg	0	mg	0
Zinc	15	mg	4	mg	23
Iron	10	mg	5	mg	54
Manganese	(2.5–5.0)	mg	4	mg	82
Copper	(2.0–3.0)	mg	0.49	mg	16

AMOUNT PER SERVING		CALORIES PER SERVING	% OF MEAL
Fat	3 grams	29	9
Proteins	12 grams	47	14
Carbohydrates	65 grams	260	77
Cholesterol	0 mg		
Amino acid (essential)			101–145
Fiber	2 grams		

Key: USRDA = Recommended Dietary Allowance
　　　IU = International Unit
　　　mg = milligrams
　　　μg = micrograms
NOTE: The numbers with arrows exceed 100 percent of required USRDA.

Pork Apple Love Affair

Ingredients:

1 lb boneless pork loin,
    cut in ½-inch cubes
4 apples, cored and sliced
1 tsp vegetable oil
2 Tbs whole wheat flour
½ cup apple cider
½ cup low-sodium
    chicken broth
½ cup brown sugar
2 Tbs lite soy sauce

Preparation: Sauté

Time: 25 minutes

Calories: 684 per serving

Serves: 5

Directions

Heat oil in a large skillet. Add pork loin cubes and brown on all sides. Add the sliced apples and sauté for 3 minutes. Add apple cider; reduce heat. Cover and simmer for 10 minutes. Mix broth with sugar and ¼ cup apple cider, whole wheat flour, soy sauce, and salt and pepper to season. Add this to skillet; cook over medium heat until sauce thickens. Stir occasionally. Serve with 1 cup cooked broccoli with pimento and sliced cucumber in a cup of plain yogurt with scallions if desired. Very high levels of B_1, potassium, and iron and tremendous EAA are recorded.

TIP: When eating oat bran, do not overeat, as a little goes a long way, and overeating is not a particularly good idea. Remember, when adding more fiber to your diet that the recommendation is to increase intake slowly and drink more water.

MYTH: You can determine if one has a fever by feeling the forehead.

FACT: This method is not considered to be very accurate, according to medical authorities. For a more accurate reading, use a thermometer and leave it in place at least 3 minutes.

Nutrients Contained in: Pork Apple Love Affair

VITAMINS USRDA			ONE SERVING GIVES YOU APPROXIMATELY		APPROXIMATE PERCENTAGE OF USRDA
A	5,000	IU	59	IU	1
B$_1$	1.4	mg	2	mg	137◄
B$_2$	1.6	mg	0.46	mg	33
B$_3$	16	mg	7	mg	43
B$_5$	10	mg	1	mg	10
B$_6$	2.2	mg	0.67	mg	30
B$_{12}$	3	μg	0.87	μg	29
C	60	mg	6	mg	10
D	400	IU	30	IU	7
E	15	IU	2	IU	10
K	500	μg	13	μg	2
Folic Acid	400	μg	24	μg	5

MINERALS USRDA			ONE SERVING GIVES YOU APPROXIMATELY		APPROXIMATE PERCENTAGE OF USRDA
Sodium	(1,100–3,000)	mg	572	mg	57
Calcium	1,000	mg	77	mg	9
Phosphorus	(800–1,000)	mg	409	mg	51
Potassium	(1,875–5,625)	mg	1,020	mg	127◄
Magnesium	400	μg	103	μg	29
Selenium	200	μg	57	μg	28
Iodine	150	mg	0	mg	0
Zinc	15	mg	2	mg	13
Iron	10	mg	9	mg	88
Manganese	(2.5–5.0)	mg	0.08	mg	1
Copper	(2.0–3.0)	mg	0.07	mg	2

AMOUNT PER SERVING		CALORIES PER SERVING	% OF MEAL
Fat	15 grams	138	20
Proteins	40 grams	162	24
Carbohydrates	96 grams	384	56
Cholesterol	100 mg		
Amino acid (essential)			234–695
Fiber	3 grams		

Key: USRDA = Recommended Dietary Allowance
      IU = International Unit
      mg = milligrams
      μg = micrograms
NOTE: The numbers with arrows exceed 100 percent of required USRDA.

Pork and Prunes

Ingredients:

4 boneless pork chops,
   1-inch thick
1 cup prunes
1 tsp lemon juice
2 Tbs tamari sauce
2 Tbs shallots, minced
2 Tbs brown sugar
1/2 tsp marjoram

Preparation: Broil

Time: 1 hour, 30 minutes

Calories: 432 per serving

Serves: 4

Directions

Preheat broiler. Combine tamari sauce, sugar, and shallots with lemon juice. Marinate the chops in this mixture for about an hour or more. Remove, saving marinade. Place prunes on top of chops. Sprinkle marjoram over all. Put chops in broiler, brush with marinade, and broil for 15 minutes on each side 5 inches from heat. Serve with cup of brown rice sprinkled with sesame seeds and a cup of broccoli if desired.

TIP: Psyllium, which has eight times as much soluble fiber as oat bran, is now being added to some cereals. It comes from the husk of an Indian-grown seed grain and has been used for some time in over-the-counter bulk laxatives.

MYTH: Organic food is always better than processed food.

FACT: According to nutritionists at the National Institutes of Health, organic foods can contain toxic substances and metals from soil and water. The advice given for maximum nutrition is to eat a balanced diet with a variety of foods.

Nutrients Contained in: Pork and Prunes

VITAMINS USRDA			ONE SERVING GIVES YOU APPROXIMATELY		APPROXIMATE PERCENTAGE OF USRDA
A	5,000	IU	485	IU	9
B$_1$	1.4	mg	0.97	mg	80
B$_2$	1.6	mg	0.36	mg	25
B$_3$	16	mg	6	mg	35
B$_5$	10	mg	0.86	mg	8
B$_6$	2.2	mg	0.57	mg	25
B$_{12}$	3	µg	0.86	µg	28
C	60	mg	6	mg	10
D	400	IU	15	IU	3
E	15	IU	0.20	IU	1
K	500	µg	0	µg	0
Folic Acid	400	µg	6	µg	1

MINERALS USRDA			ONE SERVING GIVES YOU APPROXIMATELY		APPROXIMATE PERCENTAGE OF USRDA
Sodium	(1,100–3,000)	mg	67	mg	6
Calcium	1,000	mg	29	mg	3
Phosphorus	(800–1,000)	mg	248	mg	30
Potassium	(1,875–5,625)	mg	563	mg	70
Magnesium	400	µg	38	µg	10
Selenium	200	µg	17	µg	8
Iodine	150	mg	0	mg	0
Zinc	15	mg	2	mg	15
Iron	10	mg	2	mg	17
Manganese	(2.5–5.0)	mg	0.07	mg	1
Copper	(2.0–3.0)	mg	0.19	mg	6

AMOUNT PER SERVING		CALORIES PER SERVING	% OF MEAL
Fat	29 grams	259	60
Proteins	21 grams	83	19
Carbohydrates	22 grams	90	21
Cholesterol	81 mg		
Amino acid (essential)			236–328
Fiber	1 gram		

Key: USRDA = Recommended Dietary Allowance
    IU = International Unit
    mg = milligrams
    µg = micrograms
NOTE: The numbers with arrows exceed 100 percent of required USRDA.

Scotch Pearl Soup

Ingredients:

- 1 cup pearl barley
- 1 cup lentils
- 2 cloves garlic, minced
- 2 cups parsnips, peeled and chopped
- 8 shiitake mushrooms
- 2 Tbs lemon juice
- ⅓ cup rice bran
- 1 celery stalk, diced
- 4 potatoes, diced
- 1 bay leaf
- 1 large onion, chopped
- ¼ tsp chili powder
- tahini sauce to taste

Preparation: Boil

Time: 2 hours

Calories: 523 per serving

Serves: 4

Directions

Place barley in a saucepan and cook slowly for 30 minutes; add potatoes and lentils and cook another half-hour; add parsnips, rice, bran, celery, bay leaf, onions, chili powder, lemon juice, and mushrooms and cook another half-hour. Serve hot. This dish is high in fiber, potassium, B_3, B_6, and EAA.

TIP: Both kinds of fiber, soluble and insoluble, are described jointly as dietary fiber. The best sources of soluble fiber from oats are oatmeal and oat bran. A half cup of cooked blackeye peas has about 4 grams of fiber. Beans of every kind as well as peas and lentils are excellent sources.

MYTH: You should get a complete checkup every year.

FACT: Most medical authorities now say that a complete annual physical for everyone is a waste of time and money. The advice is to get a complete exam every five years after age 40, every two years after age 60, and every year after 75.

Nutrients Contained in: Scotch Pearl Soup

VITAMINS USRDA			ONE SERVING GIVES YOU APPROXIMATELY		APPROXIMATE PERCENTAGE OF USRDA
A	5,000	IU	24	IU	0
B$_1$	1.4	mg	0.50	mg	41
B$_2$	1.6	mg	0.14	mg	9
B$_3$	16	mg	9	mg	54
B$_5$	10	mg	1	mg	14
B$_6$	2.2	mg	0.89	mg	40
B$_{12}$	3	μg	0	μg	0
C	60	mg	21	mg	34
D	400	IU	0	IU	0
E	15	IU	1	IU	8
K	500	μg	0	μg	0
Folic Acid	400	μg	88	μg	21

MINERALS USRDA			ONE SERVING GIVES YOU APPROXIMATELY		APPROXIMATE PERCENTAGE OF USRDA
Sodium	(1,100–3,000)	mg	30	mg	3
Calcium	1,000	mg	77	mg	9
Phosphorus	(800–1,000)	mg	273	mg	34
Potassium	(1,875–5,625)	mg	1,231	mg	153◄
Magnesium	400	μg	156	μg	44
Selenium	200	μg	4	μg	1
Iodine	150	mg	0	mg	0
Zinc	15	mg	3	mg	22
Iron	10	mg	4	mg	44
Manganese	(2.5–5.0)	mg	0.26	mg	5
Copper	(2.0–3.0)	mg	0.38	mg	12

AMOUNT PER SERVING		CALORIES PER SERVING	% OF MEAL
Fat	2 grams	21	4
Proteins	15 grams	61	12
Carbohydrates	110 grams	441	84
Cholesterol	0 mg		
Amino acid (essential)			117–288
Fiber	3 grams		

Key: USRDA = Recommended Dietary Allowance
    IU = International Unit
    mg = milligrams
    μg = micrograms
NOTE: The numbers with arrows exceed 100 percent of required USRDA.

North African Stew

Ingredients:

1 cup couscous
1 cup lentils
½ head cabbage, shredded
1 green pepper, chopped
1 cup tomato paste
1 cup water
¼ cup apple juice
1 cup green onion, chopped
1 tsp vegetable oil
⅛ tsp cayenne pepper

Preparation: Sauté and simmer

Time: 55 minutes

Calories: 232 per serving

Serves: 4

Directions

Cook couscous according to package instructions, about 5 minutes. Set aside. Place lentils in a saucepan and cover with water. Bring to boil, reduce heat, and simmer for about 35 minutes. Drain and set aside. Heat oil in a large skillet and sauté peppers, cabbage, and onions. Add the tomato paste and water and apple juice. Bring to a boil and simmer for about 5 minutes. Sprinkle cayenne pepper on lentils and mix with the couscous. Pour tomato paste mixture over all and serve. Check the chart for high amounts of vitamins C and A, magnesium, EAA, and iron.

TIP: There are two types of fiber, soluble and insoluble. Insoluble is found in wheat bran, whole grains, beans, fruits, and vegetables. It goes through the digestive system adding bulk and softness aiding elimination. Researchers at the Northwestern University Medical School report that diets high in insoluble fiber seem to alleviate constipation and irritable bowel syndrome.

MYTH: Butter should be put on a burn to ease the pain.

FACT: Doctors say products such as butter tend to deepen the area of injury and can delay healing and lead to infection. Soap and cool water is suggested as a better approach to treating minor burns.

Nutrients Contained in: North African Stew

VITAMINS USRDA			ONE SERVING GIVES YOU APPROXIMATELY		APPROXIMATE PERCENTAGE OF USRDA
A	5,000	IU	3,636	IU	72
B$_1$	1.4	mg	0.32	mg	26
B$_2$	1.6	mg	0.22	mg	15
B$_3$	16	mg	3	mg	20
B$_5$	10	mg	0.90	mg	8
B$_6$	2.2	mg	0.28	mg	12
B$_{12}$	3	μg	0	μg	0
C	60	mg	117	mg	195◄
D	400	IU	0	IU	0
E	15	IU	3	IU	22
K	500	μg	50	μg	10
Folic Acid	400	μg	79	μg	19

MINERALS USRDA			ONE SERVING GIVES YOU APPROXIMATELY		APPROXIMATE PERCENTAGE OF USRDA
Sodium	(1,100–3,000)	mg	48	mg	4
Calcium	1,000	mg	104	mg	13
Phosphorus	(800–1,000)	mg	167	mg	30
Potassium	(1,875–5,625)	mg	543	mg	20
Magnesium	400	μg	1,097	μg	137◄
Selenium	200	μg	51	μg	14
Iodine	150	mg	14	mg	7
Zinc	15	mg	0.84	mg	5
Iron	10	mg	5	mg	50
Manganese	(2.5–5.0)	mg	0.22	mg	4
Copper	(2.0–3.0)	mg	0.19	mg	6

AMOUNT PER SERVING		CALORIES PER SERVING	% OF MEAL
Fat	2 grams	21	9
Proteins	10 grams	40	17
Carbohydrates	43 grams	171	74
Cholesterol	0 mg		
Amino acid (essential)			73–245
Fiber	2 grams		

Key: USRDA = Recommended Dietary Allowance
     IU = International Unit
    mg = milligrams
    μg = micrograms
NOTE: The numbers with arrows exceed 100 percent of required USRDA.

Peppers and Prunes

Ingredients:

- 2 large bell peppers
- 1 cup prunes, pitted and chopped
- 1 onion, chopped
- 4 cloves garlic, chopped finely
- $\frac{1}{8}$ tsp crushed red pepper
- 1 $\frac{1}{2}$ cup parsnips, chopped
- 1 cup red lentils
- 2 Tbs dill
- $\frac{1}{2}$ tsp cumin
- 1 cup low-sodium chicken broth

Preparation: Broil

Time: 1 hour

Calories: 170 per serving

Serves: 4

Directions

Cut peppers in half lengthwise and remove seeds. Place in broiler cut side down and broil about 6 minutes or until soft. Remove from broiler. Use nonstick spray for skillet, and sauté onion, parsnips, and garlic about 5 minutes. Add crushed red pepper, cumin, lentils, and chicken broth. Bring to a boil, cover, and simmer 30 minutes. During last 5 minutes stir in dill and prunes. Spoon this mixture in pepper halves and heat for a minute before serving. Good amount of vitamins C and E, iron, and fiber are recorded.

TIP: Researchers in the 1960s said prunes stimulated the intestines and now modern researchers are agreeing. A study similar to the Boston University School of Medicine study in the 1960s found that after measuring the daily output of fluid of a number of subjects, prune juice was confirmed as the most potent food of a variety eaten to stimulate intestinal fluid output.

MYTH: The slogan that says "laxatives are safe and gentle" has validity.

FACT: Consumers Union of the United States says research indicates that when used regularly, all laxatives tend to cause a weakening of bowel functioning and create dependence.

Nutrients Contained in: Peppers and Prunes

VITAMINS USRDA			ONE SERVING GIVES YOU APPROXIMATELY		APPROXIMATE PERCENTAGE OF USRDA
A	5,000	IU	632	IU	12
B$_1$	1.4	mg	0.10	mg	8
B$_2$	1.6	mg	0.12	mg	8
B$_3$	16	mg	1	mg	8
B$_5$	10	mg	0.83	mg	8
B$_6$	2.2	mg	0.38	mg	17
B$_{12}$	3	μg	0.04	μg	1
C	60	mg	56	mg	92
D	400	IU	0	IU	0
E	15	IU	2	IU	10
K	500	μg	0	μg	0
Folic Acid	400	μg	38	μg	9

MINERALS USRDA			ONE SERVING GIVES YOU APPROXIMATELY		APPROXIMATE PERCENTAGE OF USRDA
Sodium	(1,100–3,000)	mg	105	mg	10
Calcium	1,000	mg	56	mg	6
Phosphorus	(800–1,000)	mg	97	mg	12
Potassium	(1,875–5,625)	mg	572	mg	71
Magnesium	400	μg	48	μg	13
Selenium	200	μg	4	μg	1
Iodine	150	mg	0	mg	0
Zinc	15	mg	0.81	mg	5
Iron	10	mg	2	mg	24
Manganese	(2.5–5.0)	mg	0.18	mg	3
Copper	(2.0–3.0)	mg	0.30	mg	9

AMOUNT PER SERVING		CALORIES PER SERVING	% OF MEAL
Fat	1 gram	5	3
Proteins	6 grams	25	15
Carbohydrates	35 grams	140	82
Cholesterol	0 mg		
Amino acid (essential)			49–188
Fiber	2 grams		

Key: USRDA = Recommended Dietary Allowance
     IU = International Unit
     mg = milligrams
     μg = micrograms
NOTE: The numbers with arrows exceed 100 percent of required USRDA.

Double Rice

Ingredients:

1 cup brown rice
2 cups hot water
1 cup low-sodium
   chicken broth
1 cup onion, chopped
½ cup green peppers,
   seeded and chopped
4 shiitake mushrooms,
   chopped
1 cup peas
⅓ cup rice bran
1 Tbs Worcestershire sauce
1 tsp vegetable oil

Preparation: Sauté and bake

Time: 1 hour, 15 minutes

Calories: 300 per serving

Serves: 4

Directions

Preheat oven to 400° F. Sauté onion and pepper in oil until soft. Add rice, mushrooms, peas, and Worcestershire sauce and heat through for a minute. Turn all ingredients including mushrooms into a baking dish. Cover and bake, stirring occasionally, for about 1 hour.

TIP: Harvard Medical School publications say that people with basically normal bowel function going through temporary discomfort with constipation can probably be helped by increasing their dietary fiber intake, drinking plenty of water, and engaging in moderate amounts of exercise.

MYTH: Waste products need to be eliminated regularly; otherwise, the body will suffer contamination.

FACT: Physicians say that the frequency of bowel movements vary among healthy people, from three a day to three a week. The report is that if you have comfortable movements and do not feel bloated, you are not constipated.

Nutrients Contained in: Double Rice

VITAMINS USRDA			ONE SERVING GIVES YOU APPROXIMATELY		APPROXIMATE PERCENTAGE OF USRDA
A	5,000	IU	310	IU	6
B$_1$	1.4	mg	0.48	mg	40
B$_2$	1.6	mg	0.14	mg	9
B$_3$	16	mg	8	mg	47
B$_5$	10	mg	0.60	mg	6
B$_6$	2.2	mg	0.67	mg	30
B$_{12}$	3	μg	0.08	μg	2
C	60	mg	26	mg	43
D	400	IU	0	IU	0
E	15	IU	1	IU	7
K	500	μg	110	μg	22
Folic Acid	400	μg	48	μg	12

MINERALS USRDA			ONE SERVING GIVES YOU APPROXIMATELY		APPROXIMATE PERCENTAGE OF USRDA
Sodium	(1,100–3,000)	mg	460	mg	42
Calcium	1,000	mg	37	mg	4
Phosphorus	(800–1,000)	mg	167	mg	20
Potassium	(1,875–5,625)	mg	495	mg	26
Magnesium	400	μg	128	μg	32
Selenium	200	μg	20	μg	10
Iodine	150	mg	0	mg	0
Zinc	15	mg	3	mg	20
Iron	10	mg	3	mg	31
Manganese	(2.5–5.0)	mg	1	mg	40
Copper	(2.0–3.0)	mg	0.19	mg	9

AMOUNT PER SERVING		CALORIES PER SERVING	% OF MEAL
Fat	3 grams	26	9
Proteins	10 grams	38	13
Carbohydrates	59 grams	236	78
Cholesterol	0 mg		
Amino acid (essential)			54–90
Fiber	1 gram		

Key: USRDA = Recommended Dietary Allowance
    IU = International Unit
    mg = milligrams
    μg = micrograms
NOTE: The numbers with arrows exceed 100 percent of required USRDA.

VEGETABLES RANKED IN THE HIGHEST ORDER FOR DIETARY FIBER MILLIGRAMS GIVEN EQUAL AMOUNTS FOR ½ CUP

	DIETARY FIBER (MILLIGRAMS)	PERCENTAGE OF USRDA
Beans, kidney, canned	10.0	35.7
Beans, pinto, cooked	9.4	33.6
Beans, lima, cooked	7.4	26.4
Beans, baked, pork/sauce	6.0	21.4
Beans, fava, canned	6.0	21.4
Peas, blackeye, canned	5.7	20.4
Peas, frozen	5.7	20.4
Peas, canned, low salt	5.0	17.9
Beans, baked, plain	5.0	17.9
Parsnips, cooked	4.9	17.5
Corn, cooked, ½ cup	4.7	16.8
Potato, baked, with skin	4.4	15.7
Corn on the cob, cooked	3.9	13.9
Broccoli, cooked	3.8	13.6
Potato, sweet	3.7	13.2
Corn, canned	3.3	11.8
Brussels sprouts, frozen	3.2	11.4
Spinach, frozen	3.1	11.1
Beans, mung, cooked	3.0	10.7
Carrots, canned	2.9	10.4

CHAPTER TEN

Healing and Preventive Recipes for Cataracts

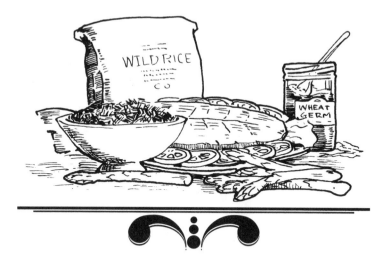

I have learned silence from the talkative, tolerance from the intolerant, and kindness from the unkind; yet strange, I am ungrateful to these teachers.
—Kahil Gibran

Foods that contain antioxidant nutrients are identified as being effective in warding off cataracts. Dr. Allen Taylor, head of nutrition and vision research at the U.S. Department of Agriculture's Nutrition Research Center at Tufts University, indicates that poor nutrition is often associated with cataract formation. USDA researchers have found that eating vitamin-rich fruits and vegetables helps to lower the risk of aging-related cataracts.

Singled out as effective antioxidant fighters are vitamins C and E. The current Recommended Daily Allowance (USRDA) for vitamin E is 15 milligrams for men and 12 milligrams for women; 3 ounces of wheat germ will give you about this much. It is estimated, however, that the median intake of vitamin E is lower than the USRDA, ranging between 7.4 and 9 milligrams.

Naturally, the recipes have been formulated to give you as much of vitamins E and C that you can get from eating without taking a supplement. If you find that you want to take vitamin E supplements, it is always advisable to check with your physician. In the meantime, enjoy such tasty delights as Dandy Halibut, Untamed Wild Rice (107 percent of RDA for vitamin E), and Elegant Asparagus. All the meals will provide you with ample amounts of vitamins E, C, A, B, and B_{12}, all antioxidant fighters.

There can be some confusion about vitamin E measurements as milligrams are sometimes used rather than International Units. In 1968 vitamin E was identified as an essential vitamin by the Food and Nutrition Board of the National Research Council. The body cannot manufacture its own vitamin E and must obtain it through foods. In 1968, the Food and Drug Administration set 30 IU as the Recommended Daily Allowance. In 1980 the Food and Nutrition Board of the National Research Council recommended 15 IU for adult men and 12 IU for adult women. The recipe nutritional charts use 15 IU.

RECOMMENDED DIETARY ALLOWANCES
FOR VITAMIN E

GROUP/AGE	VITAMIN E (MILLIGRAMS)
Infants 0–6 months	3
Infants 6–12 months	4
Children 1–3 years	5
Children 4–6 years	6
Children 7–10 years	7
Males 11–14 years	8
Males 15+ years	10
Females 11+ years	8
Pregnant women	10
Nursing women	11

Dandy Halibut

Ingredients:

1 ¾ lb halibut fillets
¼ dandelion, chopped
1 cup canned tomatoes
1 onion, finely chopped
¼ tsp basil
1 bay leaf
1 tsp dill
cayenne pepper
1 lime, sliced
red pepper, seeded
and diced
Tabasco sauce

Preparation: Bake

Time: 25 minutes

Calories: 215 per serving

Serves: 4

Directions

Preheat oven to 400° F. Put fillets in a baking pan. Sprinkle a little cayenne pepper on fillets. Toss the onion and red pepper around the fish. Spread the tomatoes over fish. Add the dandelion and bay leaf. Place thin slices of the lime over the fish and then the basil. Bake in oven for about 15 minutes. Test with a fork on the thickest part, and if fish flakes easily, it's ready. Sprinkle dill and diced red pepper over fillets and serve with a little Tabasco sauce. Observe the high percentage of EAA and vitamins A and B_3 (niacin).

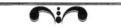

TIP: Researchers saturated eye lenses with vitamin E and then exposed them to sunlight. The vitamin E protected the lenses, which experienced only one-fifth the damage compared to lenses not protected in this way. Dr. Patrick Quillin pointed out that the *dissolving* ozone layer protects us from ultraviolet light.

MYTH: The label on foods that say "no cholesterol" means low in fat.

FACT: No food that comes from plants have cholesterol; this nutrient comes only from animal sources. Products made from vegetable oil will not have cholesterol, but could contain high amounts of saturated fats.

Nutrients Contained in: Dandy Halibut

VITAMINS USRDA			ONE SERVING GIVES YOU APPROXIMATELY		APPROXIMATE PERCENTAGE OF USRDA
A	5,000	IU	1,133	IU	22
B_1	1.4	mg	0.18	mg	14
B_2	1.6	mg	0.17	mg	11
B_3	16	mg	17	mg	107◄
B_5	10	mg	0.60	mg	6
B_6	2.2	mg	0.93	mg	42
B_{12}	3	μg	2	μg	66
C	60	mg	34	mg	57
D	400	IU	88	IU	22
E	15	IU	3	IU	18
K	500	μg	0	μg	0
Folic Acid	400	μg	33	μg	8

MINERALS USRDA			ONE SERVING GIVES YOU APPROXIMATELY		APPROXIMATE PERCENTAGE OF USRDA
Sodium	(1,100–3,000)	mg	219	mg	21
Calcium	1,000	mg	48	mg	6
Phosphorus	(800–1,000)	mg	626	mg	78
Potassium	(1,875–5,625)	mg	595	mg	74
Magnesium	400	μg	55	μg	15
Selenium	200	μg	0.18	μg	0
Iodine	150	mg	0	mg	0
Zinc	15	mg	2	mg	10
Iron	10	mg	2	mg	20
Manganese	(2.5–5.0)	mg	0.04	mg	7
Copper	(2.0–3.0)	mg	0.48	mg	16

AMOUNT PER SERVING		CALORIES PER SERVING	% OF MEAL
Fat	3 grams	24	11
Proteins	43 grams	171	80
Carbohydrates	5 grams	20	9
Cholesterol	100 mg		
Amino acid (essential)			246–597
Fiber	5 grams		

Key: USRDA = Recommended Dietary Allowance
    IU = International Unit
    mg = milligrams
    μg = micrograms
NOTE: The numbers with arrows exceed 100 percent of required USRDA.

Munchy Mollusks

Ingredients:

1 lb scallops
1 green pepper, seeded and sliced crosswise
½ cup shallots, minced
1 tsp celery seed
1 Tbs sour cream
2 ounces grated Romano cheese
1 cup black fungus mushrooms
2 Tbs rice bran
1 cucumber
½ tsp onion powder
   cayenne pepper
1 tsp lite soy sauce

Preparation: Bake

Time: 30 minutes

Calories: 430 per serving

Serves: 4

Directions

Preheat oven to 400° F. Steam scallops 1 to 2 minutes. Heat soy sauce in saucepan and add the mushrooms, green pepper, celery seed, shallots, and onion powder. Simmer for about 3 minutes. Add scallops and simmer for 2 minutes. Pour this mixture into a large baking dish, sprinkle rice bran and then the cheese. Bake scallops for 15 minutes. Chop cucumber in coarse pieces, add sour cream, mix well, and serve with scallops. Check the chart and observe the tremendous amount of vitamins and important minerals this meal gives.

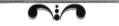

TIP: Dr. G. Edwin Bunce and Dr. John Hess of the Virginia Polytechnic Institute say that while cataracts in the elderly may not always be prevented, oxidative damage can be controlled earlier in life by using ultraviolet-absorbing sunglasses and wearing a brimmed hat. They add that vitamin E in the diet on a regular basis may help delay and slow the advance of cataracts.

MYTH: It is not safe for older people to lift weights.

FACT: William Evans, chief of the Human Physiology Laboratory at the U.S. Department of Agriculture's Human Nutrition Research Center says if it is done properly, weight-lifting doesn't increase heart rate or blood pressure and can be done without potential danger.

Nutrients Contained in: Munchy Mollusks

VITAMINS USRDA			ONE SERVING GIVES YOU APPROXIMATELY		APPROXIMATE PERCENTAGE OF USRDA
A	5,000	IU	1,396	IU	27
B_1	1.4	mg	0.14	mg	11
B_2	1.6	mg	0.52	mg	37
B_3	16	mg	65	mg	405◄
B_5	10	mg	0.28	mg	2
B_6	2.2	mg	1	mg	50
B_{12}	3	μg	51	μg	1,712◄
C	60	mg	19	mg	32
D	400	IU	0	IU	0
E	15	IU	2	IU	10
K	500	μg	1	μg	0
Folic Acid	400	μg	120	μg	30

MINERALS USRDA			ONE SERVING GIVES YOU APPROXIMATELY		APPROXIMATE PERCENTAGE OF USRDA
Sodium	(1,100–3,000)	mg	421	mg	42
Calcium	1,000	mg	234	mg	29
Phosphorus	(800–1,000)	mg	821	mg	102◄
Potassium	(1,875–5,625)	mg	1,363	mg	170◄
Magnesium	400	μg	110	μg	31
Selenium	200	μg	0.09	μg	0
Iodine	150	mg	0	mg	0
Zinc	15	mg	11	mg	70
Iron	10	mg	2	mg	24
Manganese	(2.5–5.0)	mg	0.05	mg	1
Copper	(2.0–3.0)	mg	0.07	mg	2

AMOUNT PER SERVING		CALORIES PER SERVING	% OF MEAL
Fat	7 grams	61	14
Proteins	50 grams	200	46
Carbohydrates	42 grams	169	40
Cholesterol	373 mg		
Amino acid (essential)			Over 100
Fiber	1 gram		

Key: USRDA = Recommended Dietary Allowance

IU = International Unit

mg = milligrams

μg = micrograms

NOTE: The numbers with arrows exceed 100 percent of required USRDA.

Savory Baked Chicken

Ingredients:

1 ¾ lb or 4 chicken breasts, halved, skinless
2 tomatoes, quartered
12 shiitake mushrooms
1 large onion, quartered
½ cup apple cider
juice of one lemon
½ cup wheat germ
½ cup nonfat yogurt
3 oz skimmed-milk mozzarella cheese
½ tsp thyme
½ oregano
dash cayenne pepper

Preparation: Bake
Time: 55 minutes
Calories: 328 per serving
Serves: 4

Directions

Preheat oven to 300° F. Use a shallow baking dish and place breasts snugly together in dish. Mix yogurt and wheat germ, adding apple juice slowly. Pour over chicken covering well. Then tuck in quarters of tomatoes and onion and mushrooms. Sprinkle oregano, thyme, and lemon over chicken and bake in oven for about 40 minutes. Near the end of baking time, sprinkle shredded mozzarella cheese over chicken and serve.

TIP: According to Dr. Patrick Quillin, writing in *Healing Nutrients*, a riboflavin deficiency (B₂) can lead to cataracts, especially in the elderly. Dr. Linus Pauling added that one of riboflavin's functions is to keep eyes healthy.

MYTH: Particular personality types are subject to high blood pressure.

FACT: Dr. Leonard Syme of the University of California at Berkeley says there's no evidence that any particular personality type is subject to high blood pressure. He says, however, that psychological and social stress may contribute to chronic hypertension.

Nutrients Contained in: Savory Baked Chicken

VITAMINS USRDA			ONE SERVING GIVES YOU APPROXIMATELY		APPROXIMATE PERCENTAGE OF USRDA
A	5,000	IU	707	IU	14
B_1	1.4	mg	0.32	mg	26
B_2	1.6	mg	0.26	mg	18
B_3	16	mg	9	mg	53
B_5	10	mg	0.72	mg	7
B_6	2.2	mg	0.49	mg	22
B_{12}	3	µg	0.29	µg	9
C	60	mg	21	mg	34
D	400	IU	0	IU	0
E	15	IU	0.82	IU	5
K	500	µg	4	µg	0
Folic Acid	400	µg	112	µg	27

MINERALS USRDA			ONE SERVING GIVES YOU APPROXIMATELY		APPROXIMATE PERCENTAGE OF USRDA
Sodium	(1,100–3,000)	mg	120	mg	12
Calcium	1,000	mg	144	mg	17
Phosphorus	(800–1,000)	mg	337	mg	42
Potassium	(1,875–5,625)	mg	672	mg	84
Magnesium	400	µg	106	µg	30
Selenium	200	µg	4	µg	2
Iodine	150	mg	0	mg	0
Zinc	15	mg	6	mg	41
Iron	10	mg	2	mg	21
Manganese	(2.5–5.0)	mg	3	mg	58
Copper	(2.0–3.0)	mg	0.16	mg	5

AMOUNT PER SERVING		CALORIES PER SERVING	% OF MEAL
Fat	7 grams	63	19
Proteins	21 grams	86	26
Carbohydrates	45 grams	179	55
Cholesterol	51 mg		
Amino acid (essential)			222–422
Fiber	0 grams		

Key: USRDA = Recommended Dietary Allowance
    IU = International Unit
    mg = milligrams
    µg = micrograms
NOTE: The numbers with arrows exceed 100 percent of required USRDA.

Untamed Wild Rice

Ingredients:

1 cup wild rice
2 tomatoes, finely chopped
¼ cup shallots, minced
¼ cup tomato paste
½ cup sunflower seeds
8 shiitake mushrooms, chopped
½ cup green pepper, seeded and diced
¼ tsp basil
½ tsp chili powder
1 tsp Adobo (Goya product) seasoning
1 cup water
1 cup low-sodium chicken broth

Preparation: Simmer

Time: 55 minutes

Calories: 410 per serving

Serves: 4

Directions

Pour rice into a large iron skillet. Add the tomato paste, water, chicken broth, chopped tomatoes, shallots, mushrooms, green pepper, and all seasonings. Mix all ingredients. Simmer covered for 40 minutes or until rice is dry. Add sunflower seeds 5 minutes before removing skillet from the flame. Wild rice triples in volume during cooking. Loads of vitamin E are found in this dish.

TIP: Linus Pauling, the famous vitamin C advocate, says there is ample evidence linking a low intake of vitamin C to cataract formation. He says vitamin C is important for good eye health as the concentration of vitamin C in the aqueous humor is very high. He adds that early cataracts are caused by exposure of the mother or the child to toxic substances, by malnutrition, and by certain diseases. He says that sunlight, high-energy radiation, infections, diabetes, and poor nutrition causes senile cataracts.

MYTH: Roaches are a sign of dirt and careless housekeeping.

FACT: USDA Agricultural Research Service entomologist Richard Brenner says that the cleanest kitchens can have roaches. He says there are 200 to 1,000 in hiding and they can live on nothing for as long as three weeks. They like warm, dark places and avoid the light. Brenner says airflow will drive them away.

Nutrients Contained in: Untamed Wild Rice

VITAMINS USRDA			ONE SERVING GIVES YOU APPROXIMATELY		APPROXIMATE PERCENTAGE OF USRDA
A	5,000	IU	2,190	IU	43
B_1	1.4	mg	0.62	mg	51
B_2	1.6	mg	0.16	mg	11
B_3	16	mg	6	mg	40
B_5	10	mg	0.96	mg	9
B_6	2.2	mg	0.53	mg	24
B_{12}	3	μg	0	μg	0
C	60	mg	31	mg	51
D	400	IU	0	IU	0
E	15	IU	16	IU	107◄
K	500	μg	5	μg	1
Folic Acid	400	μg	38	μg	9

MINERALS USRDA			ONE SERVING GIVES YOU APPROXIMATELY		APPROXIMATE PERCENTAGE OF USRDA
Sodium	(1,100–3,000)	mg	24	mg	2
Calcium	1,000	mg	65	mg	8
Phosphorus	(800–1,000)	mg	292	mg	36
Potassium	(1,875–5,625)	mg	768	mg	95
Magnesium	400	μg	81	μg	23
Selenium	200	μg	20	μg	9
Iodine	150	mg	0	mg	0
Zinc	15	mg	4	mg	26
Iron	10	mg	3	mg	34
Manganese	(2.5–5.0)	mg	1	mg	25
Copper	(2.0–3.0)	mg	0.49	mg	16

AMOUNT PER SERVING		CALORIES PER SERVING	% OF MEAL
Fat	10 grams	87	21
Proteins	12 grams	47	11
Carbohydrates	69 grams	276	68
Cholesterol	0 mg		
Amino acid (essential)			86–129
Fiber	2 grams		

Key: USRDA = Recommended Dietary Allowance
IU = International Unit
mg = milligrams
μg = micrograms
NOTE: The numbers with arrows exceed 100 percent of required USRDA.

Poor Man's Octopus

Ingredients:
- 2 lb squid
- 1 ½ cup onions, chopped
- 4 cloves garlic, minced
- 2 tomatoes
- ¼ cup parsley
- ½ cup water
- 1 tsp vegetable oil
- Tabasco sauce

Preparation: Simmer

Time: 1 ½ hours

Calories: 291 per serving

Serves: 4

Directions

Clean squid by removing intestines; cut off the head and wash. Cut in ½-inch rings. Heat the oil and sauté the onions and garlic. Add the squid, tomatoes, and a ½ cup of water. Season with pepper and Tabasco sauce. Cover and simmer for an hour. Serve with pasta. Sprinkle parsley over all. See chart for very high amounts of B_{12} and potassium.

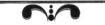

TIP: Researchers at the University of Western Ontario and others suggest that exposure to ultraviolet light is a major cause of cataracts. In some subsequent studies, vitamin E taken in large amounts helped to slow the formation of cataracts in animals exposed to ultraviolet light.

MYTH: Once you reach a certain age, it's too late to lower your cholesterol levels as the damage has already been done.

FACT: A study published in the *New England Journal of Medicine* indicates that you can benefit from lowering your cholesterol even if you already have cardiovascular disease. After following the health of over 2,000 men aged 40 to 69, researchers were able to conclude that lowering cholesterol is effective in reducing risk of death even if you have had a heart attack.

Nutrients Contained in: Poor Man's Octopus

VITAMINS USRDA			ONE SERVING GIVES YOU APPROXIMATELY		APPROXIMATE PERCENTAGE OF USRDA
A	5,000	IU	3,251	IU	65
B$_1$	1.4	mg	0.09	mg	7
B$_2$	1.6	mg	0.35	mg	24
B$_3$	16	mg	7	mg	46
B$_5$	10	mg	0.24	mg	2
B$_6$	2.2	mg	1	mg	46
B$_{12}$	3	μg	44	μg	1,470◄
C	60	mg	22	mg	37
D	400	IU	0	IU	0
E	15	IU	4	IU	27
K	500	μg	15	μg	1
Folic Acid	400	μg	44	μg	11

MINERALS USRDA			ONE SERVING GIVES YOU APPROXIMATELY		APPROXIMATE PERCENTAGE OF USRDA
Sodium	(1,100–3,000)	mg	885	mg	88
Calcium	1,000	mg	67	mg	8
Phosphorus	(800–1,000)	mg	40	mg	5
Potassium	(1,875–5,625)	mg	1,115	mg	139◄
Magnesium	400	μg	84	μg	23
Selenium	200	μg	2	μg	0
Iodine	150	mg	0	mg	0
Zinc	15	mg	12	mg	79
Iron	10	mg	2	mg	22
Manganese	(2.5–5.0)	mg	0.19	mg	3
Copper	(2.0–3.0)	mg	0.10	mg	3

AMOUNT PER SERVING		CALORIES PER SERVING	% OF MEAL
Fat	15 grams	42	14
Proteins	50 grams	198	68
Carbohydrates	13 grams	51	18
Cholesterol	528 mg		
Amino acid (essential)			Very high
Fiber	1 gram		

Key: USRDA = Recommended Dietary Allowance
    IU = International Unit
    mg = milligrams
    μg = micrograms
NOTE: The numbers with arrows exceed 100 percent of required USRDA.

Clam Special

Ingredients:

24 clams on the half shell
4 cloves garlic, minced
2 stalks celery, finely chopped
2 Tbs horseradish
½ cup scallions, minced
   juice of one lemon
½ cup mushrooms, chopped fine
½ tsp vegetable oil

Preparation: Bake

Time: 15 minutes

Calories: 377 per serving

Serves: 4

Directions

Preheat oven to 450° F. Heat oil in a saucepan and add garlic, celery, and scallions. Sauté for 2 to 3 minutes. Spoon this mixture over the half-shell clams and top with a few drops of soy sauce and the chopped mushrooms. Bake in oven for about 5 minutes. Add horseradish to each before serving. Percentage of vitamins B_{12} and B_2 (riboflavin) is very high.

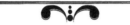

TIP: Free radicals try to destroy the structural proteins, enzymes, and membranes in the cells of the eye's lens. The body uses its antioxidants and enzymes to defend itself. The defenses break down over time and the harm builds up. This accumulated battering by the free radicals is thought to be one of the foremost causes of cataracts in older people, according to researchers such as Dr. James Robertson of the University of Western Canada.

MYTH: Store-bought reading glasses are not safe or effective.

FACT: A committee of the American Academy of Ophthalmology says that store-bought lenses must meet or exceed most standards set for lenses. They conclude that these nonprescription glasses are safe and effective and that no damage will be done to the eyes of those wearing them.

Nutrients Contained in: Clam Special

VITAMINS USRDA			ONE SERVING GIVES YOU APPROXIMATELY		APPROXIMATE PERCENTAGE OF USRDA
A	5,000	IU	2,961	IU	59
B$_1$	1.4	mg	0.62	mg	52
B$_2$	1.6	mg	1	mg	87
B$_3$	16	mg	9	mg	56
B$_5$	10	mg	0.05	mg	0
B$_6$	2.2	mg	0.61	mg	27
B$_{12}$	3	μg	252	μg	8,400◄
C	60	mg	58	mg	96
D	400	IU	0	IU	0
E	15	IU	0.25	IU	1
K	500	μg	0	μg	0
Folic Acid	400	μg	85	μg	21

MINERALS USRDA			ONE SERVING GIVES YOU APPROXIMATELY		APPROXIMATE PERCENTAGE OF USRDA
Sodium	(1,100–3,000)	mg	308	mg	30
Calcium	1,000	mg	254	mg	31
Phosphorus	(800–1,000)	mg	112	mg	13
Potassium	(1,875–5,625)	mg	1,729	mg	216◄
Magnesium	400	μg	57	μg	16
Selenium	200	μg	0.08	μg	0
Iodine	150	mg	0	mg	0
Zinc	15	mg	7	mg	49
Iron	10	mg	32	mg	315◄
Manganese	(2.5–5.0)	mg	0.03	mg	0
Copper	(2.0–3.0)	mg	0.03	mg	1

AMOUNT PER SERVING		CALORIES PER SERVING	% OF MEAL
Fat	5 grams	45	12
Proteins	67 grams	267	71
Carbohydrates	16 grams	65	17
Cholesterol	174 mg		
Amino acid (essential)			Very high
Fiber	0 grams		

Key: USRDA = Recommended Dietary Allowance
IU = International Unit
mg = milligrams
μg = micrograms
NOTE: The numbers with arrows exceed 100 percent of required USRDA.

Perch Fry

Ingredients:

2 lb perch, dressed
2 Tbs whole wheat flour
½ cup wheat germ
1 tsp vegetable oil
1 lemon, sliced
1 tsp chervil
1 Tbs horseradish
1 tsp allspice
¼ tsp black pepper
1 tsp dill

Preparation: Fry

Time: 20 minutes

Calories: 451 per serving

Serves: 4

Directions

Roll fish in a mixture of the flour and wheat germ. Heat the oil in an iron skillet, add spices and brown fish on each side, no more than 4 or 5 minutes on each side. Serve with dill, horseradish and lemon slices. Amounts of vitamin E and B_2 are good; B_{12} is

over 100 percent.

TIP: Molecules that cannot pair up with others or that are unstable can cause problems in the processing of oxygen on the cellular level. The process is much more complex than this, but what we need to know is that these molecules are referred to as free radicals, molecules that can damage our cells and cause cancers and other diseases. Free radical fighters that help to protect us are called antioxidants. Vitamins C, E, and A are antioxidants.

MYTH: Brown eggs are healthier for us than white eggs.

FACT: The egg industry says that brown eggs are just the same as white eggs. The color of the shell makes no difference, as the color depends on the breed of chicken that lays the eggs.

Nutrients Contained in: Perch Fry

VITAMINS USRDA			ONE SERVING GIVES YOU APPROXIMATELY		APPROXIMATE PERCENTAGE OF USRDA
A	5,000	IU	842	IU	16
B_1	1.4	mg	0.45	mg	37
B_2	1.6	mg	0.36	mg	25
B_3	16	mg	5	mg	31
B_5	10	mg	0.25	mg	2
B_6	2.2	mg	0.60	mg	27
B_{12}	3	μg	3	μg	106◄
C	60	mg	26	mg	42
D	400	IU	0	IU	0
E	15	IU	7	IU	49
K	500	μg	0	μg	0
Folic Acid	400	μg	51	μg	12

MINERALS USRDA			ONE SERVING GIVES YOU APPROXIMATELY		APPROXIMATE PERCENTAGE OF USRDA
Sodium	(1,100–3,000)	mg	280	mg	28
Calcium	1,000	mg	87	mg	10
Phosphorus	(800–1,000)	mg	599	mg	74
Potassium	(1,875–5,625)	mg	690	mg	86
Magnesium	400	μg	95	μg	27
Selenium	200	μg	3	μg	1
Iodine	150	mg	0	mg	0
Zinc	15	mg	4	mg	26
Iron	10	mg	4	mg	42
Manganese	(2.5–5.0)	mg	3	mg	57
Copper	(2.0–3.0)	mg	0.13	mg	4

AMOUNT PER SERVING		CALORIES PER SERVING	% OF MEAL
Fat	24 grams	213	48
Proteins	37 grams	146	32
Carbohydrates	23 grams	92	20
Cholesterol	132 mg		
Amino acid (essential)			Over 100
Fiber	0 grams		

Key: USRDA = Recommended Dietary Allowance
    IU = International Unit
    mg = milligrams
    μg = micrograms
NOTE: The numbers with arrows exceed 100 percent of required USRDA.

Elegant Asparagus

Ingredients:

20 spears asparagus
2 Tbs Jack cheese
2 Tbs whole wheat
   flour
1 tsp margarine
1 cup skimmed milk
¼ cup chopped dill
½ cup toasted almonds,
   chopped
1 shredded wheat biscuit
¼ tsp chili powder

Preparation: Boil and bake

Time: 45 minutes

Calories: 179 per serving

Serves: 4

Directions

Preheat oven to 400° F. Wash asparagus thoroughly as this vegetable can contain sand in its scales. Trim bottoms of stalks and peel stems. Boil in an asparagus steamer if available with the stem bottoms in the water and the tips steaming. Or boil the spears in a skillet on top of aluminum foil wads placed in bottom of pan and covered with an aluminum sheet punctured with holes. Drain asparagus and place in a baking dish. Top with the crunched shredded wheat biscuit. Melt the margarine, blend in the flour, stir in the milk, and bring to a boil. Stir and cook for 2 minutes. Add the chili powder and cheese and stir to melt the cheese. Pour over asparagus and sprinkle with almonds. Bake 15 minutes. Sprinkle with dill and serve.

TIP: Cataract researchers say that just as iron exposed to air gets rusty, similar offenses occur in the eye lens as it is exposed to oxygen and light throughout life. That's why antioxidants found in various foods seem to act like rust inhibitors or cataract lens inhibitors.

MYTH: Foods that are labeled "diet" and "dietetic" are low in calories.

FACT: These labels just indicate that a food contains fewer calories than the regular product. So it doesn't necessarily mean that the food is low in calories. The FDA says that "low calorie" would indicate a food that had no more than 40 calories per serving.

Nutrients Contained in: Elegant Asparagus

VITAMINS USRDA			ONE SERVING GIVES YOU APPROXIMATELY		APPROXIMATE PERCENTAGE OF USRDA
A	5,000	IU	815	IU	16
B_1	1.4	mg	0.28	mg	23
B_2	1.6	mg	0.33	mg	23
B_3	16	mg	2	mg	11
B_5	10	mg	0.51	mg	5
B_6	2.2	mg	0.30	mg	13
B_{12}	3	μg	0.24	μg	8
C	60	mg	21	mg	34
D	400	IU	25	IU	6
E	15	IU	5	IU	34
K	500	μg	50	μg	10
Folic Acid	400	μg	105	μg	26

MINERALS USRDA			ONE SERVING GIVES YOU APPROXIMATELY		APPROXIMATE PERCENTAGE OF USRDA
Sodium	(1,100–3,000)	mg	74	mg	7
Calcium	1,000	mg	174	mg	21
Phosphorus	(800–1,000)	mg	285	mg	35
Potassium	(1,875–5,625)	mg	494	mg	61
Magnesium	400	μg	80	μg	22
Selenium	200	μg	0.18	μg	0
Iodine	150	mg	3	mg	2
Zinc	15	mg	2	mg	15
Iron	10	mg	2	mg	18
Manganese	(2.5–5.0)	mg	2	mg	38
Copper	(2.0–3.0)	mg	0.25	mg	8

AMOUNT PER SERVING		CALORIES PER SERVING	% OF MEAL
Fat	8 grams	73	41
Proteins	10 grams	41	23
Carbohydrates	16 grams	65	36
Cholesterol	8 mg		
Amino acid (essential)			129–144
Fiber	1 gram		

Key: USRDA = Recommended Dietary Allowance
　　　IU = International Unit
　　　mg = milligrams
　　　μg = micrograms
NOTE: The numbers with arrows exceed 100 percent of required USRDA.

Yam What I Yam

Ingredients:

4 medium yams
1 cup pineapple juice
2 tsp grated orange rind
2 Tbs flour
3 tsp vegetable oil
6 Tbs honey
$\frac{1}{3}$ cup brown sugar
$\frac{1}{4}$ tsp salt

Preparation: Bake and boil

Time: 45 minutes

Calories: 444 per serving

Serves: 4

Directions

Preheat oven to 400° F. Boil yams for 20 minutes and then peel them. Place the yams in a baking dish. Combine the remaining ingredients in a small pan and bring to a boil, stirring. When syrup forms, pour over the potatoes and bake for about 25 minutes, spooning liquid over potatoes occasionally. Potassium and B_2 are in good amounts here.

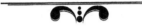

TIP: Vitamin E is an antioxidant with the potential for fighting cancer, heart disease, and cataracts, report scientists. You will get all three of these antiaging benefits from dark leafy greens, such as spinach, kale, and Swiss chard.

MYTH: Yams are identical to sweet potatoes.

FACT: True yams have a neutral starchy flavor, and the sweet potato is sweeter and has a deeper orange color. The true yam is reported to have originated in Asia and can reach sizes in the hundreds of pounds. Sweet potato is a close relative of the morning glory and are the root of a tropical vine. Yams are tubers that grow beneath the soil at the root of a vine and come from a plant distinct from that of the sweet potato.

Nutrients Contained in: Yam What I Yam

VITAMINS USRDA			ONE SERVING GIVES YOU APPROXIMATELY		APPROXIMATE PERCENTAGE OF USRDA
A	5,000	IU	9	IU	0
B$_1$	1.4	mg	0.31	mg	25
B$_2$	1.6	mg	1	mg	87
B$_3$	16	mg	2	mg	13
B$_5$	10	mg	0.81	mg	8
B$_6$	2.2	mg	0.80	mg	36
B$_{12}$	3	μg	0	μg	0
C	60	mg	33	mg	55
D	400	IU	0	IU	0
E	15	IU	0.06	IU	0
K	500	μg	0	μg	0
Folic Acid	400	μg	67	μg	16

MINERALS USRDA			ONE SERVING GIVES YOU APPROXIMATELY		APPROXIMATE PERCENTAGE OF USRDA
Sodium	(1,100–3,000)	mg	27	mg	2
Calcium	1,000	mg	16	mg	2
Phosphorus	(800–1,000)	mg	154	mg	19
Potassium	(1,875–5,625)	mg	2,309	mg	288◄
Magnesium	400	μg	100	μg	28
Selenium	200	μg	0	μg	0
Iodine	150	mg	0	mg	0
Zinc	15	mg	0.68	mg	4
Iron	10	mg	2	mg	20
Manganese	(2.5–5.0)	mg	0.64	mg	12
Copper	(2.0–3.0)	mg	0.70	mg	23

AMOUNT PER SERVING		CALORIES PER SERVING	% OF MEAL
Fat	1 gram	7	2
Proteins	8 grams	30	6
Carbohydrates	102 grams	407	92
Cholesterol	2 mg		
Amino acid (essential)			32–41*
Fiber	3 grams		

Key: USRDA = Recommended Dietary Allowance

IU = International Unit

mg = milligrams

μg = micrograms

NOTE: The numbers with arrows exceed 100 percent of required USRDA.

*Complementary food—1 cup pea pods raises EAA to 97–222%.

Roots of Another Kind

Ingredients:

3 cups raw sweet potatoes, grated
1/2 cup molasses
2 tsp cinnamon
1 tsp ground ginger
1 banana
2 Tbs vegetable oil
1/2 tsp cream of tartar
1/4 tsp baking soda
1/2 tsp salt

Preparation: Bake and simmer

Time: 55 minutes

Calories: 438 per serving

Serves: 4

Directions

Preheat oven to 400° F. Combine potatoes, molasses, ginger, cinnamon, and banana in a 3-quart saucepan. Combine the cream of tartar and baking soda, stirring to mix. Combine this and the oil with all the ingredients. Simmer for 10 minutes stirring all the while. Pour into a 9-inch baking pan and bake for 25 minutes, stirring every 10 minutes. Smooth over the top and take out when brown. Cut into squares and serve. Contains voluminous amounts of vitamins A, B_2, and E; potassium; and iron.

TIP: Current Recommended Dietary Allowance for vitamin E is 15 milligrams for men and 12 milligrams for women. This is about the equivalent of 3 ounces of wheat germ. A study of 12,000 adults found that median intakes of E are lower than the USRDA. This recipe gives you about 11 percent of the USRDA.

MYTH: Large doses of mineral oil will relieve constipation.

FACT: A report from Johns Hopkins says that mineral oil is not a good choice as 4 teaspoons can interfere with the absorption of vitamins A, D, and K.

Nutrients Contained in: Roots of Another Kind

VITAMINS USRDA			ONE SERVING GIVES YOU APPROXIMATELY		APPROXIMATE PERCENTAGE OF USRDA
A	5,000	IU	42,023	IU	840◄
B$_1$	1.4	mg	0.26	mg	21
B$_2$	1.6	mg	0.47	mg	33
B$_3$	16	mg	3	mg	15
B$_5$	10	mg	1	mg	13
B$_6$	2.2	mg	0.76	mg	34
B$_{12}$	3	µg	0	µg	0
C	60	mg	45	mg	74
D	400	IU	0	IU	0
E	15	IU	11	IU	73
K	500	µg	0.55	µg	0
Folic Acid	400	µg	32	µg	8

MINERALS USRDA			ONE SERVING GIVES YOU APPROXIMATELY		APPROXIMATE PERCENTAGE OF USRDA
Sodium	(1,100–3,000)	mg	282	mg	28
Calcium	1,000	mg	286	mg	35
Phosphorus	(800–1,000)	mg	106	mg	13
Potassium	(1,875–5,625)	mg	564	mg	70
Magnesium	400	µg	32	µg	9
Selenium	200	µg	51	µg	25
Iodine	150	mg	50	mg	33
Zinc	15	mg	0.70	mg	4
Iron	10	mg	6	mg	60
Manganese	(2.5–5.0)	mg	0.87	mg	17
Copper	(2.0–3.0)	mg	0.43	mg	14

AMOUNT PER SERVING		CALORIES PER SERVING	% OF MEAL
Fat	7 grams	66	15
Proteins	4 grams	17	4
Carbohydrates	89 grams	355	81
Cholesterol	0 mg		
Amino acid (essential)			48–70
Fiber	2 grams		

Key: USRDA = Recommended Dietary Allowance
IU = International Unit
mg = milligrams
µg = micrograms
NOTE: The numbers with arrows exceed 100 percent of required USRDA.

Red Miners and Mangoes

Ingredients:

1 lb kidney beans, dried
6 chicken livers, cut into pieces
1 mango, peeled and sliced
1 cup spring onion, chopped coarsely
3 tomatoes, chopped finely
1 cup water
4 cloves garlic, chopped
½ tsp black pepper
¼ tsp chili powder
   dash cayenne
1 tsp Adobo (Goya product) seasoning

Preparation: Bake and boil

Time: 2 hours

Calories: 194 per serving

Serves: 6

Directions

Preheat the oven to 300° F. Wash beans and let stand 6 to 8 hours. Save soaking water. When beans have soaked, bring to a boil and simmer, covered, for about 1 hour. Drain beans and put into a baking dish. Place tomatoes, mango slices, livers, onion, and seasonings in a large saucepan with 1 cup of water. Bring to a boil. Add to beans and mix thoroughly. Bake for about 2 hours or less. Check chart for vitamins E, C, and B_2; potassium; iron; and a jackpot of EAA.

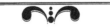

TIP: Researchers at the State University of New York at Stony Brook, Long Island, New York, found after studying about 1,400 ophthalmology patients ages 40 to 79 years old that those who ate foods rich in antioxidants such as beta-carotene and vitamins C and E on a regular basis were 25 to 33 percent less likely to have cataracts than were the other patients.

MYTH: Stress causes an aching back and other back pains.

FACT: The American Academy of Orthopaedic Surgeons reports that stress does not cause lower back pain. The Academy report indicates that if you already have a back problem to begin with, stress can aggravate that situation, but stress alone cannot cause an aching back.

Nutrients Contained in: Red Miners and Mangoes

VITAMINS USRDA			ONE SERVING GIVES YOU APPROXIMATELY		APPROXIMATE PERCENTAGE OF USRDA
A	5,000	IU	9,132	IU	182◀
B$_1$	1.4	mg	0.21	mg	17
B$_2$	1.6	mg	0.75	mg	53
B$_3$	16	mg	4	mg	25
B$_5$	10	mg	2	mg	22
B$_6$	2.2	mg	0.28	mg	12
B$_{12}$	3	μg	7	μg	245◀
C	60	mg	60	mg	100◀
D	400	IU	5	IU	1
E	15	IU	3	IU	20
K	500	μg	33	μg	6
Folic Acid	400	μg	244	μg	61

MINERALS USRDA			ONE SERVING GIVES YOU APPROXIMATELY		APPROXIMATE PERCENTAGE OF USRDA
Sodium	(1,100–3,000)	mg	36	mg	3
Calcium	1,000	mg	65	mg	8
Phosphorus	(800–1,000)	mg	243	mg	30
Potassium	(1,875–5,625)	mg	698	mg	87
Magnesium	400	μg	22	μg	6
Selenium	200	μg	0.35	μg	0
Iodine	150	mg	0	mg	0
Zinc	15	mg	0.30	mg	2
Iron	10	mg	6	mg	55
Manganese	(2.5–5.0)	mg	0.16	mg	3
Copper	(2.0–3.0)	mg	0.52	mg	17

AMOUNT PER SERVING		CALORIES PER SERVING	% OF MEAL
Fat	2 grams	17	9
Proteins	14 grams	57	29
Carbohydrates	30 grams	120	62
Cholesterol	140 mg		
Amino acid (essential)			287–499
Fiber	2 grams		

Key: USRDA = Recommended Dietary Allowance

　　　IU = International Unit

　　mg = milligrams

　　μg = micrograms

NOTE: The numbers with arrows exceed 100 percent of required USRDA.

Handsome Beets

Ingredients:

8 small beets
2 Tbs whole wheat flour
$\frac{1}{2}$ cup orange juice
2 Tbs lime juice
1 Tbs chopped dill
1 Tbs horseradish
$\frac{1}{2}$ tsp brown sugar
$\frac{1}{2}$ tsp margarine

Preparation: Boil

Time: 40 minutes

Calories: 66 per serving

Serves: 4

Directions

Wash beets but do not peel. Place beets in a pan and just cover with boiling water. Simmer slowly for about 20 minutes. Peel beets and slice. Combine the flour and sugar in a saucepan. Stir in the orange juice, lime juice, and margarine. Bring to a boil blending for 2 minutes. Add the dill and horseradish and pour over beets. This relative of the chard has small amounts of vitamin E and vitamin B_2 (riboflavin).

TIP: Dr. Allen Taylor, cataract researcher with Tufts University, says that reducing calories in the diet may be beneficial in the fight against cataracts. He says animal studies show that reducing calories by 21 percent delayed the onset of cataracts.

MYTH: The cause of obesity is psychological.

FACT: Dr. Albert J. Stunkard, a professor of psychiatry at the University of Pennsylvania, says that several studies have shown that fat people don't manifest any more psychological disturbance than thin people. One study even found that those who were obese were less anxious and depressed than were those people of normal weight.

Nutrients Contained in: Handsome Beets

VITAMINS USRDA			ONE SERVING GIVES YOU APPROXIMATELY		APPROXIMATE PERCENTAGE OF USRDA
A	5,000	IU	77	IU	1
B_1	1.4	mg	0.08	mg	6
B_2	1.6	mg	0.03	mg	2
B_3	16	mg	0.52	mg	3
B_5	10	mg	0.20	mg	2
B_6	2.2	mg	0.04	mg	1
B_{12}	3	μg	0	μg	0
C	60	mg	26	mg	43
D	400	IU	0	IU	0
E	15	IU	0.05	IU	0
K	500	μg	0	μg	0
Folic Acid	400	μg	72	μg	18

MINERALS USRDA			ONE SERVING GIVES YOU APPROXIMATELY		APPROXIMATE PERCENTAGE OF USRDA
Sodium	(1,100–3,000)	mg	57	mg	5
Calcium	1,000	mg	28	mg	3
Phosphorus	(800–1,000)	mg	44	mg	5
Potassium	(1,875–5,625)	mg	416	mg	51
Magnesium	400	μg	44	μg	12
Selenium	200	μg	0.60	μg	0
Iodine	150	mg	0	mg	0
Zinc	15	mg	0.38	mg	2
Iron	10	mg	1	mg	14
Manganese	(2.5–5.0)	mg	0.24	mg	4
Copper	(2.0–3.0)	mg	0.09	mg	3

AMOUNT PER SERVING		CALORIES PER SERVING	% OF MEAL
Fat	0 grams	2	2
Proteins	2 grams	7	11
Carbohydrates	14 grams	57	87
Cholesterol	0 mg		
Amino acid (essential)			13–17*
Fiber	1 gram		

Key: USRDA = Recommended Dietary Allowance

IU = International Unit

mg = milligrams

μg = micrograms

NOTE: The numbers with arrows exceed 100 percent of required USRDA.

*Complementary food—1 cup peas raises EAA to 88–120%.

Kale and Gobble

Ingredients:

6 cups kale, cut into small pieces
½ cup white meat turkey, diced
½ tsp salt
1 cup onion
½ tsp black pepper
1 tsp rice bran
dash cayenne pepper
1 tsp vegetable oil

Preparation: Steam and sauté

Time: 20 minutes

Calories: 99 per serving

Serves: 4

Directions

Make sure kale is washed clean of sand and grit. Steam kale for about 6 minutes. Sauté onion in heated oil for 2 minutes, add turkey pieces, and sauté until brown. Add kale, pepper, rice bran, salt, and pepper and simmer for about 7 minutes. See chart for amounts of vitamins E and A and potassium.

TIP: A Tufts University study found that beta-carotenes plus vitamin C may help prevent the formation of cataracts. Subjects who consumed only 3 ½ servings or fewer of vegetables a day were reported to have developed cataracts five times more frequently than those who ate more servings.

MYTH: Juicing the seeds from fruits such as apples causes arsenic poisoning as apples contain arsenic.

FACT: According to Varro Tyler, dean of the School of Pharmacy and Pharmacal Sciences at Purdue University, it is unlikely that this could happen drinking homemade juice, although large quantities of hydrogen cyanide which apples contain could be toxic.

Nutrients Contained in: Kale and Gobble

VITAMINS USRDA			ONE SERVING GIVES YOU APPROXIMATELY		APPROXIMATE PERCENTAGE OF USRDA
A	5,000	IU	8,855	IU	177◄
B₁	1.4	mg	0.15	mg	12
B₂	1.6	mg	0.15	mg	10
B₃	16	mg	2	mg	10
B₅	10	mg	0.99	mg	9
B₆	2.2	mg	0.41	mg	18
B₁₂	3	μg	0.05	μg	1
C	60	mg	131	mg	218◄
D	400	IU	0	IU	0
E	15	IU	12	IU	82
K	500	μg	0	μg	0
Folic Acid	400	μg	40	μg	9

MINERALS USRDA			ONE SERVING GIVES YOU APPROXIMATELY		APPROXIMATE PERCENTAGE OF USRDA
Sodium	(1,100–3,000)	mg	180	mg	18
Calcium	1,000	mg	151	mg	18
Phosphorus	(800–1,000)	mg	96	mg	12
Potassium	(1,875–5,625)	mg	571	mg	71
Magnesium	400	μg	49	μg	14
Selenium	200	μg	4	μg	1
Iodine	150	mg	0	mg	0
Zinc	15	mg	0.70	mg	4
Iron	10	mg	2	mg	21
Manganese	(2.5–5.0)	mg	0.83	mg	16
Copper	(2.0–3.0)	mg	0.32	mg	10

AMOUNT PER SERVING		CALORIES PER SERVING	% OF MEAL
Fat	2 grams	15	16
Proteins	7 grams	26	26
Carbohydrates	15 grams	58	58
Cholesterol	7 mg		
Amino acid (essential)			78–102
Fiber	2 grams		

Key: USRDA = Recommended Dietary Allowance

   IU = International Unit

   mg = milligrams

   μg = micrograms

NOTE: The numbers with arrows exceed 100 percent of required USRDA.

Grainy Turnips

Ingredients:

3 cups yellow turnips, peeled and thinly sliced
2 stalks celery, chopped
½ cup scallion, coarsely chopped
1 cup boiling water
1 cup Swiss chard
½ tsp black pepper
1 tsp vegetable oil
½ tsp thyme
¼ Nutrigrain corn cereal
2 Tbs Parmesan cheese, grated
2 Tbs flour
1 Tbs Romano cheese, grated
salt

Preparation: Boil and sauté

Time: 45 minutes

Calories: 107 per serving

Serves: 4

Directions

Put turnips in a large saucepan and add the water. Bring to a boil and let turnips simmer for about 20 minutes. They should be just tender enough for a fork to pierce. Heat the oil in a skillet and sauté the onion for a minute; then add the celery and chard and cook for about 3 minutes. Now add the thyme, pepper, and a little salt to taste. Add the cooked turnips with its liquid to the seasoned ingredients. Mix the flour with 3 Tbs of water. Stir until it mixes and add it and the Parmesan cheese into the vegetables. Heat, until all ingredients thicken. Cook for about 2 minutes. Pour into a casserole dish. Sprinkle the Nutrigrain flakes and the grated Romano cheese and put briefly under a preheated broiler for a few minutes.

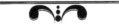

TIP: A U.S. Department of Agriculture study showed people who reported eating less than 1 and a ½ servings of fruit or less than 2 servings of vegetables a day were 3 and a ½ times more likely to develop lens clouding cataracts than were those who said they ate more. Epidemiologist Paul F. Jacques with the USDA Human Nutrition Research Center says that you may delay the usual aging of the lens by eating a healthy diet. He cites carotenoid such as vitamin E as a possible key.

MYTH: Women should not engage in strenuous exercise during menstruation.

FACT: A report in *The Physician and Sports Medicine* says this is not so. Vigorous exercise during a period can enhance well-being and health.

Nutrients Contained in: Grainy Turnips

VITAMINS USRDA			ONE SERVING GIVES YOU APPROXIMATELY		APPROXIMATE PERCENTAGE OF USRDA
A	5,000	IU	1,303	IU	26
B_1	1.4	mg	0.16	mg	13
B_2	1.6	mg	0.18	mg	13
B_3	16	mg	2	mg	11
B_5	10	mg	0.36	mg	3
B_6	2.2	mg	0.23	mg	10
B_{12}	3	μg	0.38	μg	12
C	60	mg	30	mg	50
D	400	IU	0	IU	0
E	15	IU	2	IU	12
K	500	μg	0	μg	0
Folic Acid	400	μg	43	μg	10

MINERALS USRDA			ONE SERVING GIVES YOU APPROXIMATELY		APPROXIMATE PERCENTAGE OF USRDA
Sodium	(1,100–3,000)	mg	266	mg	26
Calcium	1,000	mg	135	mg	16
Phosphorus	(800–1,000)	mg	106	mg	13
Potassium	(1,875–5,625)	mg	339	mg	42
Magnesium	400	μg	31	μg	8
Selenium	200	μg	0.83	μg	0
Iodine	150	mg	0	mg	0
Zinc	15	mg	0.44	mg	2
Iron	10	mg	1	mg	11
Manganese	(2.5–5.0)	mg	0.14	mg	2
Copper	(2.0–3.0)	mg	0.10	mg	3

AMOUNT PER SERVING		CALORIES PER SERVING	% OF MEAL
Fat	4 grams	33	30
Proteins	5 grams	19	18
Carbohydrates	14 grams	55	52
Cholesterol	5 mg		
Amino acid (essential)			54–68*
Fiber	2 grams		

Key: USRDA = Recommended Dietary Allowance

IU = International Unit

mg = milligrams

μg = micrograms

NOTE: The numbers with arrows exceed 100 percent of required USRDA.

*Complementary food—1 tablespoon of Brewer's yeast raises EAA to 391–446%.

Hammy Spinach

Ingredients:

4 cups spinach, chopped
¼ lb ham, sliced
½ cup low-sodium
   chicken broth
1 onion, chopped
½ cup cooked lima beans
¼ cup pimentos
4 cloves garlic, chopped
1 tsp ground nutmeg
   black pepper
1 tsp chervil
   juice of one lemon

Preparation: Cook

Time: 20 minutes

Calories: 184 per serving

Serves: 4

Directions

Cut ham into small pieces and cook in a little broth for about 1 or 2 minutes. Drain ham and set aside. Cook the onion and garlic in the same pan. Add the spinach. Cover and cook about 4 to 6 minutes. Don't overcook spinach as this sometimes produces a flavor, too strong for many palates. Add the beans, pimentos, chervil, nutmeg, and lemon juice and heat for a few minutes. Check your chart and see the high amounts in at least seven important minerals and vitamins.

TIP: Harvard University Professor of Nutrition Paul Jacques showed that those with higher blood and dietary levels of vitamins E and C and beta-carotene had the lowest incidence of cataracts. His study centered on the reduction in risk of getting cataracts with people who have high antioxidant protective factors in their diet.

MYTH: You should throw away all moldy vegetables.

FACT: The U.S. Department of Agriculture says firm vegetables such as cabbage and carrots can be eaten if you cut away small spots of mold from the surface. Soft vegetables, however, like tomatoes, cucumber, and lettuce should be thrown away.

Nutrients Contained in: Hammy Spinach

VITAMINS USRDA			ONE SERVING GIVES YOU APPROXIMATELY		APPROXIMATE PERCENTAGE OF USRDA
A	5,000	IU	14,825	IU	296◄
B$_1$	1.4	mg	0.48	mg	39
B$_2$	1.6	mg	0.52	mg	37
B$_3$	16	mg	3	mg	16
B$_5$	10	mg	0.49	mg	4
B$_6$	2.2	mg	0.64	mg	28
B$_{12}$	3	μg	0.23	μg	7
C	60	mg	23	mg	38
D	400	IU	8	IU	1
E	15	IU	6	IU	38
K	500	μg	180	μg	36
Folic Acid	400	μg	325	μg	81

MINERALS USRDA			ONE SERVING GIVES YOU APPROXIMATELY		APPROXIMATE PERCENTAGE OF USRDA
Sodium	(1,100–3,000)	mg	505	mg	50
Calcium	1,000	mg	262	mg	32
Phosphorus	(800–1,000)	mg	215	mg	26
Potassium	(1,875–5,625)	mg	1,218	mg	152◄
Magnesium	400	μg	213	μg	61
Selenium	200	μg	36	μg	18
Iodine	150	mg	0	mg	0
Zinc	15	mg	2	mg	15
Iron	10	mg	8	mg	80
Manganese	(2.5–5.0)	mg	3	mg	68
Copper	(2.0–3.0)	mg	0.46	mg	15

AMOUNT PER SERVING		CALORIES PER SERVING	% OF MEAL
Fat	4 grams	40	22
Proteins	15 grams	59	32
Carbohydrates	21 grams	85	46
Cholesterol	16 mg		
Amino acid (essential)			174–221
Fiber	2 grams		

Key: USRDA = Recommended Dietary Allowance

IU = International Unit

mg = milligrams

μg = micrograms

NOTE: The numbers with arrows exceed 100 percent of required USRDA.

FOODS RANKED IN THE HIGHEST ORDER FOR VITAMIN E
PERCENTAGES FOR VEGETABLES EQUAL ½ CUP PERCENTAGES
FOR NUTS AND SEEDS EQUAL 1 OUNCE

	VITAMIN E (MILLIGRAMS)	PERCENTAGE OF USRDA
Potato, sweet	5.5	68.7
Beans, kidney, canned	4.4	55.0
Beans, pinto, cooked	4.1	51.2
Beans, lima, cooked	4.1	51.2
Beans, lima, canned	4.0	50.0
Beets, cooked	2.0	25.6
Spinach	1.9	23.7
Turnip, cooked	1.8	22.5
Tofu	1.8	22.5
Asparagus, canned	1.8	22.5
Beans, mung, cooked	1.2	15.0
Sunflower kernels	14.8	185.0
Almonds	5.0	63.0
Filberts	4.1	51.2
Peanuts, unsalted	3.1	38.7
Cashews	3.1	38.7
Brazil nuts	2.2	27.5
Peanut butter	1.9	23.7
Cashews, unsalted	1.1	13.7

Note: For conversion purposes, one IU equals 0.7 milligrams.

CHAPTER ELEVEN

Recipes to Enhance Fertility

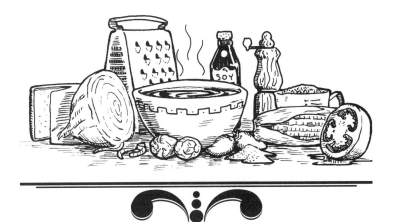

That so few dare to be eccentric marks
the chief danger of the time.
—John Stuart Mill

To maximize conditions for fertility, women should be careful not to lose too much weight. Scientists report that females must store enough body fat to maintain normal menstrual cycles to ensure the ability to give birth. Excessive fatness produces the same negatives as excessive thinness or being undernourished.

Among more direct nutritional concerns that affect fertility is the evidence that scientists have accumulated regarding insufficient vitamin C intake, which can cause genetic damage to sperm that might lead to birth defects and genetic diseases. Dr. Bruce N. Ames, a Berkeley, California, researcher, says that a lowering of vitamin C intake to a certain level causes sperm to be mutated.

A deficiency of zinc has also been found to contribute to impotence as well as lower sperm count in men; this is said to be the most common cause of infertility in males. Vitamin E is nicknamed the "antisterility" vitamin, and it is reported to be beneficial in both male and female reproduction. Look for the many reports in the Tip section that describe the results of research and study. In the meantime, use the recipes that have been designed to make certain that you get your requisite vitamins E and C and zinc.

While there are no guarantees, proper diet may help some people improve their odds of having a child.

RECOMMENDED DIETARY ALLOWANCES FOR ZINC

GROUP/AGE	ZINC (MILLIGRAMS)
Infants 0–6 months	3
Infants 6–12 months	5
Children 1–10 years	10
Males 11+ years	15
Females 11+ years	15
Pregnant women	20
Nursing women	25

Vegetable and Grain Medley

Ingredients:

1 cup bulgur
2 cups water
½ cup wheat germ
2 Tbs rice bran
12 Brussels sprouts
1 red pepper, seeded
   and chopped
2 onions, chopped
1 cup of corn
1 parsnip, peeled and chopped
1 Tbs low-salt soy sauce
1 tsp savory
2 tsp lime juice
1 ½ cups canned tomatoes
   cayenne pepper
½ ounce Romano cheese

Preparation: Boil and simmer

Time: 1 hour

Calories: 320 per serving

Serves: 4

Directions

Cook bulgur by adding to 2 cups water and bringing to a boil. Simmer for 10 minutes, remove from heat, and set aside for 30 minutes. Steam Brussels sprouts for 7 minutes. Add chopped pepper, parsnip, and onions to tomatoes and seasonings and simmer. Add bulgur, wheat germ, and rice bran, cook gently for 30 minutes. During the last 15 minutes, add corn and Brussels sprouts. Remove from heat, and bake at 350 degrees for 20 minutes. Add lime juice and cayenne pepper; sprinkle cheese over pan and serve. This dish is chock full of vitamins C and K, folic acid, magnesium, and iron.

TIP: Dr. Thomas Moore, director of perinatal medicine at the University of California at San Diego, says the most common fear of having a baby with a birth defect is exaggerated. He says it's true, the risk at age 35 is double that at age 25, but that represents only a 1 percent risk. He says that means that 99 percent of babies born to women at 35 and 97 percent at age 40 are chromosomally normal.

MYTH: Certain foods, being difficult to digest, will make you lose weight.

FACT: Nutritionists say this is not true. The calories your body burns in triggering the digestive cycle are almost nonexistent compared with the calories in the food itself.

Nutrients Contained in:
Vegetable and Grain Medley

VITAMINS USRDA			ONE SERVING GIVES YOU APPROXIMATELY		APPROXIMATE PERCENTAGE OF USRDA
A	5,000	IU	886	IU	17
B$_1$	1.4	mg	0.59	mg	49
B$_2$	1.6	mg	0.27	mg	19
B$_3$	16	mg	4	mg	23
B$_5$	10	mg	1	mg	11
B$_6$	2.2	mg	0.45	mg	20
B$_{12}$	3	μg	0.04	μg	1
C	60	mg	83	mg	138◄
D	400	IU	0	IU	0
E	15	IU	2	IU	12
K	500	μg	452	μg	90
Folic Acid	400	μg	153	μg	38

MINERALS USRDA			ONE SERVING GIVES YOU APPROXIMATELY		APPROXIMATE PERCENTAGE OF USRDA
Sodium	(1,100–3,000)	mg	74	mg	7
Calcium	1,000	mg	115	mg	14
Phosphorus	(800–1,000)	mg	407	mg	50
Potassium	(1,875–5,625)	mg	786	mg	98
Magnesium	400	μg	114	μg	32
Selenium	200	μg	28	μg	14
Iodine	150	mg	0	mg	0
Zinc	15	mg	3	mg	21
Iron	10	mg	4	mg	38
Manganese	(2.5–5.0)	mg	3	mg	68
Copper	(2.0–3.0)	mg	0.42	mg	14

AMOUNT PER SERVING		CALORIES PER SERVING	% OF MEAL
Fat	4 grams	35	11
Proteins	13 grams	54	17
Carbohydrates	58 grams	231	72
Cholesterol	4 mg		
Amino acid (essential)			139–168
Fiber	2 grams		

Key: USRDA = Recommended Dietary Allowance

IU = International Unit

mg = milligrams

μg = micrograms

NOTE: The numbers with arrows exceed 100 percent of required USRDA.

Deep Baked Greenery

Ingredients:

2 cups kale, chopped
⅓ cup rice bran
½ cup pearl barley
1 cup mustard greens, chopped
½ cup scallions, chopped
1 cup turnip greens, chopped
½ cantaloupe
1 Tbs caraway seeds
1 tsp lemon juice
1 tsp basil
cayenne pepper

Preparation: Bake

Time: 1 hour, 10 minutes

Calories: 237 per serving

Serves: 4

Directions

Preheat oven to 400° F. Steam kale, mustard greens, and turnip greens together for 5 minutes. Combine with caraway seeds, scallions, lemon juice, dash of cayenne pepper, and basil. Pour all the ingredients into a deep baking dish. Bake for 45 minutes until barley is soft. Serve with cantaloupe slices. Good vitamin C percentages, vitamin A, iron, and potassium are recorded.

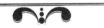

TIP: Dr. Gertrude Berkowitz, a perinatal epidemiologist at Mount Sinai Medical School in New York, says that some women may have no trouble becoming pregnant, but then lose the fetus within the pregnancy's first three months. She says the chance of miscarriage for any birth is approximately 15 percent; after age 35, she says, the risk doubles.

MYTH: Drinking liquids while exercising causes cramps.

FACT Since inadequate fluid intake will lead to dehydration, you should drink before, during, and after exercise to make up for the fluid loss that occurs with physical stress.

Nutrients Contained in: Deep Baked Greenery

	VITAMINS USRDA		ONE SERVING GIVES YOU APPROXIMATELY		APPROXIMATE PERCENTAGE OF USRDA
A	5,000	IU	8,210	IU	164◄
B$_1$	1.4	mg	0.59	mg	48
B$_2$	1.6	mg	0.29	mg	20
B$_3$	16	mg	5	mg	30
B$_5$	10	mg	0.48	mg	4
B$_6$	2.2	mg	0.58	mg	26
B$_{12}$	3	μg	0	μg	0
C	60	mg	87	mg	145◄
D	400	IU	0	IU	0
E	15	IU	4	IU	26
K	500	μg	93	μg	18
Folic Acid	400	μg	100	μg	24

	MINERALS USRDA		ONE SERVING GIVES YOU APPROXIMATELY		APPROXIMATE PERCENTAGE OF USRDA
Sodium	(1,100–3,000)	mg	38	mg	3
Calcium	1,000	mg	155	mg	19
Phosphorus	(800–1,000)	mg	283	mg	35
Potassium	(1,875–5,625)	mg	804	mg	100◄
Magnesium	400	μg	143	μg	40
Selenium	200	μg	0.09	μg	0
Iodine	150	mg	0	mg	0
Zinc	15	mg	3	mg	19
Iron	10	mg	5	mg	50
Manganese	(2.5–5.0)	mg	3	mg	61
Copper	(2.0–3.0)	mg	0.22	mg	7

AMOUNT PER SERVING		CALORIES PER SERVING	% OF MEAL
Fat	4 grams	34	14
Proteins	10 grams	41	14
Carbohydrates	41 grams	162	72
Cholesterol	0 mg		
Amino acid (essential)			92–115
Fiber	1 gram		

Key: USRDA = Recommended Dietary Allowance

IU = International Unit

mg = milligrams

μg = micrograms

NOTE: The numbers with arrows exceed 100 percent of required USRDA.

Whole Steamed Flounder

Ingredients:

2 lb flounder
3 tomatoes, coarsely chopped
2 cloves garlic, sliced thin
½ tsp brown sugar
1 onion, chopped fine
1 Tbs lime juice
1 tsp parsley, chopped
3 tsp arrowroot
1 Tbs ginger slices
1 cup low-sodium chicken broth
lettuce leaves

Preparation: Steam
Time: 35 minutes
Calories: 319 per serving
Serves: 4

Directions

Have fish cleaned and scaled leaving the head intact. Wash and pat dry and let stand for 10 minutes. Make a few diagonal slits on both sides of fish about 1 inch apart. Peel and shred ginger root; insert ginger and garlic slices in slits. Place fish wrapped in lettuce leaves on steamer and steam for about 15 minutes. Fish is done when you can flake the flesh with a fork. Be careful not to overcook. When fish is cooked, remove from steamer. Mix the sugar, arrowroot, onion, lime juice, and tomatoes with the chicken broth and cook over medium heat for about 5 minutes. Drain liquid from fish into sauce mixture and blend. Pour over fish, garnish with parsley, and serve. Very

high amount of vitamin B_{12} is recorded.

TIP: Health and life-style habits are important factors connected with fertility. Doctors say that older women tend to be overweight or develop diabetes, both of which can be obstacles to fertility. In addition smokers reach menopause a full four years earlier than nonsmokers, shortening the time an over-35-year-old woman has left on her biological clock.

MYTH: Women who work have a higher risk for cardioartery disease (CAD) than do those who are not in the workplace.

FACT: Researchers say data on women in the workplace have never shown women to have higher rates of CAD.

Nutrients Contained in: Whole Steamed Flounder

VITAMINS USRDA			ONE SERVING GIVES YOU APPROXIMATELY		APPROXIMATE PERCENTAGE OF USRDA
A	5,000	IU	2,127	IU	42
B$_1$	1.4	mg	0.29	mg	23
B$_2$	1.6	mg	0.37	mg	26
B$_3$	16	mg	7	mg	43
B$_5$	10	mg	0.29	mg	2
B$_6$	2.2	mg	0.64	mg	29
B$_{12}$	3	µg	6	µg	185◄
C	60	mg	31	mg	51
D	400	IU	0	IU	0
E	15	IU	3	IU	22
K	500	µg	8	µg	1
Folic Acid	400	µg	16	µg	3

MINERALS USRDA			ONE SERVING GIVES YOU APPROXIMATELY		APPROXIMATE PERCENTAGE OF USRDA
Sodium	(1,100–3,000)	mg	451	mg	45
Calcium	1,000	mg	75	mg	9
Phosphorus	(800–1,000)	mg	40	mg	5
Potassium	(1,875–5,625)	mg	1,158	mg	144◄
Magnesium	400	µg	156	µg	44
Selenium	200	µg	0.93	µg	0
Iodine	150	mg	0	mg	0
Zinc	15	mg	2	mg	11
Iron	10	mg	2	mg	19
Manganese	(2.5–5.0)	mg	0.17	mg	3
Copper	(2.0–3.0)	mg	0.11	mg	3

AMOUNT PER SERVING		CALORIES PER SERVING	% OF MEAL
Fat	6 grams	53	17
Proteins	58 grams	231	72
Carbohydrates	9 grams	35	11
Cholesterol	160 mg		
Amino acid (essential)			Very high
Fiber	1 gram		

Key: USRDA = Recommended Dietary Allowance

IU = International Unit

mg = milligrams

µg = micrograms

NOTE: The numbers with arrows exceed 100 percent of required USRDA.

Oyster Salsa

Ingredients:

24 oysters on the half shell
1 6-ounce can tomato paste
1/4 cup water
2 cloves garlic, minced
2 small chile peppers, minced
2 Tbs horseradish
1/2 cup onions, chopped finely
3 Tbs lime juice

Preparation: No cooking required

Time: 15 minutes

Calories: 386 per serving

Serves: 4

Directions

Chill oysters in the refrigerator until ready to serve. Combine water and tomato paste and mix well; add peppers, horseradish, onions, garlic, and lime juice and refrigerate for an hour or so covered. When ready to serve, spoon small amount of salsa mixture on top of oysters. Notice the whopping amounts of zinc, iron, and vitamins C, B_2, D, and B_{12}.

TIP: Studies now indicate that women in the 30-year-old and 40-year-old age range have almost as good a chance as younger women of conceiving and delivering a healthy baby. Fetal monitoring and fertility techniques have improved the odds. Dr. Jouko K. Halme, associate professor of obstetrics and gynecology at the University of North Carolina at Chapel Hill, says 74 out of 100 women 35 or older have a good chance at motherhood.

MYTH: Routine circumcision is a must for all babies.

FACT: The American Academy of Pediatrics, the American College of Obstetrics and Gynecology, and the Pediatric Urologists Association say this procedure is no longer considered to be routinely beneficial.

Nutrients Contained in: Oyster Salsa

VITAMINS USRDA			ONE SERVING GIVES YOU APPROXIMATELY		APPROXIMATE PERCENTAGE OF USRDA
A	5,000	IU	3,730	IU	74
B₁	1.4	mg	0.84	mg	70
B₂	1.6	mg	1	mg	79
B₃	16	mg	7	mg	45
B₅	10	mg	0.09	mg	0
B₆	2.2	mg	0.02	mg	0
B₁₂	3	µg	90	µg	3,000◄
C	60	mg	270	mg	449◄
D	400	IU	300	IU	75
E	15	IU	5	IU	33
K	500	µg	3	µg	0
Folic Acid	400	µg	55	µg	13

MINERALS USRDA			ONE SERVING GIVES YOU APPROXIMATELY		APPROXIMATE PERCENTAGE OF USRDA
Sodium	(1,100–3,000)	mg	586	mg	58
Calcium	1,000	mg	248	mg	30
Phosphorus	(800–1,000)	mg	27	mg	3
Potassium	(1,875–5,625)	mg	1,435	mg	179◄
Magnesium	400	µg	296	µg	84
Selenium	200	µg	6	µg	3
Iodine	150	mg	0	mg	0
Zinc	15	mg	456	mg	3,040◄
Iron	10	mg	35	mg	345◄
Manganese	(2.5–5.0)	mg	0.05	mg	1
Copper	(2.0–3.0)	mg	0.04	mg	1

AMOUNT PER SERVING		CALORIES PER SERVING	% OF MEAL
Fat	12 grams	110	29
Proteins	43 grams	173	45
Carbohydrates	26 grams	103	26
Cholesterol	276 mg		
Amino acid (essential)			4–7˙
Fiber	2 grams		

Key: USRDA = Recommended Dietary Allowance

     IU = International Unit

     mg = milligrams

     µg = micrograms

NOTE: The numbers with arrows exceed 100 percent of required USRDA.

˙Complementary food—1 ounce mozzarella cheese raises EAA to 79–342%.

Chicken Breast Deluxe with Bean Sprouts

Ingredients:

2 chicken breasts, boned, cut in half
2 Tbs whole wheat flour
$\frac{1}{4}$ tsp salt
1 tsp vegetable oil
3 cloves garlic, chopped
4 small white turnips, peeled and cut into strips
2 cups broccoli, cut into bite-size pieces
$\frac{1}{2}$ cup low-sodium chicken broth
$\frac{1}{2}$ cup apple juice
1 cup bean sprouts
$\frac{1}{2}$ tsp chili powder
1 tsp chervil

Preparation: Bake and sauté

Time: 55 minutes

Calories: 128 per serving

Serves: 4

Directions

Preheat oven to 400° F. Combine flour, salt, and chili powder and dip chicken in flour mixture, coating all sides. Heat oil in skillet; cook chicken until lightly brown all over. Remove and place in baking dish; bake about 15 minutes; check with a fork to make certain chicken is tender. Add garlic and turnips to skillet and cook about 5 minutes. Stir in broccoli and cook 7 minutes. Add apple juice and chicken broth; heat to boiling and add bean sprouts. Reduce heat and cook for 3 minutes. Sprinkle with chervil and serve with chicken. This dish is high in vitamins C, K, and B_3 and iron.

TIP: Dr. Richard Taylor, an obstetrician-gynecologist in Atlanta, has found that vitamin B_6 is a crucial element to fertility. A deficiency of B_6 allows estrogen to accumulate in the system. As estrogen levels rise, progesterone levels fall, he says, which may be why women with low B_6 levels are chronic aborters. He recommends a balanced diet to help ensure a healthy and safe pregnancy.

MYTH: Vitamin B_{12} shots give people energy.

FACT: B_{12} shots are effective for people who have a condition known as pernicious anemia, which comes about from an inability to absorb B_{12} from food. B_{12} injections have no particular value for people not suffering from this disorder, according to public health nutrition authorities at the University of California, Berkeley.

Nutrients Contained in: Chicken Breast Deluxe with Bean Sprouts

VITAMINS USRDA			ONE SERVING GIVES YOU APPROXIMATELY		APPROXIMATE PERCENTAGE OF USRDA
A	5,000	IU	693	IU	13
B_1	1.4	mg	0.16	mg	13
B_2	1.6	mg	0.16	mg	11
B_3	16	mg	5	mg	31
B_5	10	mg	0.74	mg	7
B_6	2.2	mg	0.37	mg	16
B_{12}	3	μg	0.17	μg	5
C	60	mg	59	mg	97
D	400	IU	0	IU	0
E	15	IU	0.52	IU	3
K	500	μg	150	μg	30
Folic Acid	400	μg	62	μg	15

MINERALS USRDA			ONE SERVING GIVES YOU APPROXIMATELY		APPROXIMATE PERCENTAGE OF USRDA
Sodium	(1,100–3,000)	mg	179	mg	17
Calcium	1,000	mg	55	mg	6
Phosphorus	(800–1,000)	mg	129	mg	16
Potassium	(1,875–5,625)	mg	487	mg	60
Magnesium	400	μg	43	μg	12
Selenium	200	μg	0.50	μg	0
Iodine	150	mg	0	mg	0
Zinc	15	mg	0.85	mg	5
Iron	10	mg	2	mg	15
Manganese	(2.5–5.0)	mg	0.19	mg	3
Copper	(2.0–3.0)	mg	0.09	mg	2

AMOUNT PER SERVING		CALORIES PER SERVING	% OF MEAL
Fat	1 gram	10	8
Proteins	12 grams	48	37
Carbohydrates	18 grams	70	55
Cholesterol	29 mg		
Amino acid (essential)			150–176
Fiber	2 grams		

Key: USRDA = Recommended Dietary Allowance

IU = International Unit

mg = milligrams

μg = micrograms

NOTE: The numbers with arrows exceed 100 percent of required USRDA.

Turkey Lentil Bake

Ingredients:

1 lb boned turkey breast, sliced
1 cup lentils
12 small white onions, peeled and sliced
½ cup scallions, chopped
1 Tbs whole wheat flour
½ cup wheat germ
1 cup tomato paste
½ cup rice
1 tsp marjoram
½ tsp chili powder
2 tsp lime juice
1 tsp chervil

Preparation: Boil and bake

Time: 1 hour, 20 minutes

Calories: 326 per serving

Serves: 4

Directions

Preheat oven to 400° F. Use a large pot and pour lentils in after washing them. Add the onions, chili powder, and marjoram. Add water to cover, bring to boil, reduce heat, and simmer, covered, for about 25 minutes. Remove the onions and drain lentils, saving liquid; add chervil and lime juice. Mix the cooked lentils with the sliced turkey and scallions and turn into a baking pan with a drop of water in the bottom. Put tomato paste in a saucepan, add the flour and stir. Add the 1 ½ cups lentil liquid and stir; add wheat germ and rice. Pour over lentils in the baking pan. Bake for 35 minutes and serve. This meal gives you a good start on zinc and vitamins B_5, B_6, and C needs to meet USRDAs.

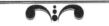

TIP: French researchers found that B vitamins play a part in fertility. This finding stemmed from research giving female rats a diet deficient in vitamin B_5 (pantothenic acid) and then allowing them to mate. The rats did conceive, but the developing fetuses spontaneously aborted. Pantothenic acid is necessary for the health of every cell in the body, and the Food and Nutrition Board suggests up to 10 milligrams daily as a requirement for adults.

MYTH: It is unsafe to eat from an open jar of mayonnaise left in the refrigerator more than a month.

FACT: According to producers, you can keep an open jar of mayonnaise up to a year as long as the temperature is sufficient. Its high acid content is one of its safety assets.

Nutrients Contained in: Turkey Lentil Bake

VITAMINS USRDA			ONE SERVING GIVES YOU APPROXIMATELY		APPROXIMATE PERCENTAGE OF USRDA
A	5,000	IU	2,234	IU	44
B_1	1.4	mg	0.54	mg	44
B_2	1.6	mg	0.29	mg	20
B_3	16	mg	6	mg	39
B_5	10	mg	4	mg	41
B_6	2.2	mg	0.60	mg	27
B_{12}	3	μg	0.19	μg	6
C	60	mg	36	mg	60
D	400	IU	0	IU	0
E	15	IU	0.85	IU	5
K	500	μg	3	μg	0
Folic Acid	400	μg	79	μg	19

MINERALS USRDA			ONE SERVING GIVES YOU APPROXIMATELY		APPROXIMATE PERCENTAGE OF USRDA
Sodium	(1,100–3,000)	mg	157	mg	15
Calcium	1,000	mg	57	mg	7
Phosphorus	(800–1,000)	mg	362	mg	45
Potassium	(1,875–5,625)	mg	1,038	mg	129◄
Magnesium	400	μg	92	μg	26
Selenium	200	μg	4	μg	1
Iodine	150	mg	0	mg	0
Zinc	15	mg	4	mg	25
Iron	10	mg	6	mg	60
Manganese	(2.5–5.0)	mg	3	mg	57
Copper	(2.0–3.0)	mg	0.27	mg	9

AMOUNT PER SERVING		CALORIES PER SERVING	% OF MEAL
Fat	7 grams	61	19
Proteins	22 grams	88	27
Carbohydrates	44 grams	177	54
Cholesterol	0 mg		
Amino acid (essential)			264–454
Fiber	2 grams		

Key: USRDA = Recommended Dietary Allowance

　　　　IU = International Unit

　　　　mg = milligrams

　　　　μg = micrograms

NOTE: The numbers with arrows exceed 100 percent of required USRDA.

Roots and Fruits

Ingredients:

- 4 white turnips, peeled and cut into strips
- 1 large pear, cored and diced
- 2 apples, cored and diced
- 1 tsp vegetable oil
- $\frac{1}{2}$ cup scallions, chopped
- 2 Tbs cilantro, chopped
- $\frac{1}{4}$ cup chard, chopped
- $\frac{1}{4}$ cup maple syrup
- $\frac{1}{2}$ cup walnuts, chopped
- $\frac{1}{8}$ tsp cayenne pepper

Preparation: Sauté

Time: 30 minutes

Calories: 197 per serving

Serves: 4

Directions

Cook peeled turnips strips in boiling water for about 10 minutes. In a large skillet heat the oil, add the pear, apples, and scallions, and cook for 5 minutes. Stir in the turnips, chard, and maple syrup and cook on medium heat for 10 minutes. Stir in cilantro and pepper, cover, and let stand for a few minutes. Sprinkle with walnuts and serve.

TIP: It was in 1974 that the USDA recognized zinc as an essential mineral and the USRDA was established as 15 milligrams. The Beltsville Human Nutrition Research Center in Maryland announced that adults are getting less than the 15 milligrams required, citing that average intake was 9.9 milligrams. They say since zinc affects both fertility and resistance to disease, adequate intake is a necessity.

MYTH: Raw ground beef that turns brown after a day or two of refrigeration is safe to eat.

FACT: The color of the beef doesn't matter according to the USDA as much as the amount of oxygen with which it comes into contact. The general rule is not to keep the raw ground beef in the refrigerator longer than two days.

Nutrients Contained in: Roots and Fruits

VITAMINS USRDA			ONE SERVING GIVES YOU APPROXIMATELY		APPROXIMATE PERCENTAGE OF USRDA
A	5,000	IU	219	IU	4
B_1	1.4	mg	0.07	mg	6
B_2	1.6	mg	0.05	mg	3
B_3	16	mg	0.41	mg	2
B_5	10	mg	0.27	mg	2
B_6	2.2	mg	0.16	mg	7
B_{12}	3	μg	0	μg	0
C	60	mg	20	mg	32
D	400	IU	0	IU	0
E	15	IU	0.71	IU	4
K	500	μg	0	μg	0
Folic Acid	400	μg	18	μg	4

MINERALS USRDA			ONE SERVING GIVES YOU APPROXIMATELY		APPROXIMATE PERCENTAGE OF USRDA
Sodium	(1,100–3,000)	mg	86	mg	8
Calcium	1,000	mg	73	mg	9
Phosphorus	(800–1,000)	mg	59	mg	7
Potassium	(1,875–5,625)	mg	311	mg	38
Magnesium	400	μg	25	μg	7
Selenium	200	μg	4	μg	1
Iodine	150	mg	0	mg	0
Zinc	15	mg	0.24	mg	1
Iron	10	mg	0.87	mg	8
Manganese	(2.5–5.0)	mg	0.21	mg	4
Copper	(2.0–3.0)	mg	0.17	mg	5

AMOUNT PER SERVING		CALORIES PER SERVING	% OF MEAL
Fat	7 grams	65	33
Proteins	2 grams	8	4
Carbohydrates	31 grams	124	63
Cholesterol	20 mg		
Amino acid (essential)			18–31*
Fiber	2 grams		

Key: USRDA = Recommended Dietary Allowance

IU = International Unit

mg = milligrams

μg = micrograms

NOTE: The numbers with arrows exceed 100 percent of required USRDA.

*Complementary food—1 cup lima beans raises EAA to 146–229%.

Barley, Tofu, and Shiitake Mushroom Soup

Ingredients:

1 cup pearl barley
1 cup dried navy beans
2 cups water
7 cups low-sodium
   chicken broth
1 tsp vegetable oil
2 cloves garlic, chopped
1 cup onion, chopped coarse
2 stalks celery, chopped coarse
8 shiitake mushrooms
2 2″-by-5″ pieces of tofu
$\frac{1}{2}$ cup wheat germ
$\frac{1}{2}$ tsp savory
2 Tbs lemon juice
1 tsp chervil
1 Tbs lite soy sauce

Preparation: Boil and sauté

Time: 1 hour, 15 minutes

Calories: 567 per serving
(as main meal)

Serves: 4

Directions

Soak beans and barley over night or use fast method of bringing to boil, turning off heat, and soaking for an hour or so. Simmer beans for half-hour and set aside. Using a large pot, bring chicken broth to a boil; add barley and navy beans with liquid from barley; cook, covered, about 45 minutes or less if barley is tender. Cut tofu in tiny cubes and add to pot during last 10 minutes of cooking. While that is cooking, heat oil in a skillet, add garlic and onions and mushrooms, and sauté 5 minutes. Add celery and sauté for 4 minutes. Add contents of skillet to barley/bean pot. Season with lemon juice, chervil, and soy sauce.

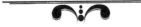

TIP: Dr. Joel L. Marmar of Cherry Hill, New Jersey, has studied the effect of zinc on fertility. He found that 10 to 15 percent of the infertile population had low zinc levels. Zinc apparently enhances the swimming ability of sperm, giving it strength to reach a woman's Fallopian tube and penetrate the egg.

MYTH: There are a number of aphrodisiacs that can stimulate the sex drive.

FACT: The FDA reports that over-the-counter drugs sold as aphrodisiacs are not effective and advises that one should receive professional medical care for a remedy for sexual problems related to performance or low interest.

Nutrients Contained in: Barley, Tofu, and Shiitake Mushroom Soup

VITAMINS USRDA			ONE SERVING GIVES YOU APPROXIMATELY		APPROXIMATE PERCENTAGE OF USRDA
A	5,000	IU	38	IU	0
B_1	1.4	mg	0.51	mg	42
B_2	1.6	mg	0.38	mg	27
B_3	16	mg	13	mg	83
B_5	10	mg	0.30	mg	2
B_6	2.2	mg	0.29	mg	13
B_{12}	3	μg	0.60	μg	20
C	60	mg	6	mg	10
D	400	IU	0	IU	0
E	15	IU	2	IU	14
K	500	μg	0	μg	0
Folic Acid	400	μg	115	μg	28

MINERALS USRDA			ONE SERVING GIVES YOU APPROXIMATELY		APPROXIMATE PERCENTAGE OF USRDA
Sodium	(1,100–3,000)	mg	1,599	mg	159◄
Calcium	1,000	mg	167	mg	20
Phosphorus	(800–1,000)	mg	478	mg	59
Potassium	(1,875–5,625)	mg	1,338	mg	167◄
Magnesium	400	μg	172	μg	49
Selenium	200	μg	4	μg	2
Iodine	150	mg	0	mg	0
Zinc	15	mg	6	mg	42
Iron	10	mg	6	mg	64
Manganese	(2.5–5.0)	mg	3	mg	58
Copper	(2.0–3.0)	mg	0.12	mg	4

AMOUNT PER SERVING		CALORIES PER SERVING	% OF MEAL
Fat	9 grams	85	15
Proteins	27 grams	106	19
Carbohydrates	94 grams	376	66
Cholesterol	2 mg		
Amino acid (essential)			226–357
Fiber	2 grams		

Key: USRDA = Recommended Dietary Allowance

IU = International Unit

mg = milligrams

μg = micrograms

NOTE: The numbers with arrows exceed 100 percent of required USRDA.

Shrimp Vegetable Stew

Ingredients:

1 lb shrimp, shelled and deveined
1 cup onion, chopped
1 stalk celery, chopped
1 cup parsnips, peeled and sliced
1 3-ounce can tomato paste
3 cups tomato juice
1 cup green beans
1 cup okra
1 cup peas
1 potato, cut into small cubes
3 Tbs sesame seeds
½ tsp chili powder
1 tsp Adobo (Goya product) seasoning
1 tsp Worcestershire sauce

Preparation: Simmer
Time: 30 minutes
Calories: 311 per serving
Serves: 4

Directions

Use a large Dutch oven and add spices and seasonings. Mix tomato paste with small can of water, add to pot, and cook for 3 to 4 minutes. Add onions, parsnips, beans, okra, peas, and potato and cook for about 10 minutes on low heat. Add all other ingredients and the shrimp, stir well and simmer for about 8 minutes. You will find very high levels of vitamins C, E, and K and folic acid. Also check the mineral column of the chart, and you will see this is an extremely powerful meal.

TIP: Researchers at the Department of Obstetrics and Gynecology at the University of Texas Medical Branch indicate that vitamin C also affects fertility. This vitamin helps correct the problem of "sticky sperm," which clumps sperm together, preventing sperm from traveling singly up the Fallopian tube. Conception, as a result, cannot occur, according to studies.

MYTH: Intense thinking, studying, and mental problem solving can burn up many calories.

FACT: Think again, as nutritionists imply that this is wishful thinking. The energy requirement of thinking is microscopic.

Nutrients Contained in: Shrimp Vegetable Stew

VITAMINS USRDA			ONE SERVING GIVES YOU APPROXIMATELY		APPROXIMATE PERCENTAGE OF USRDA
A	5,000	IU	4,243	IU	84
B$_1$	1.4	mg	0.48	mg	39
B$_2$	1.6	mg	0.40	mg	28
B$_3$	16	mg	11	mg	65
B$_5$	10	mg	2	mg	18
B$_6$	2.2	mg	0.66	mg	29
B$_{12}$	3	μg	1	μg	37
C	60	mg	86	mg	142◄
D	400	IU	125	IU	31
E	15	IU	2	IU	11
K	500	μg	196	μg	39
Folic Acid	400	μg	99	μg	24

MINERALS USRDA			ONE SERVING GIVES YOU APPROXIMATELY		APPROXIMATE PERCENTAGE OF USRDA
Sodium	(1,100–3,000)	mg	581	mg	58
Calcium	1,000	mg	178	mg	22
Phosphorus	(800–1,000)	mg	409	mg	51
Potassium	(1,875–5,625)	mg	1,826	mg	228◄
Magnesium	400	μg	121	μg	34
Selenium	200	μg	45	μg	22
Iodine	150	mg	45	mg	30
Zinc	15	mg	3	mg	20
Iron	10	mg	8	mg	80
Manganese	(2.5–5.0)	mg	0.84	mg	16
Copper	(2.0–3.0)	mg	1	mg	34

AMOUNT PER SERVING		CALORIES PER SERVING	% OF MEAL
Fat	2 grams	17	6
Proteins	32 grams	129	41
Carbohydrates	41 grams	165	53
Cholesterol	188 mg		
Amino acid (essential)			197–560
Fiber	3 grams		

Key: USRDA = Recommended Dietary Allowance

IU = International Unit

mg = milligrams

μg = micrograms

NOTE: The numbers with arrows exceed 100 percent of required USRDA.

Seedy Cabbage

Ingredients:

1 small head green cabbage, shredded
1 apple, cored and sliced
1 papaya, peeled and sliced
¼ cup sunflower seeds
½ cup apple juice
1 onion, sliced
juice of one lemon
1 tsp chervil
½ tsp vegetable oil

Preparation: Sauté

Time: 1 hour, 10 minutes

Calories: 170 per serving

Serves: 4

Directions

Heat large saucepan and sauté onion, apples, and papaya in vegetable oil for about 3 minutes. Add apple juice, juice of lemon, sunflower seeds, and chervil. Cook, uncovered, over high heat for 2 minutes. Lower heat, cover, and cook for about 15 minutes. This is a very good source for vitamins C and E.

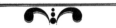

TIP: Vitamin E is present in small amounts in wheat germ, polyunsaturated oils, whole grains, seeds, nuts, and eggs according to nutritionists at the Council for Responsible Nutrition. One should check with a physician before adding vitamin E to the diet that exceeds what is received from natural intake of food.

MYTH: You want to avoid gaining weight during pregnancy as this will lessen the chance of complications during this period.

FACT: Information from the National Institute of Child Health and Human Development indicates this is a misconception and that the healthiest babies are born to women who gain 20 pounds or more.

Nutrients Contained in: Seedy Cabbage

VITAMINS USRDA			ONE SERVING GIVES YOU APPROXIMATELY		APPROXIMATE PERCENTAGE OF USRDA
A	5,000	IU	1,697	IU	33
B$_1$	1.4	mg	0.29	mg	24
B$_2$	1.6	mg	0.09	mg	6
B$_3$	16	mg	1	mg	7
B$_5$	10	mg	0.52	mg	5
B$_6$	2.2	mg	0.32	mg	14
B$_{12}$	3	µg	0	µg	0
C	60	mg	106	mg	176◄
D	400	IU	0	IU	0
E	15	IU	9	IU	59
K	500	µg	50	µg	10
Folic Acid	400	µg	73	µg	18

MINERALS USRDA			ONE SERVING GIVES YOU APPROXIMATELY		APPROXIMATE PERCENTAGE OF USRDA
Sodium	(1,100–3,000)	mg	25	mg	2
Calcium	1,000	mg	96	mg	12
Phosphorus	(800–1,000)	mg	123	mg	15
Potassium	(1,875–5,625)	mg	696	mg	87
Magnesium	400	µg	35	µg	9
Selenium	200	µg	2	µg	1
Iodine	150	mg	0	mg	0
Zinc	15	mg	0.81	mg	5
Iron	10	mg	2	mg	16
Manganese	(2.5–5.0)	mg	0.47	mg	9
Copper	(2.0–3.0)	mg	0.24	mg	7

AMOUNT PER SERVING		CALORIES PER SERVING	% OF MEAL
Fat	5 grams	43	25
Proteins	5 grams	18	11
Carbohydrates	27 grams	109	64
Cholesterol	0 mg		
Amino acid (essential)			42–62*
Fiber	2 grams		

Key: USRDA = Recommended Dietary Allowance

IU = International Unit

mg = milligrams

µg = micrograms

NOTE: The numbers with arrows exceed 100 percent of required USRDA.

*Complementary food—1 cup peas raises EAA to 122-158%.

Sprouting Peppers

Ingredients:

- 4 green bell peppers
- ½ cup alfalfa sprouts
- 1 cup bean sprouts
- ¼ cup scallions, chopped
- ⅓ cup rice bran
- 1 egg white, beaten
- 2 oz pine nuts
- 2 Tbs sesame seeds
- 2 Tbs Swiss cheese
  cayenne pepper

Preparation: Bake

Time: 50 minutes

Calories: 428 per serving

Serves: 4

Directions

Preheat oven to 400° F. Slice the top off the peppers and remove seeds. Place peppers in boiling water for a few minutes. Remove. Combine sprouts, scallions, rice bran, beaten egg white, nuts, seeds, and cheese with a dash of cayenne pepper. Fill peppers with mixture. Place stuffed peppers in a baking pan or dish. Bake for about 25 minutes. Very high percentages of all EAA are recorded.

TIP: Dr. James Milten at Nutritional Bases of Reproduction conducted a study with 50 men who were given 30 milligrams of vitamin E twice daily. The effect of vitamin E on male sperm in this instance showed an increase in the concentration of male reproductive cells in the seminal fluid in 23 of them. In 17 of the subjects there was an increase in volume of seminal fluid and fewer abnormal formations among cells.

MYTH: Low back pain is commonly caused by unequal leg length.

FACT: Based upon studies conducted in Wales, it was shown that this condition does not necessarily cause low back pain.

Nutrients Contained in: Sprouting Peppers

VITAMINS USRDA			ONE SERVING GIVES YOU APPROXIMATELY		APPROXIMATE PERCENTAGE OF USRDA
A	5,000	IU	739	IU	14
B₁	1.4	mg	0.63	mg	52
B₂	1.6	mg	0.21	mg	15
B₃	16	mg	6	mg	39
B₅	10	mg	0.80	mg	7
B₆	2.2	mg	0.66	mg	29
B₁₂	3	μg	0.24	μg	7
C	60	mg	88	mg	145◄
D	400	IU	15	IU	3
E	15	IU	2	IU	13
K	500	μg	0	μg	0
Folic Acid	400	μg	31	μg	7

MINERALS USRDA			ONE SERVING GIVES YOU APPROXIMATELY		APPROXIMATE PERCENTAGE OF USRDA
Sodium	(1,100–3,000)	mg	49	mg	4
Calcium	1,000	mg	179	mg	22
Phosphorus	(800–1,000)	mg	364	mg	45
Potassium	(1,875–5,625)	mg	499	mg	62
Magnesium	400	μg	135	μg	38
Selenium	200	μg	22	μg	10
Iodine	150	mg	0	mg	0
Zinc	15	mg	4	mg	24
Iron	10	mg	4	mg	41
Manganese	(2.5–5.0)	mg	0.93	mg	18
Copper	(2.0–3.0)	mg	0.52	mg	17

AMOUNT PER SERVING		CALORIES PER SERVING	% OF MEAL
Fat	19 grams	168	39
Proteins	14 grams	55	13
Carbohydrates	51 grams	205	48
Cholesterol	13 mg		
Amino acid (essential)			195–228
Fiber	2 grams		

Key: USRDA = Recommended Dietary Allowance

IU = International Unit

mg = milligrams

μg = micrograms

NOTE: The numbers with arrows exceed 100 percent of required USRDA.

Baked Potatoes with Skin and Wheat Germ

Ingredients:

4 potatoes with skin
½ cup wheat germ
2 Tbs sour cream
1 tsp Brewer's yeast
2 Tbs Parmesan cheese
1 tsp margarine
1 tsp chives
1 tsp Adobo (Goya product) seasoning
¼ tsp sesame seeds

Preparation: Bake

Time: 1 hour

Calories: 444 per serving

Serves: 4

Directions

Preheat oven to 425° F. Wash potatoes. Cut potatoes into thin slices without separating slices or going all the way through potato. Place potatoes in baking dish; sprinkle with margarine, wheat germ, yeast, chives, and seasoning. Bake for about 40 minutes. Remove from oven and sprinkle with cheese and sesame seeds; bake for another 10 minutes until cheese melts and potatoes can be easily pierced with a fork. Remove and spread sour cream evenly among the potatoes and serve. This dish is very high in vitamin B_1, phosphorus, potassium, and folic acid.

TIP: A study involving the effects of vitamin E on 100 infertile couples with a history of miscarriages showed that a group with 144 conceptions without a single live birth conceived 79 children after daily intake of 100 units of vitamin E by the males and 200 by the females. This was a study conducted by Dr. R. Bayer, a West German physician.

MYTH: Baldness is often a result of poor circulation in the scalp.

FACT: Dermatologists involved in research of the scalp say there is no evidence to support the idea that improving blood flow to the scalp will cure baldness.

Nutrients Contained in: Baked Potatoes with Skin and Wheat Germ

VITAMINS USRDA			ONE SERVING GIVES YOU APPROXIMATELY		APPROXIMATE PERCENTAGE OF USRDA
A	5,000	IU	77	IU	1
B$_1$	1.4	mg	1	mg	124◄
B$_2$	1.6	mg	0.48	mg	34
B$_3$	16	mg	8	mg	47
B$_5$	10	mg	2	mg	22
B$_6$	2.2	mg	1	mg	45
B$_{12}$	3	μg	0.77	μg	25
C	60	mg	27	mg	44
D	400	IU	0	IU	0
E	15	IU	0.06	IU	0
K	500	μg	3	μg	0
Folic Acid	400	μg	297	μg	74

MINERALS USRDA			ONE SERVING GIVES YOU APPROXIMATELY		APPROXIMATE PERCENTAGE OF USRDA
Sodium	(1,100–3,000)	mg	86	mg	8
Calcium	1,000	mg	102	mg	12
Phosphorus	(800–1,000)	mg	523	mg	65
Potassium	(1,875–5,625)	mg	1,178	mg	147◄
Magnesium	400	μg	150	μg	42
Selenium	200	μg	0.50	μg	0
Iodine	150	mg	0	mg	0
Zinc	15	mg	6	mg	37
Iron	10	mg	6	mg	55
Manganese	(2.5–5.0)	mg	3	mg	66
Copper	(2.0–3.0)	mg	1	mg	44

AMOUNT PER SERVING		CALORIES PER SERVING	% OF MEAL
Fat	14 grams	124	28
Proteins	16 grams	64	14
Carbohydrates	64 grams	256	58
Cholesterol	5 mg		
Amino acid (essential)			209–305
Fiber	2 grams		

Key: USRDA = Recommended Dietary Allowance
    IU = International Unit
    mg = milligrams
    μg = micrograms
NOTE: The numbers with arrows exceed 100 percent of required USRDA.

Spirit of Corn with Broccoli and Almonds

Ingredients:

- 2 cups broccoli, cut into small pieces
- 16 asparagus spears, cut into quarters
- ½ cup wheat germ
- 1 cup corn
- 1 cup onions, cut into big pieces
- 1 cup brown rice
- 2 Tbs tahini sauce
- 1 tsp vegetable oil
- ½ cup chopped almonds
- 2 Tbs lemon juice

Preparation: Sauté

Time: 20 minutes

Calories: 457 per serving

Serves: 4

Directions

Heat oil in large skillet; add broccoli, asparagus pieces, onions, wheat germ, corn, and almonds. Stir-fry over medium heat until vegetables are al dente or crisp. Blend tahini sauce with lemon juice and stir into vegetables. Follow instructions on package and cook the brown rice. Serve with the vegetables. See chart for high percentages of vitamins C, K, and B_1 and zinc.

TIP: Researchers at the USDA Human Nutrition Center in Grand Forks, North Dakota, found that after five weeks of a zinc-deficient diet, ejaculate levels dropped by one third in males involved in the study. This would suggest that zinc USRDAs should be met if fatherhood is on the menu.

MYTH: Surimi is not real fish.

FACT: Surimi is a paste made from minced fresh fish and then seasoned and steamed or broiled. Usually it is a blend of a type of cod (or pollock) and surimi, which is then packaged for consumer purchase.

Nutrients Contained in: Spirit of Corn
with Broccoli and Almonds

VITAMINS USRDA			ONE SERVING GIVES YOU APPROXIMATELY		APPROXIMATE PERCENTAGE OF USRDA
A	5,000	IU	1,301	IU	26
B$_1$	1.4	mg	.76	mg	63
B$_2$	1.6	mg	0.42	mg	30
B$_3$	16	mg	6	mg	35
B$_5$	10	mg	2	mg	16
B$_6$	2.2	mg	.73	mg	33
B$_{12}$	3	μg	0	μg	0
C	60	mg	65	mg	107◀
D	400	IU	0	IU	0
E	15	IU	6	IU	41
K	500	μg	192	μg	38
Folic Acid	400	μg	174	μg	43

MINERALS USRDA			ONE SERVING GIVES YOU APPROXIMATELY		APPROXIMATE PERCENTAGE OF USRDA
Sodium	(1,100–3,000)	mg	39	mg	3
Calcium	1,000	mg	123	mg	15
Phosphorus	(800–1,000)	mg	505	mg	63
Potassium	(1,875–5,625)	mg	873	mg	109◀
Magnesium	400.	μg	163	μg	46
Selenium	200	μg	21	μg	10
Iodine	150	mg	0	mg	0
Zinc	15	mg	5	mg	30
Iron	10	mg	4	mg	44
Manganese	(2.5–5.0)	mg	4	mg	83
Copper	(2.0–3.0)	mg	0.51	mg	17

AMOUNT PER SERVING		CALORIES PER SERVING	% OF MEAL
Fat	12 grams	111	24
Proteins	16 grams	63	14
Carbohydrates	71 grams	283	62
Cholesterol	0 mg		
Amino acid (essential)			171–211
Fiber	3 grams		

Key: USRDA = Recommended Dietary Allowance
      IU = International Unit
      mg = milligrams
      μg = micrograms
NOTE: The numbers with arrows exceed 100 percent of required USRDA.

Tuna Under Onion, Garlic, and Mushrooms

Ingredients:

4	6 to 7 oz tuna steaks
1	tsp vegetable oil
3	Tbs lemon juice
3	Tbs tomato juice
1	cup onion, coarsely chopped
2	cucumbers, chopped
4	cloves garlic, sliced
12	black fungus mushrooms
1/4	cup mint leaves, chopped
	cayenne pepper

Preparation: Bake

Time: 20 minutes

Calories: 425 per serving

Serves: 4

Directions

Preheat oven to 400°F. Moisten baking pan or dish with 2 Tbs water or chicken broth. Rub the oil on tuna sides. Set tuna in baking dish. Cover with the onions, cucumbers, garlic, mushrooms, and lemon juice. Cover and bake no more than 10 minutes or until tuna flakes with touch of a fork. Sprinkle with mint and tomato juice. Contains high amounts of vitamins E, B_{12}, and B_3, selenium, and EAA.

TIP: Researchers say that vitamin E is a nutrient that seems to aid fertility. They studied the effects of vitamin E on fertility at a large horse breeding facility in Oshawa, Canada, giving it daily to the entire herd, including old mares and older stallions. After treatment with vitamin E, 71 percent of the pregnancies resulted in births.

MYTH: Newborns and the very young do not have the neurological sensitivity to feel pain the way adults do during surgical treatment.

FACT: Dr. Myron Yaster, director of pain services at the Children's Center of Johns Hopkins Hospital in Baltimore, says this belief no longer holds. A number of studies has indicated that babies do react to pain as they were observed under standard anesthesia. Babies and young children are not, however, able to verbalize their needs when they are in pain.

Nutrients Contained in: Tuna Under Onion, Garlic, and Mushrooms

VITAMINS USRDA			ONE SERVING GIVES YOU APPROXIMATELY		APPROXIMATE PERCENTAGE OF USRDA
A	5,000	IU	232	IU	4
B$_1$	1.4	mg	0.13	mg	10
B$_2$	1.6	mg	0.14	mg	10
B$_3$	16	mg	27	mg	165◄
B$_5$	10	mg	0.43	mg	4
B$_6$	2.2	mg	0.84	mg	38
B$_{12}$	3	μg	3	μg	86
C	60	mg	12	mg	20
D	400	IU	15	IU	3
E	15	IU	6	IU	41
K	500	μg	1	μg	0
Folic Acid	400	μg	71	μg	17

MINERALS USRDA			ONE SERVING GIVES YOU APPROXIMATELY		APPROXIMATE PERCENTAGE OF USRDA
Sodium	(1,100–3,000)	mg	910	mg	91
Calcium	1,000	mg	39	mg	4
Phosphorus	(800–1,000)	mg	439	mg	54
Potassium	(1,875–5,625)	mg	969	mg	52
Magnesium	400	μg	104	μg	29
Selenium	200	μg	116	μg	57
Iodine	150	mg	0	mg	0
Zinc	15	mg	4	mg	27
Iron	10	mg	3	mg	27
Manganese	(2.5–5.0)	mg	0.19	mg	3
Copper	(2.0–3.0)	mg	0.18	mg	6

AMOUNT PER SERVING		CALORIES PER SERVING	% OF MEAL
Fat	5 grams	49	12
Proteins	56 grams	222	52
Carbohydrates	38 grams	154	36
Cholesterol	64 mg		
Amino acid (essential)			299–999
Fiber	1 gram		

Key: USRDA = Recommended Dietary Allowance

IU = International Unit

mg = milligrams

μg = micrograms

NOTE: The numbers with arrows exceed 100 percent of required USRDA.

Stuffed Red Dynamos

Ingredients:

4 red peppers
½ cup low-sodium chicken broth
½ cup shallots, minced
1 tsp vegetable oil
3 cloves garlic, chopped
½ cup baker's cheese or skim milk cottage cheese
½ tsp oregano
1 egg white
½ cup millet

½ cup bulgur
1 cup water
1 ½ cups canned tomatoes
½ tsp Adobo (Goya product) seasoning
banana slices

Preparation: Boil, sauté, bake

Time: 1 hour, 10 minutes

Calories: 196 per serving

Serves: 4

Directions

Preheat oven to 400° F. Toast millet for a few minutes in a saucepan over heat, stirring occasionally. Add 1 cup boiling water, cover, and simmer for 20 minutes. Set aside. In a larger saucepan, bring the broth to a boil, add the bulgur. Cover, remove from heat, and set aside. Bulgur should absorb the broth in about 20 minutes. Remove the tops of the peppers and the seeds inside. Drop peppers in boiling water for 3 minutes; remove and let cool. Using a large skillet, place the onions, oil, garlic, oregano, and thyme in it, and sauté for about 5 minutes over medium heat. Onions should be tender. Combine the millet and the bulgur in a separate pan and add the sautéed vegetable mixture. Put baker's cheese and egg in a blender and puree until smooth. Add to the bulgur and millet. Mix all the ingredients thoroughly. Measure the filling into the peppers. Place peppers in a medium-sized baking pan or dish. Bake for 20 minutes. Top with banana slices and serve with canned tomatoes.

TIP: According to a study reported in the *Proceedings of the National Academy of Sciences,* a man whose diet is low in vitamin C may increase his chances of fathering children with birth defects and certain kinds of cancers. Eating an unbalanced diet and smoking are factors that reduce a man's vitamin C level and increase risks for DNA damage says one of the researchers, Dr. Paul Motchnik of the University of California at Berkeley.

MYTH: Vitamin C is a stimulant and should not be taken at night as it might keep one awake.

FACT: Dr. Gary Elmer, associate professor of medicinal chemistry at the School of Pharmacy of the University of Washington in Seattle says he is not aware of any published studies in any reputable journal to support such a claim. He indicated that there would be no reason biochemically for such an effect.

Nutrients Contained in: Stuffed Red Dynamos

VITAMINS USRDA			ONE SERVING GIVES YOU APPROXIMATELY		APPROXIMATE PERCENTAGE OF USRDA
A	5,000	IU	929	IU	18
B_1	1.4	mg	0.29	mg	23
B_2	1.6	mg	0.25	mg	18
B_3	16	mg	2	mg	12
B_5	10	mg	0.23	mg	2
B_6	2.2	mg	0.13	mg	5
B_{12}	3	μg	0.32	μg	10
C	60	mg	87	mg	144◄
D	400	IU	0.63	IU	0
E	15	IU	3	IU	20
K	500	μg	3	μg	0
Folic Acid	400	μg	19	μg	4

MINERALS USRDA			ONE SERVING GIVES YOU APPROXIMATELY		APPROXIMATE PERCENTAGE OF USRDA
Sodium	(1,100–3,000)	mg	326	mg	32
Calcium	1,000	mg	42	mg	5
Phosphorus	(800–1,000)	mg	169	mg	21
Potassium	(1,875–5,625)	mg	367	mg	45
Magnesium	400	μg	67	μg	19
Selenium	200	μg	1	μg	0
Iodine	150	mg	10	mg	6
Zinc	15	mg	0.49	mg	3
Iron	10	mg	3	mg	32
Manganese	(2.5–5.0)	mg	0.07	mg	1
Copper	(2.0–3.0)	mg	0.07	mg	2

AMOUNT PER SERVING		CALORIES PER SERVING	% OF MEAL
Fat	4 grams	33	17
Proteins	10 grams	41	21
Carbohydrates	31 grams	122	62
Cholesterol	3 mg		
Amino acid (essential)			107–134
Fiber	2 grams		

Key: USRDA = Recommended Dietary Allowance

IU = International Unit

mg = milligrams

μg = micrograms

NOTE: The numbers with arrows exceed 100 percent of required USRDA.

Chicken Livers with Peppers and Mushrooms

Ingredients:

12	chicken livers
1	onion, diced into small pieces
8	shiitake mushrooms
3	Tbs whole wheat flour
⅔	cup rice bran
1	green pepper, chopped
1	cup low-sodium chicken broth
½	tsp thyme
2	Tbs Italian parsley, chopped
	cayenne pepper
1	tsp vegetable oil

Preparation: Sauté

Time: 40 minutes

Calories: 362 per serving

Serves: 4

Directions

Heat oil in skillet. Add onions, peppers, and mushrooms and sauté for 5 minutes. Add chicken livers and sauté for 3 minutes. Sprinkle on flour; cook, stirring, for about 3 minutes. Add thyme, parsley, and chicken broth; simmer for 4 minutes, stirring occasionally. Season with pepper to taste. If desired, serve with 1 ½ cups cooked collard greens with 1 Tbs Parmesan cheese. Your chart will show astounding percentages of every important nutrient, including cholesterol unfortunately, which makes this dish a once-in-a-while treat.

TIP: The U.S. Department of Health suggests that a woman's body needs about 2,100 calories a day to function properly. If you're trying to become pregnant, for maximum fertility, 30 to 60 days prior to conception, daily calorie intake should reach 2,300. After conception, daily calorie intake recommended is 2,500 to 2,700.

MYTH: The government endorses water treatment units and companies.

FACT: The Environmental Protection Agency does assign certain products registration numbers, but these numbers are not endorsements or approvals made by the government. Dealers of home water units and tests who claim that their water treatment units are approved by the government cannot substantiate that claim.

Nutrients Contained in: Chicken Livers
with Peppers and Mushrooms

VITAMINS USRDA			ONE SERVING GIVES YOU APPROXIMATELY		APPROXIMATE PERCENTAGE OF USRDA
A	5,000	IU	20,118	IU	402◄
B_1	1.4	mg	0.49	mg	40
B_2	1.6	mg	2	mg	141◄
B_3	16	mg	16	mg	97
B_5	10	mg	6	mg	60
B_6	2.2	mg	1	mg	53
B_{12}	3	μg	22	μg	737◄
C	60	mg	63	mg	105◄
D	400	IU	15	IU	3
E	15	IU	3	IU	20
K	500	μg	84	μg	16
Folic Acid	400	μg	768	μg	191◄

MINERALS USRDA			ONE SERVING GIVES YOU APPROXIMATELY		APPROXIMATE PERCENTAGE OF USRDA
Sodium	(1,100–3,000)	mg	454	mg	45
Calcium	1,000	mg	42	mg	5
Phosphorus	(800–1,000)	mg	278	mg	34
Potassium	(1,875–5,625)	mg	701	mg	87
Magnesium	400	μg	116	μg	33
Selenium	200	μg	0.98	μg	0
Iodine	150	mg	0	mg	0
Zinc	15	mg	3	mg	21
Iron	10	mg	11	mg	113◄
Manganese	(2.5–5.0)	mg	0.35	mg	7
Copper	(2.0–3.0)	mg	0.43	mg	14

AMOUNT PER SERVING		CALORIES PER SERVING	% OF MEAL
Fat	6 grams	53	15
Proteins	25 grams	98	27
Carbohydrates	53 grams	211	58
Cholesterol	427 mg		
Amino acid (essential)			237–304
Fiber	1 gram		

Key: USRDA = Recommended Dietary Allowance

　　　IU = International Unit

　　　mg = milligrams

　　　μg = micrograms

NOTE: The numbers with arrows exceed 100 percent of required USRDA.

FOODS RANKED IN THE HIGHEST ORDER FOR ZINC

	ZINC (MILLIGRAMS)	PERCENTAGE OF USRDA
Meats—3-ounce portions		
Beef, shank	8.9	74.2
Beef, short ribs, lean/fat	6.6	55.0
Beef, meatballs, 1.5-inch diameter	6.4	53.4
Beef, roast rib, lean	5.9	49.2
Beef, steak, ribeye, lean	5.9	49.2
Beef, brisket, lean	5.9	49.2
Beef, steak, sirloin, lean	5.5	46.2
Calf liver	5.2	43.3
Calf liver, fried	5.2	43.6
Beef, meatloaf	5.0	41.7
Beef, steak, filet mignon	4.8	40.0
Beef, stew	4.7	39.2
Beef, top round, lean	4.6	38.3
Beef, steak, porterhouse	4.6	38.3

Same numbers are found for ground beef patty, chuck steak, shoulder steak, T-bone steak lean, and shell steak lean.

	ZINC (MILLIGRAMS)	PERCENTAGE OF USRDA
Poultry—3-ounce portions		
Turkey, dark, without skin	3.8	31.6
Chicken, liver	3.7	30.7
Chicken, diced, 1 cup	3.2	27.1

All other poultry has zinc levels below these numbers.

	ZINC (MILLIGRAMS)	PERCENTAGE OF USRDA
Seafood—3 ounces		
Oysters, raw, 6 medium	76.4	636.7
Crab, hard, steamed	6.5	54.2
Squid, boiled	3.9	32.5

All other seafood has zinc levels below these numbers.

	ZINC (MILLIGRAMS)	PERCENTAGE OF USRDA
Vegetables—1/2 cup		
Beans, baked, pork/sauce	7.4	61.7
Beans, baked, plain	1.8	15.0
Beans, fava, canned	1.5	12.5
Garbanzo, canned	1.3	10.8
Beans, pinto, cooked	1.2	10.0

All other vegetables have zinc levels below 1.2 milligrams.

CHAPTER TWELVE

Healing and Preventive Recipes for Anemia

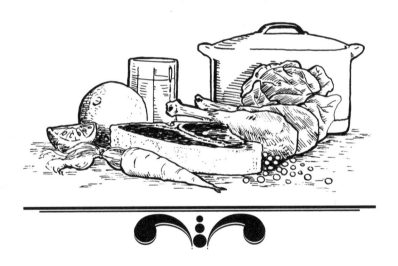

It is, in fact, nothing short of a miracle that the
modern methods of instruction have not entirely
strangled the holy curiosity of inquiry.
—Albert Einstein

One of the most important nutrients needed to combat anemia is iron. Your blood cells need iron to keep them healthy and in abundance. Without healthy blood, your body lacks sufficient oxygen, which causes one to feel tired and drained. It is no surprise that women would be the foremost sufferers of this condition because of monthly blood losses through menstruation. Dieting strenuously doesn't help either.

The best meat sources for iron are liver and red meat, but since they are very high in cholesterol, saturated fat, and calories, you should not look forward to eating them more than occasionally. You can get iron from beans, peas, and dark leafy green vegetables if you add some fish or poultry at the same meal. Extra sleep is a component in this equation also.

The foods that I have used to create recipes that are good for giving you the necessary iron include beans, all poultry, low-fat beef, tofu, seeds, and fruit. The iron known as heme iron and the most absorbable is found in meats. If you plan to get your iron from other sources such as vegetables (nonheme, which is harder to absorb than the heme), you should also consider drinking orange juice at the same meal.

The double-loaded Chicken and Beef Meet gives you 88 percent of good iron; the Steak and Vegetable Gravy dish gives you way over 100 percent of your iron needs. As vitamin C helps to boost iron absorption, you can check your chart for such meals as Fish and Peas, which offers over 100 percent of vitamin C, and Fruited Chicken, which also has an abundance of this vitamin.

RECOMMENDED DIETARY ALLOWANCES FOR IRON

GROUP/AGE	IRON (MILLIGRAMS)
Infants 0–6 months	10
Infants 6–12 months	15
Children 1–3 years	15
Children 4–10 years	10
Males 11–18 years	18
Males 19+ years	10
Females 11–50 years	18
Females 51+ years	10
Pregnant and nursing women	30–60*

*If you are in the group that needs between 30 and 60 milligrams of iron, check with your physician before taking supplements on your own.

Chicken and Beef Meet

Ingredients: 1 ½ lb chicken, cut in
           4 serving pieces
     ½ lb beef fillet, cut in
           1-inch squares
     1 tsp vegetable oil
     1 tsp margarine
     ½ tsp paprika
     1 cup onions, chopped
     2 cups bok choy, chopped
     2 Tbs ketchup
     1 cup canned tomatoes
     1 cup cooked rice
     ½ tsp sage
           cayenne pepper
     ¼ cup whole wheat flour

Preparation: Sauté and simmer

Time: 55 minutes

Calories: 515 per serving

Serves: 4

Directions

Dip chicken in flour and paprika. In a large iron skillet, sauté chicken in oil, or margarine until it is brown on both sides. Remove chicken to a large heavy pot. Brown the beef pieces in skillet used for chicken. Add beef, onions, bok choy, ketchup, and tomatoes to pot. Add cayenne pepper and sage. Simmer for 30 minutes. Add rice to pot the last 5 minutes and serve.

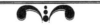

TIP: Common cuts of meat, fish, and poultry provide a form of iron called heme that is most easily absorbed by the body. Research nutritionists say that even the best nonmeat sources don't match up because they contain only nonheme iron. Red meats—beef, pork, and lamb—are the most iron-rich of the MFP (meat, fish, and poultry) group. The MFP factor boosts absorption of any nonheme iron you eat.

MYTH: Vegetarians suffer protein deficiencies.

FACT: Johanna T. Dwyer, director of the Frances Stern Nutrition Center at New England Medical Center and Tufts University, says that unless adult vegetarians are on a severe low-calorie diet (under 1,200 a day) or a bizarre diet, protein deficiency is so uncommon as to be unimportant as a concern.

Nutrients Contained in: Chicken and Beef Meet

VITAMINS USRDA			ONE SERVING GIVES YOU APPROXIMATELY		APPROXIMATE PERCENTAGE OF USRDA
A	5,000	IU	1,386	IU	27
B$_1$	1.4	mg	0.55	mg	45
B$_2$	1.6	mg	0.72	mg	51
B$_3$	16	mg	12	mg	76
B$_5$	10	mg	1	mg	10
B$_6$	2.2	mg	1	mg	56
B$_{12}$	3	μg	3	μg	84
C	60	mg	25	mg	41
D	400	IU	0	IU	0
E	15	IU	5	IU	31
K	500	μg	10	μg	2
Folic Acid	400	μg	28	μg	7

MINERALS USRDA			ONE SERVING GIVES YOU APPROXIMATELY		APPROXIMATE PERCENTAGE OF USRDA
Sodium	(1,100–3,000)	mg	461	mg	46
Calcium	1,000	mg	99	mg	12
Phosphorus	(800–1,000)	mg	363	mg	45
Potassium	(1,875–5,625)	mg	1,181	mg	147◄
Magnesium	400	μg	124	μg	35
Selenium	200	μg	31	μg	15
Iodine	150	mg	0	mg	0
Zinc	15	mg	5	mg	35
Iron	10	mg	9	mg	88
Manganese	(2.5–5.0)	mg	0.08	mg	1
Copper	(2.0–3.0)	mg	0.11	mg	3

AMOUNT PER SERVING		CALORIES PER SERVING	% OF MEAL
Fat	22 grams	202	39
Proteins	47 grams	188	37
Carbohydrates	31 grams	125	24
Cholesterol	99 mg		
Amino acid (essential)			322–844
Fiber	6 grams		

Key: USRDA = Recommended Dietary Allowance

    IU = International Unit

    mg = milligrams

    μg = micrograms

NOTE: The numbers with arrows exceed 100 percent of required USRDA.

Steak and Vegetable Gravy

Ingredients:

4 7-oz pieces of flank
  steak
1 cup chick peas,
  drained, liquid reserved
1 cup of canned kernel
  corn, drained, liquid reserved
2 cups mashed white turnips
1 packaged pea soup mix
1 tsp margarine
1 tsp vegetable oil
4 $\frac{1}{2}$ tsp arrowroot
$\frac{1}{2}$ tsp Tabasco sauce
  cayenne
$\frac{1}{2}$ tsp paprika

Preparation: Sauté

Time: 30 minutes

Calories: 780 per serving

Serves: 8

Directions

Steam turnip chunks, add margarine and paprika, and make a mash. Put chick peas in a blender and puree. Combine reserved liquid from chick peas and corn. Blend the peas into the mashed turnips until a smooth brown color emerges. Spoon in the corn kernel to this mixture. Add reserved liquid. Cut the steak on the diagonal into 2-inch strips and in a large iron skillet sauté in oil until browned. Remove steak from skillet. Blend in 4 $\frac{1}{2}$ tsp arrowroot and add 1 cup of green pea soup mix and cook to medium consistency. Add the Tabasco and cayenne. Return the steak to the sauce and simmer until done to taste. Make a large mound vegetable mixture in the center of dinner plates. Make a hole about 2-inches in diameter. Fill the hole with 1 $\frac{1}{2}$ cup of the sautéed steak and gravy and serve. Ample amounts of vitamins B_2 and E, an overload of potassium, and important iron are contained in this dish.

TIP: Most of the body's iron can be found in the blood, and women lose a large supply of iron during each menstrual period. And since many women eat less meat than men, it's harder for women to store enough iron during meals to meet the USRDA of 15 milligrams. For this reason, several million American women may be lacking sufficient iron, according to the National Center for Health Statistics.

MYTH: Most people who develop cancerous moles have red hair and freckles.

FACT: Dr. William A. Robinson, professor at University of Colorado, says a study undertaken at the university's Sciences Center in Denver disproves this.

Nutrients Contained in:
Steak and Vegetable Gravy

VITAMINS USRDA			ONE SERVING GIVES YOU APPROXIMATELY		APPROXIMATE PERCENTAGE OF USRDA
A	5,000	IU	292	IU	5
B$_1$	1.4	mg	0.53	mg	43
B$_2$	1.6	mg	1	mg	75
B$_3$	16	mg	9	mg	56
B$_5$	10	mg	2	mg	22
B$_6$	2.2	mg	1	mg	56
B$_{12}$	3	μg	4	μg	120◄
C	60	mg	11	mg	18
D	400	IU	0	IU	0
E	15	IU	4	IU	25
K	500	μg	17	μg	3
Folic Acid	400	μg	32	μg	8

MINERALS USRDA			ONE SERVING GIVES YOU APPROXIMATELY		APPROXIMATE PERCENTAGE OF USRDA
Sodium	(1,100–3,000)	mg	415	mg	41
Calcium	1,000	mg	124	mg	15
Phosphorus	(800–1,000)	mg	645	mg	80
Potassium	(1,875–5,625)	mg	1,517	mg	189◄
Magnesium	400	μg	150	μg	42
Selenium	200	μg	46	μg	22
Iodine	150	mg	0	mg	0
Zinc	15	mg	8	mg	53
Iron	10	mg	17	mg	167◄
Manganese	(2.5–5.0)	mg	0.79	mg	15
Copper	(2.0–3.0)	mg	0.49	mg	16

AMOUNT PER SERVING		CALORIES PER SERVING	% OF MEAL
Fat	33 grams	300	38
Proteins	66 grams	265	34
Carbohydrates	54 grams	215	28
Cholesterol	125 mg		
Amino acid (essential)			502–999
Fiber	39 grams		

Key: USRDA = Recommended Dietary Allowance

IU = International Unit

mg = milligrams

μg = micrograms

NOTE: The numbers with arrows exceed 100 percent of required USRDA.

Fruited Chicken

Ingredients:

4 boned chicken breast halves
¼ cup shallots, minced
1 tsp sage
½ cup pineapple juice
1 cantaloupe, peeled and cut into pieces
orange slices
⅛ tsp cayenne pepper

Preparation: Sauté and simmer

Time: 35 minutes

Calories: 125 per serving

Serves: 4

Directions

Cut the chicken breasts into chunks. In a nonstick skillet, add chicken, shallots, pepper, and pineapple juice and cook over moderate heat. When chicken turns white, add the orange slices, cantaloupe, and sage. Cover and simmer over low heat for about 7 minutes; add more juice if necessary. Serve with 1 ½ cups tossed greens, 1 sliced green pepper, and steamed mushroom slices if desired.

TIP: The recommended dietary allowances for proteins are set deliberately high by the Food and Nutrition Board of the National Research Council at the National Academy of Sciences. They are meant as a guide for nutritionists, and people should not worry if they don't eat exact amounts. Women over age 25 are advised to eat at least 50 grams of protein a day. Men over age 25 should eat 63 grams. There are about 28 grams in an ounce of meat, poultry, and fish.

MYTH: Eating protein builds muscles.

FACT: Muscle growth actually occurs only as a result of exercise.

Nutrients Contained in: Fruited Chicken

VITAMINS USRDA			ONE SERVING GIVES YOU APPROXIMATELY		APPROXIMATE PERCENTAGE OF USRDA
A	5,000	IU	4,695	IU	93
B_1	1.4	mg	0.12	mg	10
B_2	1.6	mg	0.09	mg	6
B_3	16	mg	4	mg	27
B_5	10	mg	0.56	mg	5
B_6	2.2	mg	0.38	mg	17
B_{12}	3	μg	0.13	μg	4
C	60	mg	80	mg	133◄
D	400	IU	0	IU	0
E	15	IU	0.40	IU	2
K	500	μg	0.25	μg	0
Folic Acid	400	μg	42	μg	10

MINERALS USRDA			ONE SERVING GIVES YOU APPROXIMATELY		APPROXIMATE PERCENTAGE OF USRDA
Sodium	(1,100–3,000)	mg	35	mg	3
Calcium	1,000	mg	40	mg	4
Phosphorus	(800–1,000)	mg	93	mg	11
Potassium	(1,875–5,625)	mg	608	mg	76
Magnesium	400	μg	32	μg	9
Selenium	200	μg	0.73	μg	0
Iodine	150	mg	0	mg	0
Zinc	15	mg	0.61	mg	4
Iron	10	mg	0.76	mg	7
Manganese	(2.5–5.0)	mg	0.39	mg	7
Copper	(2.0–3.0)	mg	0.11	mg	3

AMOUNT PER SERVING		CALORIES PER SERVING	% OF MEAL
Fat	1 gram	9	7
Proteins	9 grams	37	30
Carbohydrates	20 grams	79	63
Cholesterol	29 mg		
Amino acid (essential)			98–152
Fiber	1 gram		

Key: USRDA = Recommended Dietary Allowance

　　　IU = International Unit

　　　mg = milligrams

　　　μg = micrograms

NOTE: The numbers with arrows exceed 100 percent of required USRDA.

Plain and Simple Sole

Ingredients:

4	slices fillet of sole
1	cucumber, peeled, seeded, grated
2	lemons
1	Tbs nonfat yogurt
$\frac{1}{2}$	tsp chili powder
$\frac{1}{4}$	tsp onion powder
	cayenne pepper
$\frac{1}{4}$	tsp chervil

Preparation: Broil

Time: 55 minutes

Calories: 146 per serving

Serves: 4

Directions

Juice the lemons and pour juice over fish. Place fish in baking dish and let stand for about 30 minutes to marinate. Spread the fish with the yogurt and sprinkle the chili powder and onion powder on them. Put the fish under the broiler for about 7 minutes. Test to see if it flakes easily. About 2 minutes before taking out of broiler, sprinkle chervil and cayenne pepper on fish.

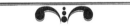

TIP: Dr. Gabe Mirkin, a sports doctor, says that clinical depression is very common in America and that tiredness is an outstanding aspect of it. Citing a large-scale population study by the National Center for Health Services Research, he found that psychological, not physical, factors are the most powerful indicators of exhaustion.

MYTH: To gain any fitness benefits, you must work out 30 to 40 minutes at a time.

FACT: This used to be the thinking, but now says a Stanford University researcher, the evidence indicates this is not true. Those who jogged for 10 minutes, three times a day, raised their oxygen uptake by 8 percent in two months. The point is that anything helps rather than no activity at all.

Nutrients Contained in: Plain and Simple Sole

VITAMINS USRDA			ONE SERVING GIVES YOU APPROXIMATELY		APPROXIMATE PERCENTAGE OF USRDA
A	5,000	IU	38	IU	0
B$_1$	1.4	mg	0.15	mg	12
B$_2$	1.6	mg	0.12	mg	8
B$_3$	16	mg	4	mg	22
B$_5$	10	mg	0.82	mg	8
B$_6$	2.2	mg	0.05	mg	2
B$_{12}$	3	μg	2	μg	53
C	60	mg	11	mg	18
D	400	IU	0	IU	0
E	15	IU	0.85	IU	5
K	500	μg	1	μg	0
Folic Acid	400	μg	34	μg	8

MINERALS USRDA			ONE SERVING GIVES YOU APPROXIMATELY		APPROXIMATE PERCENTAGE OF USRDA
Sodium	(1,100–3,000)	mg	114	mg	11
Calcium	1,000	mg	136	mg	17
Phosphorus	(800–1,000)	mg	405	mg	50
Potassium	(1,875–5,625)	mg	864	mg	108◄
Magnesium	400	μg	75	μg	21
Selenium	200	μg	51	μg	25
Iodine	150	mg	0	mg	0
Zinc	15	mg	0.78	mg	5
Iron	10	mg	2	mg	18
Manganese	(2.5–5.0)	mg	0.09	mg	1
Copper	(2.0–3.0)	mg	0.06	mg	1

AMOUNT PER SERVING		CALORIES PER SERVING	% OF MEAL
Fat	1 gram	10	7
Proteins	31 grams	122	83
Carbohydrates	4 grams	14	10
Cholesterol	0 mg		
Amino acid (essential)			178–596
Fiber	1 gram		

Key: USRDA = Recommended Dietary Allowance
    IU = International Unit
    mg = milligrams
    μg = micrograms
NOTE: The numbers with arrows exceed 100 percent of required USRDA.

Turkey's Dark Side

Ingredients:

1 lb dark meat turkey cutlets
1 Tbs whole wheat flour
½ cup low-sodium chicken broth
1 onion, chopped coarsely
1 cup zucchini, sliced
4 cloves garlic, finely chopped
1 cup cauliflower, chopped in small pieces
1 tsp ground ginger
½ tsp curry powder
1 bay leaf
1 can tomatoes
cayenne pepper
noncaloric spray

Preparation: Sauté and simmer

Calories: 206 per serving

Serves: 4

Directions

Cut turkey into strips about ½ inch wide. Roll in flour. Use a noncaloric spray and sauté the turkey in a skillet. Add a little water if pan gets dry; this will add steam to the cooking. Remove turkey after 6 minutes and add the broth to the pan; boil rapidly for a few minutes. Reduce the flame to low; add the onions, garlic, zucchini, and cauliflower; and cook until vegetables are al dente, about 3 to 4 minutes. Add the tomatoes, curry powder, ginger, bay leaf, and a dash of cayenne pepper. Cover and simmer for 8 minutes. Stir every now then. Add the turkey and heat thoroughly. This dish has high amounts of vitamin K, iron, and EAA. Serve 1 cup cooked spinach with nutmeg and lemon juice and 1 cup strawberries if desired.

TIP: Pediatricians say the human baby who is breast fed receives all the iron it needs from its mother, if the mother is fairly well fed herself. In a study done with breast-fed babies who received only their mother's milk for the first 18 months of life, the children grew and gained the right amount of weight and were not anemic.

MYTH: With menopause you will lose all desire for sex.

FACT: Dr. Brian W. Walsh, director of the menopause unit at Brigham and Women's Hospital in Boston says, there are mechanical "problems" that can create obstacles, but there are ways to bypass them. Staying active with sex and using various creams or getting testosterone treatment are available remedies that can be tried.

Nutrients Contained in: Turkey's Dark Side

VITAMINS USRDA			ONE SERVING GIVES YOU APPROXIMATELY		APPROXIMATE PERCENTAGE OF USRDA
A	5,000	IU	126	IU	2
B_1	1.4	mg	0.12	mg	10
B_2	1.6	mg	0.14	mg	9
B_3	16	mg	3	mg	15
B_5	10	mg	0.66	mg	6
B_6	2.2	mg	0.29	mg	13
B_{12}	3	μg	0.15	μg	4
C	60	mg	23	mg	38
D	400	IU	0	IU	0
E	15	IU	0.26	IU	1
K	500	μg	900	μg	180◄
Folic Acid	400	μg	36	μg	8

MINERALS USRDA			ONE SERVING GIVES YOU APPROXIMATELY		APPROXIMATE PERCENTAGE OF USRDA
Sodium	(1,100–3,000)	mg	40	mg	3
Calcium	1,000	mg	50	mg	6
Phosphorus	(800–1,000)	mg	217	mg	27
Potassium	(1,875–5,625)	mg	440	mg	55
Magnesium	400	μg	59	μg	16
Selenium	200	μg	0.95	μg	0
Iodine	150	mg	0	mg	0
Zinc	15	mg	3	mg	21
Iron	10	mg	2	mg	15
Manganese	(2.5–5.0)	mg	0.19	mg	3
Copper	(2.0–3.0)	mg	0.42	mg	13

AMOUNT PER SERVING		CALORIES PER SERVING	% OF MEAL
Fat	14 grams	122	59
Proteins	12 grams	47	23
Carbohydrates	9 grams	37	18
Cholesterol	28 mg		
Amino acid (essential)			167–258
Fiber	1 gram		

Key: USRDA = Recommended Dietary Allowance
   IU = International Unit
   mg = milligrams
   μg = micrograms
NOTE: The numbers with arrows exceed 100 percent of required USRDA.

Little Livers

Ingredients:

- 8 chicken livers
- 1 onion, chopped
- 2 cups kale, chopped
- $\frac{1}{2}$ tsp lite soy sauce
- 1 cup apple cider or juice
- 4 cloves garlic, sliced
- 1 lemon, sliced
- $\frac{1}{2}$ cup sunflower seeds
- $\frac{1}{2}$ tsp ground ginger
- 1 cup water
- 1 tsp chervil
- 1 tsp whole wheat flour
- cayenne pepper

Preparation: Cook and simmer

Time: 45 minutes

Calories: 320 per serving

Serves: 4

Directions

Steam kale for about 10 minutes. Cook onion, livers, and kale in $\frac{1}{2}$ Tsp lite soy sauce. If pan gets dry, add a little water. Sprinkle in flour, add 1 cup of water and apple cider. Add garlic and lemon; cover and simmer over low heat for 20 minutes. Ground sunflower seeds in a blender and stir into pan 5 minutes before serving. Notice the beneficial amounts of vitamins B_2, A, and E ; folic acid; and EAA from just a few small chicken livers.

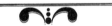

TIP: According to Dr. D. W. Edington, director of the Fitness Research Center at the University of Michigan, it takes only a little exercise for an energy boost. He says a brisk 10-minute walk can boost energy and relieve tension for a couple of hours.

MYTH: Menopause causes heart disease.

FACT: Dr. Trudy Bush, professor of epidemiology and gynecology at Johns Hopkins University in Baltimore, says this is not exactly true. What may happen is that an unhealthy life-style and eating patterns may play a more dominant role than the lack of estrogen that occurs. She looks more at smoking, high blood pressure, and sedentary habits as important factors.

Nutrients Contained in: Little Livers

VITAMINS USRDA			ONE SERVING GIVES YOU APPROXIMATELY		APPROXIMATE PERCENTAGE OF USRDA
A	5,000	IU	14,645	IU	292◄
B$_1$	1.4	mg	0.70	mg	58
B$_2$	1.6	mg	1	mg	96
B$_3$	16	mg	8	mg	47
B$_5$	10	mg	4	mg	44
B$_6$	2.2	mg	0.96	mg	43
B$_{12}$	3	μg	15	μg	490◄
C	60	mg	54	mg	89
D	400	IU	10	IU	2
E	15	IU	28	IU	187◄
K	500	μg	56	μg	11
Folic Acid	400	μg	486	μg	121◄

MINERALS USRDA			ONE SERVING GIVES YOU APPROXIMATELY		APPROXIMATE PERCENTAGE OF USRDA
Sodium	(1,100–3,000)	mg	62	mg	6
Calcium	1,000	mg	80	mg	9
Phosphorus	(800–1,000)	mg	435	mg	54
Potassium	(1,875–5,625)	mg	643	mg	80
Magnesium	400	μg	42	μg	12
Selenium	200	μg	4	μg	1
Iodine	150	mg	0	mg	0
Zinc	15	mg	2	mg	11
Iron	10	mg	8	mg	81
Manganese	(2.5–5.0)	mg	0.96	mg	19
Copper	(2.0–3.0)	mg	0.83	mg	27

AMOUNT PER SERVING		CALORIES PER SERVING	% OF MEAL
Fat	17 grams	155	48
Proteins	19 grams	78	24
Carbohydrates	22 grams	87	28
Cholesterol	200 mg		
Amino acid (essential)			244–315
Fiber	2 grams		

Key: USRDA = Recommended Dietary Allowance
     IU = International Unit
    mg = milligrams
    μg = micrograms
NOTE: The numbers with arrows exceed 100 percent of required USRDA.

Big Liver

Ingredients:

- 1 lb calf's liver
- 1 cup low-sodium chicken broth
- 4 cloves garlic, chopped
- 1 cup okra
- ½ cup wheat germ
- 8 shiitake mushrooms
- 1 tsp vegetable oil
- 1 cup tomatoes, chopped
- ¼ tsp caraway seeds
- ¼ tsp thyme
- 1 tsp basil
- 1 onion, sliced into rings
- 1 tsp lite soy sauce

Preparation: Sauté

Time: 25 minutes

Calories: 355 per serving

Serves: 4

Directions

Combine the chicken broth and tomatoes. Bring to a boil in a saucepan. Cook the onion rings, garlic, okra, wheat germ, and mushrooms in the oil until okra and onions are done. Add these ingredients to the tomato and chicken broth. Season with caraway seeds, thyme, basil, and a dash of cayenne pepper. Sauté liver in a teaspoon of lite soy sauce in a skillet over high heat for about 1 minute. Add the liver to the tomato/broth. Cover and simmer for 5 minutes. A look at the chart will astound you at the nutritional

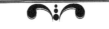

gold mine contained in liver.

TIP: Sleep researchers say when people are deprived of such time cues as alarm clocks and daylight, they usually sleep longer. They also estimate that some 80 percent of us are chronically sleep deprived. By adding just one more hour of sleep at night, you can boost waking energy dramatically, according to Dr. Timothy Roehrs at the Henry Ford Hospital's Sleep Disorders and Research Center in Detroit.

MYTH: Biomedical decline is inevitable with old age.

FACT: Dr. Franklin Williams at the Buck Geriatric Center for Research on Aging in Marin County, California, says that evidence shows most of our organs are surprisingly functional throughout later years. He found that people in their 70s seldom show intellectual decline.

Nutrients Contained in: Big Liver

VITAMINS USRDA			ONE SERVING GIVES YOU APPROXIMATELY		APPROXIMATE PERCENTAGE OF USRDA
A	5,000	IU	28,470	IU	569◄
B$_1$	1.4	mg	0.58	mg	47
B$_2$	1.6	mg	4	mg	256◄
B$_3$	16	mg	19	mg	117◄
B$_5$	10	mg	10	mg	102◄
B$_6$	2.2	mg	1	mg	51
B$_{12}$	3	μg	75	μg	2,502◄
C	60	mg	60	mg	100◄
D	400	IU	56	IU	14
E	15	IU	1	IU	8
K	500	μg	115	μg	23
Folic Acid	400	μg	378	μg	94

MINERALS USRDA			ONE SERVING GIVES YOU APPROXIMATELY		APPROXIMATE PERCENTAGE OF USRDA
Sodium	(1,100–3,000)	mg	405	mg	40
Calcium	1,000	mg	60	mg	7
Phosphorus	(800–1,000)	mg	196	mg	24
Potassium	(1,875–5,625)	mg	932	mg	116◄
Magnesium	400	μg	108	μg	30
Selenium	200	μg	56	μg	28
Iodine	150	mg	0	mg	0
Zinc	15	mg	10	mg	64
Iron	10	mg	13	mg	130◄
Manganese	(2.5–5.0)	mg	3	mg	65
Copper	(2.0–3.0)	mg	7	mg	219◄

AMOUNT PER SERVING		CALORIES PER SERVING	% OF MEAL
Fat	8 grams	72	20
Proteins	33 grams	130	37
Carbohydrates	38 grams	153	43
Cholesterol	375 mg		
Amino acid (essential)			277–541
Fiber	5 grams		

Key: USRDA = Recommended Dietary Allowance

　　　　IU = International Unit

　　　　mg = milligrams

　　　　μg = micrograms

NOTE: The numbers with arrows exceed 100 percent of required USRDA.

American Swedish Meatballs

Ingredients:

- 1 lb lean ground beef
- $\frac{1}{2}$ lb ground pork
- $\frac{1}{2}$ cup wheat germ
- 1 onion, chopped
- $\frac{1}{3}$ cup skimmed milk
- 2 egg whites, beaten
- $\frac{1}{2}$ tsp allspice
- $\frac{1}{2}$ tsp nutmeg
- $\frac{1}{2}$ cup low-sodium chicken broth
- $\frac{1}{2}$ cup cranberry sauce

Preparation: Sauté

Time: 20 minutes

Calories: 340 per serving

Serves: 5

Directions

Combine all the ingredients except broth and cranberry sauce. Create 36 small meatballs out of this mixture and brown in a large iron skillet. Once brown, remove and set aside. Add wheat germ and cranberry sauce to skillet. Stir and cook for about 2 minutes. Add broth and mix well. Return meatballs to skillet and heat through. Serve with 1 cup cooked green beans with almonds and a 5-inch watermelon wedge, which adds 68 calories and 3 grams fat, 2 grams protein, 9 grams carbohydrate, and 1 gram fiber. High amounts of iron, vitamin B_2, and EAA are obtained from this meal.

TIP: Dr. Jon Kabat-Zinn, director of the stress reduction clinic at the University of Massachusetts Medical Center, says a positive outlook can affect your energy level in a big way and regularly missing just one hour of sleep a night can cause energy problems. The advice is: Don't stint on sleep.

MYTH: You can reduce your amount of sleep without any negative consequences.

FACT: Dr. Robert H. Hicks, at San Jose State University in California, says that it's a common myth that you can reduce your amount of sleep without negative consequences. He says the average person needs about seven and a half hours of sleep each night to fight fatigue.

Nutrients Contained in:
American Swedish Meatballs

VITAMINS USRDA			ONE SERVING GIVES YOU APPROXIMATELY		APPROXIMATE PERCENTAGE OF USRDA
A	5,000	IU	102	IU	2
B_1	1.4	mg	0.95	mg	79
B_2	1.6	mg	0.44	mg	31
B_3	16	mg	11	mg	71
B_5	10	mg	1	mg	12
B_6	2.2	mg	0.78	mg	35
B_{12}	3	μg	2	μg	78
C	60	mg	4	mg	6
D	400	IU	25	IU	6
E	15	IU	1	IU	6
K	500	μg	13	μg	2
Folic Acid	400	μg	58	μg	14

MINERALS USRDA			ONE SERVING GIVES YOU APPROXIMATELY		APPROXIMATE PERCENTAGE OF USRDA
Sodium	(1,100–3,000)	mg	176	mg	17
Calcium	1,000	mg	69	mg	8
Phosphorus	(800–1,000)	mg	581	mg	72
Potassium	(1,875–5,625)	mg	1,011	mg	126◄
Magnesium	400	μg	80	μg	22
Selenium	200	μg	49	μg	24
Iodine	150	mg	6	mg	4
Zinc	15	mg	6	mg	41
Iron	10	mg	8	mg	79
Manganese	(2.5–5.0)	mg	2	mg	46
Copper	(2.0–3.0)	mg	0.18	mg	9

AMOUNT PER SERVING		CALORIES PER SERVING	% OF MEAL
Fat	12 grams	104	31
Proteins	50 grams	199	58
Carbohydrates	9 grams	37	11
Cholesterol	181 mg		
Amino acid (essential)			351-929
Fiber	19 grams		

Key: USRDA = Recommended Dietary Allowance

IU = International Unit

mg = milligrams

μg = micrograms

NOTE: The numbers with arrows exceed 100 percent of required USRDA.

Chili Turkey

Ingredients:

- 1 lb ground turkey
- 1 cup chopped onion, coarse pieces
- 4 cloves garlic, crushed
- 4 Tbs horseradish
- 1 tsp chili powder
- 1 tsp cumin
- 1 tsp sage
- 2 cups cooked kidney beans
- $\frac{1}{2}$ cup low-sodium chicken broth
- 1 cup mild salsa sauce
- 2 Tbs whole wheat flour
- $\frac{1}{4}$ cup plain yogurt
- 1 Tbs Parmesan cheese, grated
- 1 tsp vegetable oil

Preparation: Sauté and simmer

Time: 25 minutes

Calories: 256 per serving

Serves: 4

Directions

Heat oil in iron skillet. Add turkey, onions, and garlic. Cook for about 4 minutes. Add chili powder, cumin, sage, and horseradish; cook and mix until turkey is cooked through. Stir in beans and broth. Combine salsa sauce and whole wheat flour. Add to skillet and bring to a boil. Reduce heat and simmer uncovered about 10 minutes. Spoon into soup bowls and top with yogurt to taste. Sprinkle cheese over top. High amounts of iron, vitamin E, and EAA come with this meal.

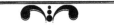

TIP: If you want to get more iron without adding a lot of calories, choose liver, lean red meat, and plant sources such as peas and beans and leafy dark green vegetables and whole grains.

MYTH: Once you reach menopause, calcium and exercise won't help your bones.

FACT: The USDA Human Nutrition Research Center on Aging at Tufts University found that postmenopausal women who have low-calcium diet can reduce bone loss by bringing their calcium intakes to USRDA levels.

Nutrients Contained in: Chili Turkey

VITAMINS USRDA			ONE SERVING GIVES YOU APPROXIMATELY		APPROXIMATE PERCENTAGE OF USRDA
A	5,000	IU	25	IU	0
B_1	1.4	mg	0.21	mg	17
B_2	1.6	mg	0.19	mg	13
B_3	16	mg	3	mg	15
B_5	10	mg	0.54	mg	5
B_6	2.2	mg	0.22	mg	10
B_{12}	3	μg	0.26	μg	8
C	60	mg	3	mg	5
D	400	IU	6	IU	1
E	15	IU	4	IU	25
K	500	μg	0	μg	0
Folic Acid	400	μg	18	μg	4

MINERALS USRDA			ONE SERVING GIVES YOU APPROXIMATELY		APPROXIMATE PERCENTAGE OF USRDA
Sodium	(1,100–3,000)	mg	176	mg	17
Calcium	1,000	mg	109	mg	13
Phosphorus	(800–1,000)	mg	247	mg	30
Potassium	(1,875–5,625)	mg	624	mg	77
Magnesium	400	μg	30	μg	8
Selenium	200	μg	0.80	μg	0
Iodine	150	mg	7	mg	4
Zinc	15	mg	2	mg	11
Iron	10	mg	3	mg	34
Manganese	(2.5–5.0)	mg	0.06	mg	1
Copper	(2.0–3.0)	mg	0.43	mg	14

AMOUNT PER SERVING		CALORIES PER SERVING	% OF MEAL
Fat	6 grams	58	23
Proteins	18 grams	72	28
Carbohydrates	32 grams	126	49
Cholesterol	30 mg		
Amino acid (essential)			253–569
Fiber	3 grams		

Key: USRDA = Recommended Dietary Allowance
      IU = International Unit
      mg = milligrams
      μg = micrograms
NOTE: The numbers with arrows exceed 100 percent of required USRDA.

Cruciferous Cabbage Roll

Ingredients:

1	lb lean ground beef
1	head green cabbage
$\frac{1}{3}$	cup rice bran
$\frac{1}{4}$	cup sesame seeds
1	onion, chopped
3	cloves garlic, chopped
1	red pepper, seeded and chopped
$\frac{1}{4}$	cup tomato paste
$\frac{1}{2}$	cup water
	cayenne pepper
$\frac{1}{4}$	tsp salt

Preparation: Bake

Time: 50 minutes

Calories: 348 per serving

Serves: 5

Directions

Mix all the ingredients except the cabbage and tomato paste in a large bowl. Trim the outer leaves of the cabbage and separate the cabbage into leaves. Steam leaves for about 1 minute. When soft, place a heaping tablespoon of the meat mixture into each cabbage leaf and roll edges of leaf around it. Put the rolls in a baking pan. Combine the tomato paste and the water and pour over the rolls. Bake about 30 minutes. See chart and ample percentages of vitamins E and B_2, potassium, and EAA contained here.

TIP: To help replace the iron lost regularly through menstruation, women are advised to get the USRDA of 18 milligrams of iron a day. This meal gives you 8 milligrams. The average American diet is reported to contain about 6 milligrams of iron per thousand calories.

MYTH: Red meat should not be included in one's diet.

FACT: Dietitians say there is no need to omit red meat in a heart-healthy diet. Lean cuts with less than 30 percent of their calories from fat are available. These include "select" grades of lean cuts such as top round and tenderloin, which are the lowest in fat.

Nutrients Contained in: Cruciferous Cabbage Roll

VITAMINS USRDA			ONE SERVING GIVES YOU APPROXIMATELY		APPROXIMATE PERCENTAGE OF USRDA
A	5,000	IU	743	IU	14
B_1	1.4	mg	0.57	mg	47
B_2	1.6	mg	0.27	mg	19
B_3	16	mg	11	mg	70
B_5	10	mg	0.99	mg	9
B_6	2.2	mg	0.81	mg	36
B_{12}	3	μg	2	μg	55
C	60	mg	96	mg	160◄
D	400	IU	5	IU	1
E	15	IU	3	IU	18
K	500	μg	87	μg	17
Folic Acid	400	μg	135	μg	33

MINERALS USRDA			ONE SERVING GIVES YOU APPROXIMATELY		APPROXIMATE PERCENTAGE OF USRDA
Sodium	(1,100–3,000)	mg	252	mg	25
Calcium	1,000	mg	130	mg	16
Phosphorus	(800–1,000)	mg	366	mg	45
Potassium	(1,875–5,625)	mg	1,263	mg	157◄
Magnesium	400	μg	120	μg	34
Selenium	200	μg	26	μg	13
Iodine	150	mg	5	mg	3
Zinc	15	mg	5	mg	32
Iron	10	mg	8	mg	76
Manganese	(2.5–5.0)	mg	0.38	mg	7
Copper	(2.0–3.0)	mg	0.28	mg	9

AMOUNT PER SERVING		CALORIES PER SERVING	% OF MEAL
Fat	10 grams	92	26
Proteins	34 grams	135	39
Carbohydrates	30 grams	121	35
Cholesterol	130 mg		
Amino acid (essential)			245–582
Fiber	2 grams		

Key: USRDA = Recommended Dietary Allowance
     IU = International Unit
    mg = milligrams
    μg = micrograms
NOTE: The numbers with arrows exceed 100 percent of required USRDA.

Fava Chicken

Ingredients:

1 ½ cup fava beans
1 cup onions, chopped
4 cups water
1 tsp vegetable oil
4 cloves garlic
¼ cup sesame seeds
1 ½ lb chicken
1 cup kasha
1 egg white, beaten lightly
¼ tsp turmeric
½ tsp ground ginger
1 ½ cups low-sodium
   chicken broth
   juice of one lemon
¼ tsp cumin
¼ tsp chili powder
   noncaloric spray

Preparation: Boil, simmer, bake

Time: 3 hours

Calories: 867 per serving

Serves: 4

Directions

Preheat oven to 350°F. Soak beans overnight. Use the same soaking water and place beans in a large saucepan. Cover and cook over medium heat for 1 hour. Using noncaloric spray or nonstick frying pan, sauté the onions until soft; add sesame seeds and garlic. Sauté for about 2 minutes. Stir in cinnamon, ginger, turmeric, and cumin. In a large casserole dish, add the onion mixture. Top this with the fava beans. Add 1 cup of broth and the juice of one lemon. Simmer on top of the stove. Cut the chicken into pieces removing skin and fat. Lay the pieces over the beans and onions. Sprinkle with chili powder. Cover and bake for about 1 hour. Check to see if chicken is tender; if not cook another 30 minutes. Put the remaining broth in a saucepan and bring to boil. Add the kasha and an egg white and stir until egg has dried on kasha. Reduce heat, cover, and simmer for about 20 minutes until soft. Cover the kasha with the beans and sesame seed mixture and add a little liquid to the kasha. Lay the chicken on top and serve. High amounts of folic acid, potassium, and vitamins B$_2$ and E are found in this meal.

TIP: Try to preserve the vitamins and minerals in your food. It is advisable to use the least possible heat, water, and cooking time. For example, folic acid is destroyed by heat. So eat vegetables raw or steam them when possible.

Nutrients Contained in: Fava Chicken

VITAMINS USRDA			ONE SERVING GIVES YOU APPROXIMATELY		APPROXIMATE PERCENTAGE OF USRDA
A	5,000	IU	651	IU	13
B$_1$	1.4	mg	1	mg	91
B$_2$	1.6	mg	0.44	mg	31
B$_3$	16	mg	10	mg	63
B$_5$	10	mg	0.87	mg	8
B$_6$	2.2	mg	1	mg	47
B$_{12}$	3	μg	0.24	μg	8
C	60	mg	23	mg	38
D	400	IU	0	IU	0
E	15	IU	2	IU	16
K	500	μg	0	μg	0
Folic Acid	400	μg	555	μg	138◀

MINERALS USRDA			ONE SERVING GIVES YOU APPROXIMATELY		APPROXIMATE PERCENTAGE OF USRDA
Sodium	(1,100–3,000)	mg	834	mg	83
Calcium	1,000	mg	421	mg	52
Phosphorus	(800–1,000)	mg	283	mg	35
Potassium	(1,875–5,625)	mg	2,598	mg	324◀
Magnesium	400	μg	322	μg	92
Selenium	200	μg	4	μg	1
Iodine	150	mg	0	mg	0
Zinc	15	mg	7	mg	46
Iron	10	mg	14	mg	136◀
Manganese	(2.5–5.0)	mg	0.58	mg	11
Copper	(2.0–3.0)	mg	0.52	mg	17

AMOUNT PER SERVING		CALORIES PER SERVING	% OF MEAL
Fat	17 grams	149	17
Proteins	59 grams	236	27
Carbohydrates	121 grams	482	56
Cholesterol	30 mg		
Amino acid (essential)			209–309
Fiber	181 grams		

Key: USRDA = Recommended Dietary Allowance

  IU = International Unit

  mg = milligrams

  μg = micrograms

NOTE: The numbers with arrows exceed 100 percent of required USRDA.

Stuffed Reds

Ingredients:

2 lbs lean chopped beef
3 cloves garlic, crushed
1 tsp chervil
1 tsp vegetable oil
1 cup cooked red lentils
4 large tomatoes
1/2 cup tomato paste
1/2 cup water
1 tsp cinnamon
1 tsp rosemary
1 tsp onion flakes
8 shiitake mushrooms
sprinkle of cayenne
pepper

Preparation: Sauté and simmer

Time: 35 minutes

Calories: 425 per serving

Serves: 4

Directions

Sauté chopped beef in half teaspoon of the oil, add garlic and chervil, and sauté until beef is brown. Add 1 cup cooked lentils. Using very firm tomatoes, slit halfway across the center of each. Scoop out the tomato flesh with a spoon. Fill the scooped-out shell with the beef mixture and close the tomato. Heat the rest of the oil in the skillet and sauté the tomatoes, rolling them gently until they become dark red all round. Remove tomatoes and place them in a large saucepan. Combine the tomato paste, chopped mushrooms, water, cinnamon, onion flakes, and rosemary and pour over tomatoes. Simmer over low flame for about 10 minutes and serve on a large platter. Surround the tomatoes with cut melon slices.

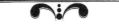

TIP: Dietitian Maudene Nelson, with Metropolitan Life's Center for Healthy Living, advises that there should be ample vitamin C in the diet as this nutrient boosts iron absorption. So when eating iron-rich foods, accompany them with some citrus fruit or strawberries, melons, or tomatoes.

MYTH: Gelatin will strengthen and grow fingernails.

FACT: Nutritional researchers say there's no truth to this claim. The collagen you get from protein-filled foods such as lean meats, lentils, and fat-free dairy products, which provide amino acids that helps the body produce its own collagen, is more effective than is collagen taken in capsule form.

Nutrients Contained in: Stuffed Reds

VITAMINS USRDA			ONE SERVING GIVES YOU APPROXIMATELY		APPROXIMATE PERCENTAGE OF USRDA
A	5,000	IU	2,485	IU	49
B_1	1.4	mg	0.45	mg	37
B_2	1.6	mg	0.32	mg	22
B_3	16	mg	15	mg	93
B_5	10	mg	2	mg	16
B_6	2.2	mg	0.75	mg	34
B_{12}	3	μg	2	μg	75
C	60	mg	38	mg	62
D	400	IU	0	IU	0
E	15	IU	3	IU	23
K	500	μg	21	μg	4
Folic Acid	400	μg	51	μg	12

MINERALS USRDA			ONE SERVING GIVES YOU APPROXIMATELY		APPROXIMATE PERCENTAGE OF USRDA
Sodium	(1,100–3,000)	mg	91	mg	9
Calcium	1,000	mg	55	mg	6
Phosphorus	(800–1,000)	mg	467	mg	58
Potassium	(1,875–5,625)	mg	1,564	mg	195◄
Magnesium	400	μg	88	μg	25
Selenium	200	μg	39	μg	19
Iodine	150	mg	0	mg	0
Zinc	15	mg	7	mg	47
Iron	10	mg	9	mg	87
Manganese	(2.5–5.0)	mg	0.18	mg	3
Copper	(2.0–3.0)	mg	0.31	mg	10

AMOUNT PER SERVING		CALORIES PER SERVING	% OF MEAL
Fat	7 grams	65	15
Proteins	48 grams	190	45
Carbohydrates	42 grams	170	40
Cholesterol	113 mg		
Amino acid (essential)			352–961
Fiber	1 gram		

Key: USRDA = Recommended Dietary Allowance
　　　IU = International Unit
　　　mg = milligrams
　　　μg = micrograms
NOTE: The numbers with arrows exceed 100 percent of required USRDA.

Onion Lover's Chicken

Ingredients:

4	chicken boned breast halves
1	lemon cut in half
2	lb small white onions, sliced
¼	cup parsley, chopped
1	bay leaf
1	tsp sage
½	cup apple juice
½	cup lemon juice
4	Tbs nonfat sour cream
½	cup plain yogurt
1	cup peas
1	cup of green beans
2	cups low-sodium chicken broth cayenne pepper

Preparation: Broil and bake

Time: 1 hour, 40 minutes

Calories: 176 per serving

Serves: 4

Directions

Preheat broiler. Rub cut lemon over chicken (remove skin if desired) and place chicken in large baking pan. Cover chicken with onions, parsley, bay leaf, sage, and cayenne pepper. Combine apple juice, lemon juice, sour cream, and yogurt and pour over chicken. Allow to marinate for 30 minutes. Remove chicken and broil until brown on both sides and half done. Remove chicken from broiler and reduce oven heat to 350°F. Simmer the mixture chicken was marinated in for about 5 minutes. Now place the chicken in the pan covering with the onion mixture. Pour the chicken broth over the mixture and bake for about 20 minutes until onions are slightly brown. Steam the peas and beans for about 8 minutes and add some strips of pimento. Place on plates and top with the chicken breasts. Cover with the onion mixture and serve. This meal has a fair amount of iron and is rich in EAA.

TIP: Dr. Henry Lukaski of the U.S. Department of Agricultural Research Service says he observed that otherwise healthy young women who were eating an iron-poor diet had iron shortages which caused them to tire easily during exercise and to feel chilled often because they produced less body heat and lost it faster.

MYTH: Grapefruit burns fat off the body.

FACT: Nutritionists say grapefruit is a good food, but it can't burn fat.

Nutrients Contained in: Onion Lover's Chicken

VITAMINS USRDA			ONE SERVING GIVES YOU APPROXIMATELY		APPROXIMATE PERCENTAGE OF USRDA
A	5,000	IU	371	IU	7
B$_1$	1.4	mg	0.19	mg	15
B$_2$	1.6	mg	0.22	mg	15
B$_3$	16	mg	6	mg	38
B$_5$	10	mg	0.65	mg	6
B$_6$	2.2	mg	0.39	mg	17
B$_{12}$	3	μg	0.48	μg	15
C	60	mg	25	mg	42
D	400	IU	13	IU	3
E	15	IU	0.63	IU	4
K	500	μg	110	μg	22
Folic Acid	400	μg	46	μg	11

MINERALS USRDA			ONE SERVING GIVES YOU APPROXIMATELY		APPROXIMATE PERCENTAGE OF USRDA
Sodium	(1,100–3,000)	mg	446	mg	44
Calcium	1,000	mg	105	mg	13
Phosphorus	(800–1,000)	mg	177	mg	22
Potassium	(1,875–5,625)	mg	525	mg	65
Magnesium	400	μg	46	μg	13
Selenium	200	μg	4	μg	1
Iodine	150	mg	13	mg	8
Zinc	15	mg	1	mg	8
Iron	10	mg	2	mg	15
Manganese	(2.5–5.0)	mg	0.31	mg	6
Copper	(2.0–3.0)	mg	0.12	mg	4

AMOUNT PER SERVING		CALORIES PER SERVING	% OF MEAL
Fat	5 grams	41	23
Proteins	15 grams	60	34
Carbohydrates	19 grams	75	43
Cholesterol	37 mg		
Amino acid (essential)			138–217
Fiber	1 gram		

Key: USRDA = Recommended Dietary Allowance

IU = International Unit

mg = milligrams

μg = micrograms

NOTE: The numbers with arrows exceed 100 percent of required USRDA.

Lean and Mean Haddock

Ingredients: 1 ½ lb whole haddock
                      1 cup onions, chopped
                      1 ½ cups cauliflower, cut
                              into pieces
                      4 cloves garlic, crushed
                      ¼ tsp red pepper flakes
                      1 tsp chervil
                          juice of one lemon
                      1 tsp horseradish
                          noncaloric spray

Preparation: Bake

Time: 25 minutes

Calories: 242 per serving

Serves: 4

Directions

Preheat oven to 450° F. Mix chervil, garlic, red pepper, and lemon juice in a small bowl. Rub the mixture over the fish. Place fish in baking pan. Bake about 10 to 15 minutes. Sauté onions and cauliflower in a pan with noncaloric spray. Spread the onions and cauliflower over fish and place on a large platter and serve. Spread horseradish over fish if desired. Serve 1 cup of cooked asparagus and 1 ½ cups honeydew melon with mint if desired. Notice the high content of iodine, potassium, vitamin K, and EAA.

TIP: Physicians at Columbia University's College of Physicians and Surgeons in New York City say that among women of childbearing age the most common dietary deficiencies are of nutrients such as iron (essential to hemoglobin formation) and vitamin B_{12} and folic acid, both of which are necessary for red blood cell production.

MYTH: You will find sorbitol, a common artificial sweetener, only in manufactured products.

FACT: Not so. Many fruits contain a natural source of sorbitol. Prunes, for example, have about 12 grams in a 3-ounce portion.

Nutrients Contained in: Lean and Mean Haddock

VITAMINS USRDA			ONE SERVING GIVES YOU APPROXIMATELY		APPROXIMATE PERCENTAGE OF USRDA
A	5,000	IU	420	IU	8
B_1	1.4	mg	0.11	mg	8
B_2	1.6	mg	0.13	mg	9
B_3	16	mg	3	mg	21
B_5	10	mg	0.30	mg	3
B_6	2.2	mg	0.42	mg	19
B_{12}	3	μg	0.20	μg	6
C	60	mg	35	mg	57
D	400	IU	0	IU	0
E	15	IU	1	IU	9
K	500	μg	1,350	μg	270◄
Folic Acid	400	μg	48	μg	11

MINERALS USRDA			ONE SERVING GIVES YOU APPROXIMATELY		APPROXIMATE PERCENTAGE OF USRDA
Sodium	(1,100–3,000)	mg	114	mg	11
Calcium	1,000	mg	41	mg	5
Phosphorus	(800–1,000)	mg	380	mg	47
Potassium	(1,875–5,625)	mg	746	mg	93
Magnesium	400	μg	58	μg	16
Selenium	200	μg	31	μg	15
Iodine	150	mg	209	mg	139◄
Zinc	15	mg	0.63	mg	4
Iron	10	mg	1	mg	11
Manganese	(2.5–5.0)	mg	0.16	mg	3
Copper	(2.0–3.0)	mg	0.05	mg	1

AMOUNT PER SERVING		CALORIES PER SERVING	% OF MEAL
Fat	10 grams	91	38
Proteins	31 grams	126	52
Carbohydrates	6 grams	25	10
Cholesterol	0 mg		
Amino acid (essential)			172–562
Fiber	1 gram		

Key: USRDA = Recommended Dietary Allowance
　　　IU = International Unit
　　　mg = milligrams
　　　μg = micrograms
NOTE: The numbers with arrows exceed 100 percent of required USRDA.

Fish and Peas

Ingredients:

4 6-ounce pieces of halibut
1 cup cooked blackeyed peas
1 cantaloupe
2 cups strawberries
2 Tbs horseradish
1/2 cup apple cider
2 Tbs honey
1 tomato, chopped fine
1 cup onion, chopped fine

Preparation: Broil

Time: 20 minutes

Calories: 434 per serving

Serves: 4

Directions

Preheat broiler. Place halibut steak pieces in preheated broiler and broil fish about 4 to 5 minutes on each side at about 6 inches from the flames. Mix the horseradish, apple cider, honey, and tomatos and spread over fish while broiling. Place peas in center of large serving plates and surround with melon chunks and strawberries. When fish is done, place the halibut on top of the peas and serve. The analysis chart indicates that this dish is loaded with important nutrients.

TIP: When hemoglobin, the factor in the red blood cells that is responsible for the rich red color of the cells, is starved for oxygen, the hemoglobin levels fall below normal. This is because your cells now are deprived of oxygen. What results is anemia. So eat meals such as this one to provide nutrition for your cells.

MYTH: Starchy foods are fattening.

FACT: Not in and of themselves. It is usually what goes with bread, potatoes, pasta, and other carbohydrate-rich foods such as fat toppings, butter, and other fat-rich accompaniments. A slice of bread, a small baked potato, or one-third cup of pasta contains fewer than 100 calories.

Nutrients Contained in: Fish and Peas

VITAMINS USRDA			ONE SERVING GIVES YOU APPROXIMATELY		APPROXIMATE PERCENTAGE OF USRDA
A	5,000	IU	5,818	IU	116◀
B$_1$	1.4	mg	0.31	mg	26
B$_2$	1.6	mg	0.34	mg	24
B$_3$	16	mg	19	mg	117◀
B$_5$	10	mg	1	mg	11
B$_6$	2.2	mg	2	mg	71
B$_{12}$	3	μg	2	μg	66
C	60	mg	109	mg	181◀
D	400	IU	88	IU	22
E	15	IU	3	IU	20
K	500	μg	9	μg	1
Folic Acid	400	μg	163	μg	40

MINERALS USRDA			ONE SERVING GIVES YOU APPROXIMATELY		APPROXIMATE PERCENTAGE OF USRDA
Sodium	(1,100–3,000)	mg	265	mg	26
Calcium	1,000	mg	93	mg	11
Phosphorus	(800–1,000)	mg	685	mg	85
Potassium	(1,875–5,625)	mg	1,500	mg	187◀
Magnesium	400	μg	122	μg	34
Selenium	200	μg	1	μg	0
Iodine	150	mg	0	mg	0
Zinc	15	mg	3	mg	16
Iron	10	mg	4	mg	37
Manganese	(2.5–5.0)	mg	0.42	mg	8
Copper	(2.0–3.0)	mg	0.61	mg	20

AMOUNT PER SERVING		CALORIES PER SERVING	% OF MEAL
Fat	4 grams	35	8
Proteins	51 grams	205	47
Carbohydrates	48 grams	194	45
Cholesterol	100 mg		
Amino acid (essential)			256–848
Fiber	7 grams		

Key: USRDA = Recommended Dietary Allowance

IU = International Unit

mg = milligrams

μg = micrograms

NOTE: The numbers with arrows exceed 100 percent of required USRDA.

CHAPTER THIRTEEN

Healing and Preventive Recipes for the Immune System

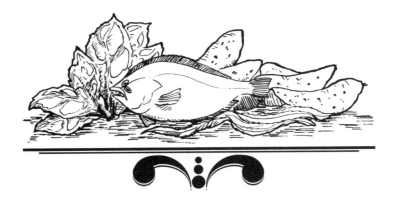

Millions of persons long for immortality who do not know
what to do with themselves on a rainy afternoon.
—Source unknown

What protects most of us from all of the conditions in the preceding chapters is a strong immune system. Dr. Jeffrey Blumberg, associate director of the USDA's Human Nutrition Research Center on Aging in Boston, has concluded that our diet is one way we can use to shape our immune function. He says that specific nutrients are effective in helping to control the immune system.

Based upon numerous reports and studies, scientists are highlighting the importance of good nutrition in warding off infection and preventing disease. Some important measures to consider come from research that says too much fat can suppress immunity, that vitamins A and C and zinc help boost the immune response, and that it is helpful to maintain normal levels of calcium, magnesium, and other nutrients. Not too surprising is the advice to eat a diet low in fats and rich in complex carbohydrates such as those found in whole grains, vegetables, especially red and yellow ones, and fruits containing high amounts of beta-carotene and vitamin C; several servings of fish a week are also recommended.

Meals in this chapter such as Halibut and Mustard Greens, Sweet Potato Brew, Citrus Baked Bluefish, Orange Spinach, and others are packed with the important nutrients just mentioned. They are healthy and delicious—reasons enough to get you started and to keep you moving toward a long and healthy life.

Halibut and Mustard Greens

Ingredients:

4 6-ounce pieces halibut steak
4 cloves garlic, minced
1 red pepper, seeded and cut in thin strips
2 cups mustard greens, chopped
2 Tbs horseradish
12 shiitake mushrooms
$\frac{1}{2}$ tsp rosemary
$\frac{1}{8}$ tsp sage
1 lemon, sliced
soy sauce

Preparation: Saute and steam

Time: 30 minutes

Calories: 342 per serving

Serves: 4

Directions

Rinse greens in cold water and steam for 10 minutes. Saute garlic for 3 minutes in a little soy sauce. Add fish and saute for 5 minutes. Add mustard greens, mushrooms, and horseradish and saute for 10 minutes. During the last 3 minutes of cooking, add rosemary, sage, and red pepper strips. Serve with lemon slices. Check nutrient chart and see how much EAA, vitamins C, B_3, and A, and potassium this meal offers.

TIP: Dr. John Bogden, director of a study conducted at the University of Medicine and Dentistry of New Jersey, says that zinc has been found to be vital to a strong immune system and severe zinc deficiencies can lead to negative effects on immunity and to serious disease. He warned, however, that zinc supplements may slow down improvement in immunity—one study found that taking daily zinc supplements does not help strengthen the immune system in healthy elderly people.

MYTH: No one should eat any food that gets more than 30 percent of its calories from fat.

FACT: The key is total day's food intake. The American Diabetes Association and others say that you can have a higher fat item in one meal or in one day if the rest of the meal or the day's food is low in fat. Then the day's total food intake will contain no more than 30 percent of its calories from fat.

Nutrients Contained in:
Halibut and Mustard Greens

VITAMINS USRDA			ONE SERVING GIVES YOU APPROXIMATELY		APPROXIMATE PERCENTAGE OF USRDA
A	5,000	IU	6,641	IU	132◄
B₁	1.4	mg	0.22	mg	18
B₂	1.6	mg	0.30	mg	21
B₃	16	mg	18	mg	112◄
B₅	10	mg	0.69	mg	6
B₆	2.2	mg	0.80	mg	36
B₁₂	3	μg	2	μg	58
C	60	mg	68	mg	113◄
D	400	IU	77	IU	19
E	15	IU	5	IU	35
K	500	μg	0	μg	0
Folic Acid	400	μg	73	μg	18

MINERALS USRDA			ONE SERVING GIVES YOU APPROXIMATELY		APPROXIMATE PERCENTAGE OF USRDA
Sodium	(1,100–3,000)	mg	130	mg	12
Calcium	1,000	mg	173	mg	21
Phosphorus	(800–1,000)	mg	584	mg	73
Potassium	(1,875–5,625)	mg	902	mg	112◄
Magnesium	400	μg	102	μg	29
Selenium	200	μg	0.18	μg	0
Iodine	150	mg	0	mg	0
Zinc	15	mg	4	mg	29
Iron	10	mg	3	mg	33
Manganese	(2.5–5.0)	mg	0.04	mg	0
Copper	(2.0–3.0)	mg	0.43	mg	14

AMOUNT PER SERVING		CALORIES PER SERVING	% OF MEAL
Fat	3 grams	24	7
Proteins	43 grams	170	50
Carbohydrates	37 grams	148	43
Cholesterol	88 mg		
Amino acid (essential)			226–755
Fiber	1 gram		

Key: USRDA = Recommended Dietary Allowance
   IU = International Unit
   mg = milligrams
   μg = micrograms
NOTE: The numbers with arrows exceed 100 percent of required USRDA.

Sweet Potato Brew

Ingredients:

- 3 cups cooked sweet potatoes, mashed
- $\frac{1}{2}$ cup orange juice
- $\frac{1}{2}$ cup apricot nectar
- 1 Tbs lemon juice
- $\frac{1}{4}$ cup wheat germ
- 1 tsp Brewer's yeast
- 1 tsp brown sugar
- 2 egg whites
- $\frac{1}{8}$ tsp cinnamon
- $\frac{1}{4}$ tsp curry powder

Preparation: Bake

Time: 45 minutes

Calories: 387 per serving

Serves: 4

Directions

Preheat oven to 400°F. Combine the orange juice, apricot nectar, curry, cinnamon, lemon juice, wheat germ, yeast, and brown sugar and add to the cooked sweet potatoes. Beat the egg whites until stiff and fold them into the sweet potato mixture. Place the entire mixture in a baking dish and bake for 20 minutes. This meal will give you high amounts of folic acid, iron, copper, vitamins C, A_1, and B_1, and EAA.

TIP: Nutritionists say that iron deficiency is the most common nutritional deficiency. Iron is considered to be essential for maintaining proper immune cell function. Dietary deficiencies of certain amino acids are also associated with reduced immune function.

MYTH: You can depend on the look and smell of ground round that has been refrigerated for a week to determine if it should be eaten.

FACT: According to the USDA, ground meats that have been stored for more than two days are highly perishable. Also guard against tight wraps, as they set the stage for bacterial growth.

Nutrients Contained in: Sweet Potato Brew

VITAMINS USRDA			ONE SERVING GIVES YOU APPROXIMATELY		APPROXIMATE PERCENTAGE OF USRDA
A	5,000	IU	42,476	IU	849◄
B$_1$	1.4	mg	2	mg	190◄
B$_2$	1.6	mg	0.96	mg	68
B$_3$	16	mg	7	mg	44
B$_5$	10	mg	3	mg	30
B$_6$	2.2	mg	0.98	mg	44
B$_{12}$	3	μg	2	μg	50
C	60	mg	59	mg	98
D	400	IU	0	IU	0
E	15	IU	5	IU	30
K	500	μg	0	μg	0
Folic Acid	400	μg	522	μg	130◄

MINERALS USRDA			ONE SERVING GIVES YOU APPROXIMATELY		APPROXIMATE PERCENTAGE OF USRDA
Sodium	(1,100–3,000)	mg	85	mg	8
Calcium	1,000	mg	93	mg	11
Phosphorus	(800–1,000)	mg	379	mg	47
Potassium	(1,875–5,625)	mg	875	mg	109◄
Magnesium	400	μg	84	μg	24
Selenium	200	μg	1	μg	0
Iodine	150	mg	0	mg	0
Zinc	15	mg	3	mg	21
Iron	10	mg	4	mg	43
Manganese	(2.5–5.0)	mg	2	mg	45
Copper	(2.0–3.0)	mg	1	mg	38

AMOUNT PER SERVING		CALORIES PER SERVING	% OF MEAL
Fat	2 grams	15	4
Proteins	13 grams	53	14
Carbohydrates	80 grams	319	82
Cholesterol	0 mg		
Amino acid (essential)			162–221
Fiber	2 grams		

Key: USRDA = Recommended Dietary Allowance

IU = International Unit

mg = milligrams

μg = micrograms

NOTE: The numbers with arrows exceed 100 percent of required USRDA.

Citrus Baked Bluefish

Ingredients:

4 6-ounce pieces of
  bluefish
1 cup parsnips, peeled
  and sliced
¼ cup apple cider
½ cup orange juice
1 tsp marjoram
½ cup apricot nectar
1 tangerine, divided
  sections
¼ tsp black pepper
1 lemon, sliced

Preparation: Bake

Time: 40 minutes

Calories: 347 per serving

Serves: 4

Directions

Preheat oven to 400°F. Boil parsnips until tender. Set aside. Clean and wash the fish. Sprinkle fish all over with pepper and marjoram. Place the fish in a large baking dish; add nectar, orange juice, and apple cider. Bake for about 10 to 15 minutes, basting often with the juice. Serve with lemon slices and tangerine sections. This dish is loaded with vitamins B_{12} and C.

TIP: A report from the *American Journal of Clinical Nutrition* says deficiencies of vitamin A, vitamin B_6, and zinc have been shown to reduce the size of the thymus (the thymus makes cells that produce antibodies and help kill harmful microorganisms) and to reduce the production of antibodies for fighting infections.

MYTH: You should try to save a broken egg if you find it in your carton when you get home from shopping.

FACT: According to the USDA raw eggs are highly susceptible to contamination if the shell is broken and discarding a cracked egg is an economy measure in the long run.

Nutrients Contained in: Citrus Baked Bluefish

VITAMINS USRDA			ONE SERVING GIVES YOU APPROXIMATELY		APPROXIMATE PERCENTAGE OF USRDA
A	5,000	IU	865	IU	17
B_1	1.4	mg	0.23	mg	19
B_2	1.6	mg	0.27	mg	19
B_3	16	mg	5	mg	31
B_5	10	mg	0.19	mg	1
B_6	2.2	mg	6	mg	200◄
B_{12}	3	µg	0	µg	0
C	60	mg	54	mg	90
D	400	IU	0	IU	0
E	15	IU	0.59	IU	3
K	500	µg	0	µg	0
Folic Acid	400	µg	81	µg	20

MINERALS USRDA			ONE SERVING GIVES YOU APPROXIMATELY		APPROXIMATE PERCENTAGE OF USRDA
Sodium	(1,100–3,000)	mg	185	mg	18
Calcium	1,000	mg	72	mg	8
Phosphorus	(800–1,000)	mg	19	mg	2
Potassium	(1,875–5,625)	mg	311	mg	38
Magnesium	400	µg	90	µg	25
Selenium	200	µg	3	µg	1
Iodine	150	mg	0	mg	0
Zinc	15	mg	1	mg	9
Iron	10	mg	2	mg	15
Manganese	(2.5–5.0)	mg	0.03	mg	0
Copper	(2.0–3.0)	mg	0.06	mg	2

AMOUNT PER SERVING		CALORIES PER SERVING	% OF MEAL
Fat	9 grams	82	24
Proteins	46 grams	184	53
Carbohydrates	20 grams	81	23
Cholesterol	124 mg		
Amino acid (essential)			Very high
Fiber	1 gram		

Key: USRDA = Recommended Dietary Allowance
IU = International Unit
mg = milligrams
µg = micrograms

NOTE: The numbers with arrows exceed 100 percent of required USRDA.

Orange Spinach

Ingredients:

- 4 cups spinach, chopped coarse
- 1 tsp margarine
- $\frac{1}{4}$ cup whole wheat flour
- $\frac{1}{4}$ cup low-fat milk
- 2 kiwi, peeled and sliced
- 1 egg
- 1 orange, peeled and cut into bite-size pieces
- 1 Tbs lemon juice
- 1 tsp grated orange rind
- $\frac{1}{4}$ cup apricot nectar
- $\frac{1}{4}$ tsp salt

Preparation: Boil

Time: 20 minutes

Calories: 166 per serving

Serves: 4

Directions

Wash spinach thoroughly and cook in its attendant water for about 5 minutes or less. Melt margarine and blend with the flour. Stir in the salt and milk and bring to a boil. Allow to thicken. Remove from heat and stir in the egg, orange rind, apricot nectar, and kiwi. Combine the spinach, orange pieces, and the sauce. This dish is high in iron, vitamin K, folic acid, vitamin A, and potassium.

TIP: Scientists at the University of California School of Medicine report that people who eat live-culture yogurt have 25 percent fewer cold symptoms than do nonyogurt eaters. They also have fewer hay-fever symptoms and less frequent instances of diarrhea. They suggest that this might be because yogurt boosts the production of immune-stimulating gamma interferon.

MYTH: Melanoma, a cancer that arises from moles, is a disease that primarily affects outdoor workers.

FACT: A report in the *Western Journal of Medicine* says that people at greater risk are those who work indoors and expose themselves every now and then to the sun.

Nutrients Contained in: Orange Spinach

VITAMINS USRDA			ONE SERVING GIVES YOU APPROXIMATELY		APPROXIMATE PERCENTAGE OF USRDA
A	5,000	IU	15,041	IU	300◀
B_1	1.4	mg	0.28	mg	23
B_2	1.6	mg	0.52	mg	36
B_3	16	mg	2	mg	9
B_5	10	mg	0.61	mg	6
B_6	2.2	mg	0.51	mg	23
B_{12}	3	μg	0.22	μg	7
C	60	mg	44	mg	73
D	400	IU	13	IU	3
E	15	IU	6	IU	37
K	500	μg	180	μg	36
Folic Acid	400	μg	292	μg	73

MINERALS USRDA			ONE SERVING GIVES YOU APPROXIMATELY		APPROXIMATE PERCENTAGE OF USRDA
Sodium	(1,100–3,000)	mg	155	mg	15
Calcium	1,000	mg	298	mg	37
Phosphorus	(800–1,000)	mg	144	mg	17
Potassium	(1,875–5,625)	mg	1,114	mg	59◀
Magnesium	400	μg	185	μg	52
Selenium	200	μg	19	μg	9
Iodine	150	mg	6	mg	3
Zinc	15	mg	2	mg	11
Iron	10	mg	7	mg	72
Manganese	(2.5–5.0)	mg	2	mg	33
Copper	(2.0–3.0)	mg	0.35	mg	11

AMOUNT PER SERVING		CALORIES PER SERVING	% OF MEAL
Fat	4 grams	35	22
Proteins	8 grams	34	20
Carbohydrates	24 grams	97	58
Cholesterol	79 mg		
Amino acid (essential)			91–99
Fiber	4 grams		

Key: USRDA = Recommended Dietary Allowance

IU = International Unit

mg = milligrams

μg = micrograms

NOTE: The numbers with arrows exceed 100 percent of required USRDA.

Onion Garlic Potatoes with Corn

Ingredients:

4 medium potatoes, diced fine
2 onions, chopped
6 cloves garlic, chopped fine
1 cup canned corn
4 Tbs nonfat sour cream
$\frac{1}{2}$ tsp caraway seeds
$\frac{1}{4}$ tsp cinnamon
1 tsp margarine
$\frac{1}{4}$ cup half and half

Preparation: Baked

Time: 1 hour, 30 minutes

Calories: 346 per serving

Serves: 4

Directions

Preheat oven to 375°F. Grease a baking dish with the margarine. Combine all the ingredients in the baking dish and bake for an hour or until vegetables are cooked.

TIP: Tufts University researchers say the immune system decline begins after puberty. This means that the immune-building power of good nutrition may have direct importance to everybody over the age of 12 or so.

MYTH: So called hot flashes are inevitable for everyone.

FACT: Dr. Cynthia Stuenkel, director of the comprehensive menopause program at the University of California at San Diego, says that while a majority of women get them, only 10 to 15 percent have flashes severe enough to interfere with their daily lives.

Nutrients Contained in:
Onion Garlic Potatoes with Corn

VITAMINS USRDA			ONE SERVING GIVES YOU APPROXIMATELY		APPROXIMATE PERCENTAGE OF USRDA
A	5,000	IU	237	IU	4
B₁	1.4	mg	0.36	mg	29
B₂	1.6	mg	0.12	mg	8
B₃	16	mg	4	mg	25
B₅	10	mg	2	mg	16
B₆	2.2	mg	0.85	mg	38
B₁₂	3	μg	0.04	μg	1
C	60	mg	35	mg	58
D	400	IU	0	IU	0
E	15	IU	0.76	IU	5
K	500	μg	4	μg	0
Folic Acid	400	μg	57	μg	14

MINERALS USRDA			ONE SERVING GIVES YOU APPROXIMATELY		APPROXIMATE PERCENTAGE OF USRDA
Sodium	(1,100–3,000)	mg	48	mg	4
Calcium	1,000	mg	57	mg	7
Phosphorus	(800–1,000)	mg	194	mg	24
Potassium	(1,875–5,625)	mg	1,098	mg	58
Magnesium	400	μg	77	μg	22
Selenium	200	μg	2	μg	1
Iodine	150	mg	0	mg	0
Zinc	15	mg	1	mg	6
Iron	10	mg	3	mg	32
Manganese	(2.5–5.0)	mg	0.66	mg	13
Copper	(2.0–3.0)	mg	0.68	mg	22

AMOUNT PER SERVING		CALORIES PER SERVING	% OF MEAL
Fat	5 grams	44	13
Proteins	7 grams	30	9
Carbohydrates	68 grams	272	78
Cholesterol	15 mg		
Amino acid (essential)			95–106
Fiber	2 grams		

Key: USRDA = Recommended Dietary Allowance

IU = International Unit

mg = milligrams

μg = micrograms

NOTE: The numbers with arrows exceed 100 percent of required USRDA.

Universal Potatoes Baked with Cabbage

Ingredients:

1 small head of cabbage, chopped fine
3 medium potatoes, cubed
1 Tbs margarine
¼ cup sesame seed
3 Tbs nonfat sour cream
¾ cup skim milk
⅓ cup rice bran
3 Tbs whole wheat flour
½ cup wheat germ
4 Tbs Parmesan cheese, grated
¼ tsp cinnamon

Preparation: Bake and boil

Time: 40 minutes

Calories: 456 per serving

Serves: 4

Directions

Preheat oven to 400° F. Boil cabbage and potatoes for about 10 minutes. Drain both and place in large baking dish. Melt margarine and blend in the flour. Slowly stir in sour cream and milk; bring to a boil. Cook for about 2 minutes. Add sesame seeds, cinnamon, and cheese, stirring to melt cheese. Pour this mixture over the cabbage and potatoes and sprinkle wheat germ and rice bran over all. Bake 15 minutes in hot oven and serve when vegetables are lightly brown. This dish is well over the USRDA for vitamin C and contains good amounts of vitamin B_1, potassium, magnesium, manganese, and iron.

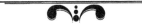

TIP: Dr. Pamela Frakter, immunologist and professor of biochemistry at Michigan State University in East Lansing, says the billions of new cells produced by our bodies live a few days and have to be replaced. The immune system consequently has a high turnover of infection-fighting cells. So, she says, the immune system may be more vulnerable to deficiencies of essential nutrients than previously thought.

MYTH: No one can predict when menopause will occur.

FACT: Epidemiologist Elizabeth Whelan, at the National Institute of Environmental Health Sciences, says menopause can occur anytime in your 40s and 50s, most commonly, however, between ages 45 and 54. She says there are clues that can help further narrow that down. Genetics is one, so that you can expect, she says, to reach menopause around the same time your mother did.

Nutrients Contained in: Universal Potatoes Baked with Cabbage

VITAMINS USRDA			ONE SERVING GIVES YOU APPROXIMATELY		APPROXIMATE PERCENTAGE OF USRDA
A	5,000	IU	465	IU	9
B$_1$	1.4	mg	0.73	mg	60
B$_2$	1.6	mg	0.34	mg	24
B$_3$	16	mg	7	mg	43
B$_5$	10	mg	1	mg	14
B$_6$	2.2	mg	1	mg	50
B$_{12}$	3	μg	0.21	μg	7
C	60	mg	75	mg	124◄
D	400	IU	19	IU	4
E	15	IU	1	IU	7
K	500	μg	52	μg	10
Folic Acid	400	μg	142	μg	35

MINERALS USRDA			ONE SERVING GIVES YOU APPROXIMATELY		APPROXIMATE PERCENTAGE OF USRDA
Sodium	(1,100–3,000)	mg	192	mg	19
Calcium	1,000	mg	229	mg	28
Phosphorus	(800–1,000)	mg	424	mg	53
Potassium	(1,875–5,625)	mg	1,311	mg	69◄
Magnesium	400	μg	192	μg	54
Selenium	200	μg	1	μg	0
Iodine	150	mg	2	mg	1
Zinc	15	mg	5	mg	32
Iron	10	mg	6	mg	59
Manganese	(2.5–5.0)	mg	3	mg	67
Copper	(2.0–3.0)	mg	0.76	mg	25

AMOUNT PER SERVING		CALORIES PER SERVING	% OF MEAL
Fat	15 grams	133	30
Proteins	16 grams	66	14
Carbohydrates	64 grams	257	56
Cholesterol	29 mg		
Amino acid (essential)			186–245
Fiber	3 grams		

Key: USRDA = Recommended Dietary Allowance

IU = International Unit

mg = milligrams

μg = micrograms

NOTE: The numbers with arrows exceed 100 percent of required USRDA.

Southern Oysters

Ingredients:
24 raw oysters
1 Tbs finely chopped shallots
2 Tbs chopped parsley
½ tsp black pepper
1 tsp low-salt soy sauce
1 tsp lemon juice
1 tsp chili powder
½ cup plain yogurt
2 shredded wheat biscuits
½ cup orange juice
grated orange peel

Preparation: Bake
Time: 40 minutes
Calories: 161 per serving
Serves: 4

Directions

Preheat oven to 400° F. Place half the oysters in baking dish. Sprinkle with pepper, parsley, soy sauce, lemon juice, and half the shredded biscuits. Make a second layer with the remaining oysters. Sprinkle remaining shredded wheat, chili powder, orange juice, grated peel, and yogurt on top. Bake for 20 minutes. Take from oven and serve. Observe large amounts of zinc, vitamin B_{12}, and vitamin C on your chart.

TIP: Immunologist William Beisel of Johns Hopkins indicates that zinc has been found to aid in the healing of wounds and is crucial to proper immune cell function. Studies show that a zinc deficiency in a fetus or infant can cause permanent damage to the immune system. Taking zinc supplements without a doctor's approval is not recommended as too much zinc can be toxic.

MYTH: Honey does not raise blood glucose to levels as high as table sugar (sucrose) does because honey is unprocessed sugar.

FACT: The American Diabetes Association says honey does raise blood glucose as quickly as sucrose and also has more calories than sucrose.

Nutrients Contained in: Southern Oysters

VITAMINS USRDA			ONE SERVING GIVES YOU APPROXIMATELY		APPROXIMATE PERCENTAGE OF USRDA
A	5,000	IU	1,201	IU	24
B_1	1.4	mg	0.23	mg	19
B_2	1.6	mg	0.37	mg	26
B_3	16	mg	2	mg	12
B_5	10	mg	0.53	mg	5
B_6	2.2	mg	0.09	mg	3
B_{12}	3	μg	15	μg	510◄
C	60	mg	66	mg	110◄
D	400	IU	75	IU	18
E	15	IU	0.98	IU	6
K	500	μg	0	μg	0
Folic Acid	400	μg	39	μg	9

MINERALS USRDA			ONE SERVING GIVES YOU APPROXIMATELY		APPROXIMATE PERCENTAGE OF USRDA
Sodium	(1,100–3,000)	mg	394	mg	39
Calcium	1,000	mg	163	mg	20
Phosphorus	(800–1,000)	mg	144	mg	17
Potassium	(1,875–5,625)	mg	488	mg	61
Magnesium	400	μg	84	μg	24
Selenium	200	μg	0	μg	0
Iodine	150	mg	26	mg	17
Zinc	15	mg	0.30	mg	512◄
Iron	10	mg	7	mg	65
Manganese	(2.5–5.0)	mg	0.40	mg	8
Copper	(2.0–3.0)	mg	0.10	mg	3

AMOUNT PER SERVING		CALORIES PER SERVING	% OF MEAL
Fat	3 grams	28	18
Proteins	12 grams	49	30
Carbohydrates	21 grams	84	52
Cholesterol	50 mg		
Amino acid (essential)			47–80
Fiber	0 grams		

Key: USRDA = Recommended Dietary Allowance

IU = International Unit

mg = milligrams

μg = micrograms

NOTE: The numbers with arrows exceed 100 percent of required USRDA.

Three Green Chicken with Walnuts and Oranges

Ingredients:

2 cups mustard greens
2 cups collard greens
1 cup turnip greens
2 lb chicken, cut into
    serving pieces
1 Tbs mustard powder
$\frac{1}{2}$ cup walnuts
1 orange, peeled and sliced
1 kiwi, peeled and sliced
$\frac{1}{2}$ cup orange juice
1 tsp low-salt soy sauce
1 cup onion, chopped
$\frac{1}{2}$ tsp savory
$\frac{1}{8}$ tsp cayenne pepper
2 tsp lemon juice

2 cups water

Preparation: Bake and boil

Time: 1 hour, 30 minutes

Calories: 256 per serving

Serves: 4

Directions

Preheat oven to 400° F. Mix soy sauce with mustard powder and rub on chicken pieces. Set aside. Trim the greens and wash in cold water. Add 2 cups of water to a large pot and add greens along with the savory, onions, and lemon juice. Bring to a boil and simmer about 40 minutes, until tender. Meanwhile, place chicken in a baking pan in oven. Bake 8 minutes; turn and bake 8 minutes more. While chicken is baking, combine orange juice, walnuts, kiwi, and orange slices in pan and bring to a boil. Reduce oven heat to 300° F, pour fruit mixture over chicken, and bake 20 minutes. Place cooked greens on a large platter; top with chicken and pan juices and serve.

TIP: This recipe is very high in vitamin A, a nutrient that can ward off infections of the eyes and the respiratory and gastrointestinal tracts. Research by the U.S. Department of Agriculture's Human Nutrition Research Center at Tufts University in Boston has shown that consumption of large amounts of beta-carotene, a vitamin A-like compound, may reduce the incidence of lung, colon, stomach, and cervical cancer.

MYTH: When you see a product that says "no cholesterol" on the label, this means your blood cholesterol level will not be affected if you eat it.

FACT: The problem here is that products marked "no cholesterol" may have saturated fat, which will raise blood cholesterol levels, say scientists.

Nutrients Contained in: Three Green Chicken with Walnuts and Oranges

VITAMINS USRDA			ONE SERVING GIVES YOU APPROXIMATELY		APPROXIMATE PERCENTAGE OF USRDA
A	5,000	IU	10,155	IU	203◄
B$_1$	1.4	mg	0.27	mg	22
B$_2$	1.6	mg	0.30	mg	21
B$_3$	16	mg	4	mg	27
B$_5$	10	mg	0.92	mg	9
B$_6$	2.2	mg	0.42	mg	19
B$_{12}$	3	μg	0.13	μg	4
C	60	mg	129	mg	214◄
D	400	IU	0	IU	0
E	15	IU	5	IU	31
K	500	μg	93	μg	18
Folic Acid	400	μg	76	μg	18

MINERALS USRDA			ONE SERVING GIVES YOU APPROXIMATELY		APPROXIMATE PERCENTAGE OF USRDA
Sodium	(1,100–3,000)	mg	73	mg	7
Calcium	1,000	mg	319	mg	39
Phosphorus	(800–1,000)	mg	176	mg	21
Potassium	(1,875–5,625)	mg	714	mg	89
Magnesium	400	μg	82	μg	23
Selenium	200	μg	6	μg	3
Iodine	150	mg	0	mg	0
Zinc	15	mg	2	mg	10
Iron	10	mg	3	mg	32
Manganese	(2.5–5.0)	mg	0.66	mg	13
Copper	(2.0–3.0)	mg	0.52	mg	17

AMOUNT PER SERVING		CALORIES PER SERVING	% OF MEAL
Fat	13 grams	114	45
Proteins	14 grams	57	22
Carbohydrates	21 grams	85	33
Cholesterol	29 mg		
Amino acid (essential)			142–218
Fiber	2 grams		

Key: USRDA = Recommended Dietary Allowance

IU = International Unit

mg = milligrams

μg = micrograms

NOTE: The numbers with arrows exceed 100 percent of required USRDA.

Halloween Chicken

Ingredients:

1 1 ¾ lb chicken, cut
   into serving pieces
1 cup pumpkin pieces
2 cloves garlic, chopped
1 cup low-sodium
   chicken broth
¼ cup Italian parsley
1 tsp vegetable oil
3 Tbs horseradish
¼ chili powder
½ cup pumpkin seeds

Preparation: Boil and simmer

Time: 55 minutes

Calories: 207 per serving

Serves: 4

Directions

Rub horseradish on chicken and brown in oil in a large skillet. Set aside. Toast the pumpkin seeds in same skillet. Add the garlic, parsley, chili powder, and pumpkin pieces and slowly stir in the broth. Bring to a boil and return chicken to pan. Cover and simmer for about 40 minutes, longer if chicken is not fully cooked. Very high amount of important vitamin E.

TIP: Wheat germ and whole-grain breads and cereals, along with vegetable oils and nuts, provide the potent antioxidant vitamin E. Vitamin E makes cells more resistant to cancer invasion by protecting cells from oxidative damage. This vitamin also promotes the production of infection-fighting white blood cells that bolster the immune response say researchers from Tufts University in Boston.

MYTH: One of the easiest ways to determine how much sugar is in a cereal box is to read the ingredients list.

FACT: According to the American Diabetes Association, you will get more accurate information by checking the carbohydrate information on the box. They suggest that you will find the grams of sucrose and other sugars listed there. Four grams or fewer of sucrose per serving is considered low in sugars.

Nutrients Contained in: Halloween Chicken

VITAMINS USRDA			ONE SERVING GIVES YOU APPROXIMATELY		APPROXIMATE PERCENTAGE OF USRDA
A	5,000	IU	999	IU	19
B$_1$	1.4	mg	0.42	mg	34
B$_2$	1.6	mg	0.15	mg	10
B$_3$	16	mg	6	mg	35
B$_5$	10	mg	0.78	mg	7
B$_6$	2.2	mg	0.45	mg	20
B$_{12}$	3	μg	0.20	μg	6
C	60	mg	10	mg	16
D	400	IU	0	IU	0
E	15	IU	17	IU	113◄
K	500	μg	1	μg	0
Folic Acid	400	μg	3	μg	0

MINERALS USRDA			ONE SERVING GIVES YOU APPROXIMATELY		APPROXIMATE PERCENTAGE OF USRDA
Sodium	(1,100–3,000)	mg	230	mg	23
Calcium	1,000	mg	52	mg	6
Phosphorus	(800–1,000)	mg	241	mg	30
Potassium	(1,875–5,625)	mg	507	mg	63
Magnesium	400	μg	28	μg	7
Selenium	200	μg	0	μg	0
Iodine	150	mg	0	mg	0
Zinc	15	mg	2	mg	10
Iron	10	mg	2	mg	22
Manganese	(2.5–5.0)	mg	0.47	mg	9
Copper	(2.0–3.0)	mg	0.45	mg	15

AMOUNT PER SERVING		CALORIES PER SERVING	% OF MEAL
Fat	13 grams	116	56
Proteins	14 grams	56	27
Carbohydrates	9 grams	35	17
Cholesterol	30 mg		
Amino acid (essential)			147–217
Fiber	1 gram		

Key: USRDA = Recommended Dietary Allowance

IU = International Unit

mg = milligrams

μg = micrograms

NOTE: The numbers with arrows exceed 100 percent of required USRDA.

Turkey and Oyster on Whole Wheat Toast

Ingredients:

18	raw oysters
12	shiitake mushrooms
1	Tbs scallions, finely chopped
2	Tbs whole wheat flour
1	cup plain yogurt
¼	tsp cinnamon
½	tsp marjoram
½	lb turkey, white meat diced
1	cup zucchini, finely chopped
2	tsp lemon juice
3	egg whites
¼	cup cream
4 to 6	slices whole wheat toast
1	tsp peanut oil

Preparation: Saute and boil

Time: 25 minutes

Calories: 335 per serving

Serves: 4

Directions

Heat oil in a skillet and saute scallions and mushrooms for about 3 minutes. Add flour to the skillet and stir for about 1 minute. Pour in the yogurt and bring to a boil; season with cinnamon and marjoram and cook for 2 minutes. Add the turkey, zucchini, and lemon juice and cook for 3 minutes. Cook longer if turkey is not done. Beat the egg whites with the cream, add a dash of cayenne pepper, and add to pan. Heat until mixture thickens a bit. Don't boil. Add the oysters and heat on low until the oysters are heated through, about 5 minutes. Spoon on top of toast and serve. This meal is a zinc atom bomb, with vitamin B_{12} very high and good amounts of iron and vitamin E.

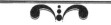

TIP: Dr. Jeffrey Blumberg of the USDA's Human Nutrition Research Center at Tufts University in Boston speaks of studies that report zinc aids in the healing of wounds and is crucial to proper immune cell function. A zinc deficiency in a fetus or infant can cause permanent damage to the immune system. Another mineral—selenium—is needed to produce antibodies and enzymes necessary for the immune system to work.

MYTH: Products that are sugar-free do not raise blood glucose.

FACT: "Sugar-free" does not mean the product is calorie free, and calories, from any source, do raise blood glucose.

Nutrients Contained in: Turkey and Oyster on Whole Wheat Toast

VITAMINS USRDA		ONE SERVING GIVES YOU APPROXIMATELY		APPROXIMATE PERCENTAGE OF USRDA
A	5,000 IU	999	IU	19
B1	1.4 mg	0.22	mg	18
B2	1.6 mg	0.39	mg	27
B3	16 mg	6	mg	36
B5	10 mg	2	mg	22
B6	2.2 mg	0.25	mg	11
B12	3 μg	12	μg	395◄
C	60 mg	37	mg	60
D	400 IU	77	IU	19
E	15 IU	0.80	IU	5
K	500 μg	0	μg	0
Folic Acid	400 μg	79	μg	19

MINERALS USRDA		ONE SERVING GIVES YOU APPROXIMATELY		APPROXIMATE PERCENTAGE OF USRDA
Sodium	(1,100–3,000) mg	143	mg	14
Calcium	1,000 mg	175	mg	21
Phosphorus	(800–1,000) mg	177	mg	22
Potassium	(1,875–5,625) mg	776	mg	97
Magnesium	400 μg	101	μg	28
Selenium	200 μg	0.73	μg	0
Iodine	150 mg	26	mg	17
Zinc	15 mg	0.30	mg	408◄
Iron	10 mg	5	mg	54
Manganese	(2.5–5.0) mg	0.09	mg	1
Copper	(2.0–3.0) mg	0.10	mg	3

AMOUNT PER SERVING		CALORIES PER SERVING	% OF MEAL
Fat	9 grams	77	23
Proteins	19 grams	76	23
Carbohydrates	45 grams	182	54
Cholesterol	131 mg		
Amino acid (essential)			95–182
Fiber	1 gram		

Key: USRDA = Recommended Dietary Allowance

IU = International Unit

mg = milligrams

μg = micrograms

NOTE: The numbers with arrows exceed 100 percent of required USRDA.

Citrus Fruit Gathering

Ingredients:

- 1 papaya, peeled and cut into chunks
- ½ cantaloupe, peeled and cut into chunks
- 1 cup strawberries, hulled
- 1 orange, cut into sections
- 1 kiwi, peeled and sliced thin
- 1 large grapefruit, peeled and cut into segments
- ½ cup apple cider mint leaves

Preparation: No cooking required

Time: 10 minutes

Calories: 161 per serving

Serves: 4

Directions

Mix the fruits together in a large bowl. Pour apple cider over fruit and sprinkle with mint leaves. Chill and serve in individual sherbert dishes. If desired, serve with four tomato halves baked with 1 ounce of shredded skim-milk mozzarella cheese. This is a powerhouse of vitamin C, potassium, and vitamin A; see chart for percentages of USRDA.

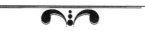

TIP: Researchers at the National Institutes of Health indicate that if you have low levels of vitamin C in your body, you are more susceptible to contracting an illness and will have a more difficult time recovering from infections. Also vitamin C may be able to, like vitamin E and beta-carotene, weaken free radicals and help fight cancerous growths.

MYTH: Foods marked "dietetic" are good choices for people with diabetes.

FACT: Consumers must be careful not to confuse dietetic with diabetic labels. A dietetic label means only that at least one ingredient has been changed. The Food and Drug Administration says that food specifically intended for people with diabetes must be labeled, "Diabetics: This product may be useful in your diet on the advice of a physician."

Nutrients Contained in: Cirtus Fruit Gathering

VITAMINS USRDA			ONE SERVING GIVES YOU APPROXIMATELY		APPROXIMATE PERCENTAGE OF USRDA
A	5,000	IU	3,900	IU	77
B$_1$	1.4	mg	0.12	mg	9
B$_2$	1.6	mg	0.13	mg	9
B$_3$	16	mg	1	mg	8
B$_5$	10	mg	0.63	mg	6
B$_6$	2.2	mg	0.36	mg	16
B$_{12}$	3	μg	0	μg	0
C	60	mg	134	mg	223◄
D	400	IU	0	IU	0
E	15	IU	0.38	IU	2
K	500	μg	4	μg	0
Folic Acid	400	μg	34	μg	8

MINERALS USRDA			ONE SERVING GIVES YOU APPROXIMATELY		APPROXIMATE PERCENTAGE OF USRDA
Sodium	(1,100–3,000)	mg	12	mg	1
Calcium	1,000	mg	70	mg	8
Phosphorus	(800–1,000)	mg	32	mg	3
Potassium	(1,875–5,625)	mg	858	mg	107◄
Magnesium	400	μg	50	μg	14
Selenium	200	μg	0.68	μg	0
Iodine	150	mg	0	mg	0
Zinc	15	mg	0.27	mg	1
Iron	10	mg	0.74	mg	7
Manganese	(2.5–5.0)	mg	0.16	mg	3
Copper	(2.0–3.0)	mg	0.10	mg	3

AMOUNT PER SERVING		CALORIES PER SERVING	% OF MEAL
Fat	1 gram	7	5
Proteins	3 grams	11	7
Carbohydrates	36 grams	143	88
Cholesterol	0 mg		
Amino acid (essential)			5–13*
Fiber	4 grams		

Key: USRDA = Recommended Dietary Allowance

IU = International Unit

mg = milligrams

μg = micrograms

NOTE: The numbers with arrows exceed 100 percent of required USRDA.

*Complementary food—1 ounce Swiss cheese raises EAA to 97–166%.

Magic Mushroom Bake

Ingredients:

- 24 shiitake mushrooms, quartered
- 2 red peppers, seeded and chopped
- ½ cup sunflower seeds
- 1 Tbs tahini sauce
- 2 cloves garlic, chopped
- juice of one lemon
- ½ tsp black pepper
- 1 tsp chervil

Preparation: Bake

Time: 35 minutes

Calories: 424 per serving

Serves: 4

Directions

Preheat oven to 425° F. Sprinkle mushrooms with lemon juice and chervil; place in a baking pan. Add red peppers, garlic, sunflower seeds, chervil, and tahini sauce to mushrooms. Bake for 10 to 15 minutes. If desired, serve with watermelon wedges. Look on the chart and see the large amounts of vitamin E, zinc, and magnesium present.

TIP: Free radicals can alter the genetic makeup of cells, predisposing tissues to cancerous growths. Vitamin E protects against cancer by blocking the action of free radicals, according to studies conducted by researchers in Finland.

MYTH: Fat found in lard, butter, and nonskim milk is more fattening than the fat found in nuts and seeds.

FACT: Fats contain 9 calories per gram, whether the fat comes from saturated or unsaturated fats. It's just that we try to avoid saturated fats which come from animal fats.

Nutrients Contained in: Magic Mushroom Bake

VITAMINS USRDA			ONE SERVING GIVES YOU APPROXIMATELY		APPROXIMATE PERCENTAGE OF USRDA
A	5,000	IU	155	IU	3
B$_1$	1.4	mg	0.44	mg	36
B$_2$	1.6	mg	0.13	mg	9
B$_3$	16	mg	8	mg	49
B$_5$	10	mg	0.29	mg	2
B$_6$	2.2	mg	0.34	mg	15
B$_{12}$	3	μg	0	μg	0
C	60	mg	48	mg	80
D	400	IU	0	IU	0
E	15	IU	16	IU	105◄
K	500	μg	0	μg	0
Folic Acid	400	μg	95	μg	23

MINERALS USRDA			ONE SERVING GIVES YOU APPROXIMATELY		APPROXIMATE PERCENTAGE OF USRDA
Sodium	(1,100–3,000)	mg	25	mg	2
Calcium	1,000	mg	56	mg	6
Phosphorus	(800–1,000)	mg	192	mg	23
Potassium	(1,875–5,625)	mg	771	mg	96
Magnesium	400	μg	82	μg	23
Selenium	200	μg	3	μg	1
Iodine	150	mg	0	mg	0
Zinc	15	mg	7	mg	47
Iron	10	mg	2	mg	21
Manganese	(2.5–5.0)	mg	0.40	mg	7
Copper	(2.0–3.0)	mg	0.42	mg	13

AMOUNT PER SERVING		CALORIES PER SERVING	% OF MEAL
Fat	11 grams	97	23
Proteins	12 grams	48	11
Carbohydrates	70 grams	279	66
Cholesterol	0 mg		
Amino acid (essential)			45–94*
Fiber	1 gram		

Key: USRDA = Recommended Dietary Allowance

　　　IU = International Unit

　　　mg = milligrams

　　　μg = micrograms

NOTE: The numbers with arrows exceed 100 percent of required USRDA.

*Complementary food—1 cup peas raises EAA to 143–174%.

Pungent Onion Stuffed with Carrots

Ingredients:

4 large onions
2 egg whites
½ cup wheat germ
½ tsp brown sugar
4 carrots, chopped fine
4 medium-thin ham slices
1 Tbs parsley, chopped
4 slices mozzarella cheese
juice of one lemon
1 tsp chervil
¼ tsp marjoram

Preparation: Steam and bake

Time: 1 hour, 15 minutes

Calories: 295 per serving

Serves: 4

Directions

Preheat oven to 400° F. Steam chopped carrots for about 10 minutes. Hollow out onions with fruit knife, leaving ½-inch shell. Chop the carved-out onion pieces and combine with carrots, wheat germ, egg, and sugar. Sprinkle hollow with lemon juice and chervil. Fill onion hollow with mixture and cover with the slices of mozzarella cheese and 1 slice of ham. Press ham around onion tops. Place in a baking dish and bake about 35 minutes.

TIP: In a study by Tufts University, it was found that the immune systems of people who took daily supplements containing many times the USRDA of vitamin E show much more capability of fighting disease than the immune systems of people who did not take vitamin E. It is important to eat foods with vitamin E, but relatively few foods contain vast amounts of the vitamin.

MYTH: Fruit juices make a good drink if you are trying to lose weight and don't raise blood glucose levels.

FACT: Nutritionists say that fruit juices raise blood glucose levels so quickly that they are often used to treat low blood glucose. Fruit juices also add calories as an 8-ounce glass of apple, grapefruit, grape, or orange juice has about 120 calories.

Nutrients Contained in: Pungent Onion Stuffed with Carrots

VITAMINS USRDA			ONE SERVING GIVES YOU APPROXIMATELY		APPROXIMATE PERCENTAGE OF USRDA
A	5,000	IU	20,384	IU	407◄
B_1	1.4	mg	0.65	mg	54
B_2	1.6	mg	0.37	mg	26
B_3	16	mg	3	mg	19
B_5	10	mg	0.74	mg	7
B_6	2.2	mg	0.61	mg	27
B_{12}	3	μg	0.43	μg	14
C	60	mg	24	mg	40
D	400	IU	8	IU	1
E	15	IU	1	IU	8
K	500	μg	100	μg	20
Folic Acid	400	μg	97	μg	24

MINERALS USRDA			ONE SERVING GIVES YOU APPROXIMATELY		APPROXIMATE PERCENTAGE OF USRDA
Sodium	(1,100–3,000)	mg	535	mg	53
Calcium	1,000	mg	219	mg	27
Phosphorus	(800–1,000)	mg	419	mg	52
Potassium	(1,875–5,625)	mg	768	mg	96
Magnesium	400	μg	86	μg	24
Selenium	200	μg	21	μg	10
Iodine	150	mg	0	mg	0
Zinc	15	mg	4	mg	26
Iron	10	mg	3	mg	27
Manganese	(2.5–5.0)	mg	3	mg	63
Copper	(2.0–3.0)	mg	0.22	mg	7

AMOUNT PER SERVING		CALORIES PER SERVING	% OF MEAL
Fat	11 grams	101	34
Proteins	19 grams	76	26
Carbohydrates	30 grams	118	40
Cholesterol	38 mg		
Amino acid (essential)			228–513
Fiber	1 gram		

Key: USRDA = Recommended Dietary Allowance

IU = International Unit

mg = milligrams

μg = micrograms

NOTE: The numbers with arrows exceed 100 percent of required USRDA.

Lean Cod Potato Stew

Ingredients:

- 4 6-ounce pieces codfish
- 1/2 cup whole wheat flour
- 1 tsp corn oil
- 3 whole tomatoes, chopped
- 1 cup tomato juice
- 1 sweet potato, peeled and sliced
- 1 white potato, peeled and sliced
- 1 cup string beans
- 1 onion, chopped
- 2 stalks celery, chopped
- 1/2 tsp black pepper

Preparation: Saute and simmer

Time: 55 minutes

Calories: 477 per serving

Serves: 4

Directions

Heat oil in iron skillet; dip fish in flour and brown lightly in skillet. Set aside. Steam potatoes for about 15 minutes. In a large pan, brown onion and celery with a little of the oil. Add tomatoes, tomato juice, potatoes, and pepper. Stir and simmer for 20 minutes. Add string beans and codfish and simmer for 15 minutes additionally. The chart shows large amounts of zinc, iodine, potassium, and vitamins A, B_6, and E.

TIP: According to Harvard Medical School in Boston and Albany Medical College in New York, omega-3 fatty acids, oils found in fish, may be able to relieve the pain and other symptoms of rheumatoid arthritis, a disease in which the body's immune system attacks its own tissues.

MYTH: Over-the-counter products sold in drugstores will make hair grow.

FACT: According to the FDA, products sold in drugstores, over the counter, or through the mail have not shown the ability to grow hair.

Nutrients Contained in: Lean Cod Potato Stew

VITAMINS USRDA			ONE SERVING GIVES YOU APPROXIMATELY		APPROXIMATE PERCENTAGE OF USRDA
A	5,000	IU	15,279	IU	305◄
B₁	1.4	mg	0.39	mg	32
B₂	1.6	mg	0.38	mg	26
B₃	16	mg	7	mg	41
B₅	10	mg	1	mg	11
B₆	2.2	mg	0.82	mg	37
B₁₂	3	μg	1	μg	40
C	60	mg	43	mg	72
D	400	IU	78	IU	19
E	15	IU	6	IU	38
K	500	μg	89	μg	17
Folic Acid	400	μg	76	μg	18

MINERALS USRDA			ONE SERVING GIVES YOU APPROXIMATELY		APPROXIMATE PERCENTAGE OF USRDA
Sodium	(1,100–3,000)	mg	197	mg	19
Calcium	1,000	mg	107	mg	13
Phosphorus	(800–1,000)	mg	476	mg	59
Potassium	(1,875–5,625)	mg	1,299	mg	162◄
Magnesium	400	μg	99	μg	28
Selenium	200	μg	45	μg	22
Iodine	150	mg	150	mg	100◄
Zinc	15	mg	22	mg	146◄
Iron	10	mg	4	mg	36
Manganese	(2.5–5.0)	mg	0.62	mg	12
Copper	(2.0–3.0)	mg	0.66	mg	22

AMOUNT PER SERVING		CALORIES PER SERVING	% OF MEAL
Fat	12 grams	107	22
Proteins	45 grams	180	38
Carbohydrates	48 grams	190	40
Cholesterol	0 mg		
Amino acid (essential)			200–570
Fiber	4 grams		

Key: USRDA = Recommended Dietary Allowance

   IU = International Unit

   mg = milligrams

   μg = micrograms

NOTE: The numbers with arrows exceed 100 percent of required USRDA.

Trout Fruit Melange

Ingredients:

- 1 ½ lb trout, cleaned and scaled
- ½ cup tomato juice
- 4 scallions
- 1 Tbs lime juice
- 1 orange, peeled and sliced
- 6 apricots, pitted and sliced
- ½ tsp vegetable oil
- ½ cup whole wheat flour
- 1 tsp low-salt soy sauce
- ½ tsp curry powder
- ½ tsp black pepper
- cayenne pepper
- curry powder

Preparation: Fry

Time: 30 minutes

Calories: 417 per serving

Serves: 4

Directions

Arrange trout in baking dish. Combine tomato juice, scallions, lime juice, soy sauce, dash of cayenne pepper, and curry powder in small bowl. Blend and mix well. Pour over fish and allow to marinate in refrigerator about 30 minutes. Mix flour with pepper. Drain fish; save the marinade liquid. Dip fish in flour and fry in oil in a large skillet over medium heat for 10 minutes per inch of fish; test by using fork to see if fish flakes. Transfer trout to platter. Add marinade to same skillet. Heat over high heat to reduce marinade. Pour over trout; top trout with apricot slices and surround with orange slices.

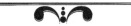

TIP: A major nutrient that is important for immune protection is, according to USDA, vitamin B_6. Adults with depleted reserves of this vitamin have fewer antibodies, the fighters that the immune system produces for protection. Check the chart to see how much this meal provides of vitamin B_6.

MYTH: A food low in salt is low in sodium.

FACT: An important distinction for people who must watch their intake of sodium is to recognize that a food low in salt is not necessarily low in sodium. Other ingredients than salt contain sodium, so check the label for sodium content.

Nutrients Contained in: Trout Fruit Melange

VITAMINS USRDA			ONE SERVING GIVES YOU APPROXIMATELY		APPROXIMATE PERCENTAGE OF USRDA
A	5,000	IU	2,484	IU	49
B_1	1.4	mg	0.33	mg	27
B_2	1.6	mg	0.16	mg	11
B_3	16	mg	5	mg	31
B_5	10	mg	0.29	mg	2
B_6	2.2	mg	0.15	mg	6
B_{12}	3	μg	0	μg	0
C	60	mg	33	mg	54
D	400	IU	0	IU	0
E	15	IU	3	IU	18
K	500	μg	0.25	μg	0
Folic Acid	400	μg	24	μg	5

MINERALS USRDA			ONE SERVING GIVES YOU APPROXIMATELY		APPROXIMATE PERCENTAGE OF USRDA
Sodium	(1,100–3,000)	mg	63	mg	6
Calcium	1,000	mg	360	mg	45
Phosphorus	(800–1,000)	mg	431	mg	53
Potassium	(1,875–5,625)	mg	360	mg	44
Magnesium	400	μg	81	μg	23
Selenium	200	μg	0.63	μg	0
Iodine	150	mg	0	mg	0
Zinc	15	mg	0.56	mg	3
Iron	10	mg	3	mg	30
Manganese	(2.5–5.0)	mg	0.08	mg	1
Copper	(2.0–3.0)	mg	0.10	mg	3

AMOUNT PER SERVING		CALORIES PER SERVING	% OF MEAL
Fat	19 grams	171	41
Proteins	39 grams	155	37
Carbohydrates	23 grams	91	22
Cholesterol	0 mg		
Amino acid (essential)			180–593
Fiber	2 grams		

Key: USRDA = Recommended Dietary Allowance
      IU = International Unit
      mg = milligrams
      μg = micrograms

NOTE: The numbers with arrows exceed 100 percent of required USRDA.

Sweet on Apricots

Ingredients:

4 sweet potatoes
$\frac{1}{2}$ cup apricot nectar
1 tsp low-salt soy sauce
6 apricots
1 tsp brown sugar
1 cup plain yogurt
$\frac{1}{2}$ cup almonds
1 tsp margarine

Preparation: Boil and bake

Time: 50 minutes

Calories: 523 per serving

Serves: 4

Directions

Preheat oven to 350° F. Place potatoes in large pot and cover with water. Bring to a boil and continue boiling for about 30 minutes. When soft, drain, peel, and mash. Add nectar, margarine, and soy sauce. Cut apricots in half, pit, and place 4 to 5 tablespoons of the sweet potato mixture on each. Top with chopped almonds. Heat sweet potatoes with topping in oven for about 10 minutes. This meal, with its bounty of nutrients, gives a tremendous boost to immunity.

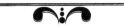

TIP: Dr. Jeffrey Blumberg at the U.S. Department of Agriculture's Human Nutrition Research Center at Tufts University in Boston says it appears that what we eat can help our immune system function better and that new research suggests that certain nutrients may actually boost your immune system and reduce the risk of illness.

MYTH: Swimming after eating will give you stomach cramps.

FACT: Swim coach authorities say this is not usually the case. They say it's not harmful to go into the water immediately after a light meal.

Nutrients Contained in: Sweet on Apricots

VITAMINS USRDA			ONE SERVING GIVES YOU APPROXIMATELY		APPROXIMATE PERCENTAGE OF USRDA
A	5,000	IU	58,247	IU	1,164◄
B₁	1.4	mg	0.24	mg	20
B₂	1.6	mg	0.69	mg	49
B₃	16	mg	3	mg	19
B₅	10	mg	2	mg	22
B₆	2.2	mg	0.95	mg	43
B₁₂	3	μg	0.32	μg	10
C	60	mg	62	mg	103◄
D	400	IU	25	IU	6
E	15	IU	8	IU	56
K	500	μg	0	μg	0
Folic Acid	400	μg	47	μg	11

MINERALS USRDA			ONE SERVING GIVES YOU APPROXIMATELY		APPROXIMATE PERCENTAGE OF USRDA
Sodium	(1,100–3,000)	mg	214	mg	21
Calcium	1,000	mg	209	mg	26
Phosphorus	(800–1,000)	mg	237	mg	29
Potassium	(1,875–5,625)	mg	1,046	mg	130◄
Magnesium	400	μg	77	μg	21
Selenium	200	μg	0.88	μg	0
Iodine	150	mg	26	mg	17
Zinc	15	mg	2	mg	12
Iron	10	mg	3	mg	29
Manganese	(2.5–5.0)	mg	1	mg	26
Copper	(2.0–3.0)	mg	0.70	mg	23

AMOUNT PER SERVING		CALORIES PER SERVING	% OF MEAL
Fat	7 grams	62	12
Proteins	11 grams	45	8
Carbohydrates	104 grams	416	80
Cholesterol	4 mg		
Amino acid (essential)			128–175
Fiber	3 grams		

Key: USRDA = Recommended Dietary Allowance
IU = International Unit
mg = milligrams
μg = micrograms

NOTE: The numbers with arrows exceed 100 percent of required USRDA.

Tuna Cabbage Jackets

Ingredients:

- 3 6.5- or 7-oz cans tuna (in water or vegetable oil)
- ¼ cup wheat germ
- 1 small head cabbage
- 2 large shredded wheat biscuits
- ¼ cup sesame seeds
- 1 tsp caraway seeds
- ¼ tsp cumin seeds
- 1 tsp peanut oil
- 4 Tbs low-fat sour cream
- 2 tsp lemon juice

Preparation: Bake

Time: 40 minutes

Calories: 406 per serving

Serves: 4

Directions

Preheat oven to 400° F. Separate and wash cabbage leaves. Combine in a large bowl the wheat germ, shredded wheat crumbled into flakes, sesame seeds, and cumin; mix thoroughly. Add and blend to this mixture sour cream, caraway seeds, lemon juice, and tuna. Fill cabbage leaves with mixture; secure with strings or picks. Coat with peanut oil and bake in a casserole dish, covered, for 8 minutes. Remove cover and bake 5 minutes more. This dish is very high in EAA, vitamins B$_3$, C, and E, and selenium.

TIP: A study conducted by the University of California at Davis in the *International Journal of Immunotherapy* reports a link between consumption of yogurt with live and active cultures and increased production of gamma interferon, which has been shown to improve the immune defense. The study followed 68 healthy adults between the ages of 20 and 40 and constituted the first large-scale clinical trial on the effects of yogurt on the immune system.

MYTH: Pretzels are junk food and should be thought of in the same way as chips and other packaged treats and snacks.

FACT: Not really, as pretzels are simply flour, water, and vegetable oil baked together. The 100 calories in an ounce of pretzels are almost without fat, unlike potato chips and pork rinds, which are deep-fried. Beware of salted pretzels, however, if you care about sodium intake. One ounce of pretzels has about 450 milligrams of salt.

Nutrients Contained in: Tuna Cabbage Jackets

VITAMINS USRDA			ONE SERVING GIVES YOU APPROXIMATELY		APPROXIMATE PERCENTAGE OF USRDA
A	5,000	IU	623	IU	12
B$_1$	1.4	mg	0.28	mg	23
B$_2$	1.6	mg	0.23	mg	16
B$_3$	16	mg	19	mg	118◄
B$_5$	10	mg	0.60	mg	5
B$_6$	2.2	mg	0.74	mg	33
B$_{12}$	3	μg	2	μg	66
C	60	mg	68	mg	113◄
D	400	IU	11	IU	2
E	15	IU	7	IU	49
K	500	μg	50	μg	10
Folic Acid	400	μg	102	μg	25

MINERALS USRDA			ONE SERVING GIVES YOU APPROXIMATELY		APPROXIMATE PERCENTAGE OF USRDA
Sodium	(1,100–3,000)	mg	681	mg	68
Calcium	1,000	mg	104	mg	12
Phosphorus	(800–1,000)	mg	524	mg	65
Potassium	(1,875–5,625)	mg	845	mg	105◄
Magnesium	400	μg	130	μg	37
Selenium	200	μg	90	μg	45
Iodine	150	mg	0	mg	0
Zinc	15	mg	3	mg	22
Iron	10	mg	4	mg	38
Manganese	(2.5–5.0)	mg	2	mg	40
Copper	(2.0–3.0)	mg	0.38	mg	12

AMOUNT PER SERVING		CALORIES PER SERVING	% OF MEAL
Fat	15 grams	132	33
Proteins	45 grams	182	45
Carbohydrates	23 grams	92	22
Cholesterol	53 mg		
Amino acid (essential)			310–829
Fiber	1 gram		

Key: USRDA = Recommended Dietary Allowance

IU = International Unit

mg = milligrams

μg = micrograms

NOTE: The numbers with arrows exceed 100 percent of required USRDA.

REFERENCES

CHAPTER ONE—CANCER

Beisel, W. R. Single nutrients and immunity. *American Journal Clinical Nutrition*, Feb. 1982, 35(Supp):417–68.

Block, Gladys. Epidemiologic evidence regarding vitamin C and cancer. *American Journal of Clinical Nutrition*, December 1991, 54(6):1310S.

Changing the American diet: impact on cancer prevention policy (editorial). *Cancer*, May 15, 1991 67(10):2671 (10).

Garland, Cedric F., et al. Can colon cancer incidence and death rates be reduced with calcium and vitamin D? *American Journal of Clinical Nutrition*, July 1991, 54(1):190S(9).

Good, R. A. and Lorenz, B. A. Nutrition, immunity, aging and cancer. *Nutrition Review,* 1988, (46):62–67.

High-fat and high-calorie diets and cancer (study). *American Journal of Epidemiology*, 1990, 131(4):612–624.

Jacob, Robert A. U.S. Department of Agriculture Western Human Nutrition Research Center, San Francisco.

Low-fat and high-fiber diet reduces risk of colon cancer in men (Federation of American Societies for Experimental Biology). *Cancer Weekly*, May 13, 1991, p. 6.

Malone, Winfred. Chemoprevention Branch of the National Cancer Institute, Bethesda, Maryland.

Michnovica, Jon J. Institute for Hormone Research, New York City.

Stampfer, Meir, et al. Study about the relationship between colon cancer and diet. National Cancer Institute and the National Heart, Lung and Blood Institute, 1991.

CHAPTER TWO—STROKE

Carotid surgery proven in sickest: Endarterectomy provided so marked an advantage in patients with severe symptomatic carotid disease that a North American stroke prevention trial quit enrolling them. *Medical World News*, March 1991, 32(3):56.

An elemental finding (nutrition and hypertension). *Harvard Health Letter*, May 1992, 17(7):5.

Khaw, Kayh-Tee and Barrett-Connor, E. High dietary potassium intake is inversely correlated with stroke rates. *The New England Journal of Medicine*, January 29, 1987.

Malter, M. G., Schriever, G., and Eilber, U. Natural killer cells, vitamins, and other blood components of vegetarian and omnivorous men. *Nutrition Cancer*, 1989, 12:271–278.

Risk of death can be reduced by foods rich in potassium. *Nutrition Health Review*, Fall 1989, 52:11.

Salt intake leads lifestyle links to hypertension in global study. *Medical World News,* August 22, 1988, 29(16):10.

Watson, R. R., Prabhala, R. H., Plezia, P. M., and Alberts, D. A. Effect of beta-carotene on lymphocyte subpopulations in elderly human: Evidence for a dose-response relationship. *American Journal of Clinical Nutrition*, 1991, 53:90–94.

CHAPTER THREE—BLOOD PRESSURE

Anderson, J.W., et al. Hypocholesterolemic effects of oat-bran and bean intake for hypercholesterolemic men. *American Journal of Clinical Nutrition*, December 1984, 40:1146–1155.

Anderson, T. W. Large-scale trials of vitamin C. *New York Academy Science*, September 1975, 30(258):498–504.

Baked potatoes may help prevent strokes. *HeartCorps*, March–April 1990, 2(5):13.

Blood pressure changes following extracorporeal shock wave lithotripsy and other forms of treatment for nephrolithiasis. *Journal of the American Medical Association,* April 4, 1990, 263(13):1789.

Borida, Arun, and Bansal, H. C. Essential oil of garlicin—prevention of arteriosclerosis. *The Lancet*, December 1973, 29:1491.

Cavallito, C. J., Buck, J. S., and Suter, C. M. Allicin: Garlic's anti-bacterial agent. *Journal of the American Chemical Society*, 1944, 66:1952–1954.

Comparative assessment of sodium intake from meals and snacks consumed by selected American and British students. *Journal of the American Dietetic Association*, January 1990, 90:97.

Hypertension prevention trial (HPT): Food pattern changes resulting from intervention on sodium, potassium, and energy intake. *Journal of the American Dietetic Association*, January 1990, 90:69.

Potassium can lower blood pressure (column), *Better Nutrition*, January 1990, 52:6.

CHAPTER FOUR—HEART DISEASE

Anderson, J., et al. Oat-bran cereal lowers serum total and LDL cholesterol in hypercholesterolemia men. *American Journal of Clinical Nutrition*, May 1990, (52):495–499.

Cardiovascular disease. *Nutrition Research Newsletter*, September 1990, 9(3):98.

Flaten, Hugo, et al. Fish-oil concentrate: Effects on variables related to cardiovascular disease. *American Journal of Clinical Nutrition*, August 1990, 52(2):300–306.

Goldbourt, Uri, and Yaari, S. Cholesterol and coronary heart disease mortality: A 23-year follow-up study of 9902 men in Israel, *Arteriosclerosis*, July–August 1990, 10(4):512–519.

Kragballe, K., et al. A low-fat supplemented with fish oil results in improvement of psoriasis. *Acta Dermatologica Venera*, 1989, (69):23–28.

Margolin, G., et al. Blood pressure lowering in elderly subjects: A double-blind crossover study of omega 3 and omega 6 fatty acids. *American Journal of Clinical Nutrition*, 1991, (53):562–572.

Mensink, R. P., and Katan, M. B. Effect of dietary trans fatty acids on high-density and low-density lipoprotein cholesterol levels in healthy subject. *New England Journal of Medicine*, August 16, 1990, 323(7):439–445.

Ornish, Dean, et al. Can lifestyle changes reverse coronary heart disease: The lifestyle heart trial. *The Lancet*, July 21, 1990, 336(8798):129–133.

Radack, Kenneth, Deck, C., and Huster, G. The comparative effects of n-3 and n-6 polyunsaturated fatty acids on plasma fibrinogen levels: A controlled clinical trial in hypertriglyceridemic subjects. *Journal American College of Nutrition*, August 1990, 9(4):352–357.

Seldeen, Tom. A mixed Australian fish diet and fish-oil supplementation. *American Journal of Clinical Nutrition*, November 1990, 52(9):825.

Thiamine deficiency in patients with congestive heart failure receiving long-term furosemide therapy: A pilot study. *American Journal of Medicine*, August 1991, 91(2):151.

Vitamin C seen to help prevent CAD (coronary artery disease). *Medical World News*, August 1991, 32(1):11.

CHAPTER FIVE—DIABETES

Adequate chromium intake could prevent most cases of mild glucose intolerance from progressing to type-II diabetes. *Federation of American Societies for Experimental Biology*, 1990, 2964:A777.

A commentary from the May–June issue of the *Diabetes Educator*: islet cell transplants. *Diabetes Educator*, September 1991.

Grundy, S. M., et al. Comparison of actions of soy protein and casein on metabolism of plasma lipoprotein and cholesterol in humans. *American Journal of Clinical Nutrition*, August 1983, 38:245–252.

New approach to diabetes prevention. ADA news release from the 52nd annual scientific sessions.

CHAPTER SIX—OSTEOPOROSIS

Food and nutrient intakes of individuals in 1 day in the United States. United States Department of Agriculture (nationwide food consumption survey), 1977–1978.

Matkovic, V., Fontana, D., Tominac, C., Goel, P., et al. Factors which influence peak bone mass formation: A study of calcium balance and the inheritance of bone mass in adolescent females. *American Journal of Clinical Nutrition*, 1990, 52:878–889.

Matkovic, V., et al. Bone status and fracture rates in two regions of Yugoslavia. *American Journal of Clinical Nutrition*, 1979, 32:540–549.

Peck, W. A., Riggs, L. B., and Bell, N. H. *Physician's Resource Manual on Osteoporosis*. Washington, D.C.: National Osteoporosis Foundation, 1987.

Pollitzer, W. S., and Anderson, J. J. B. Ethnic and genetic differences in bone mass: A review with a hereditary versus environmental perspective. *American Journal of Clinical Nutrition*, 1989, 50:1244–1259.

Resnick, N. M., and Greenspan, S. L. Older women with osteoporosis should eat foods high in calcium. *Journal of American Medical Association*, February 1989, 261:1025.

Seeman, E., Hooper, J. L., et al. Reduced bone mass in daughters of women with osteoporosis. *New England Journal of Medicine*, 1989, 320:554–558.

Tanner, J. M. *Growth at Adolescence*. Oxford: Blackwell Scientific Publications, 1962.

CHAPTER SEVEN—ARTHRITIS

Controlled trial of fasting and one year vegetarian diet in rheumatoid arthritis (International Abstracts), *Journal of the American Medical Association*, February 5, 1992, 267(5):646.

Controlled trial of fasting and one-year vegetarian diet in rheumatoid arthritis. *The Lancet*, October 12, 1991, 338(8772):899.

Diet and rheumatoid arthritis: New study shows benefit. *Health Facts*, November 16, 1991, (150):3.

The food factor in arthritis. *Arthritis Today*, September–October 1991, 5(5):22.

A ray of dietary hope for arthritis sufferers. *Tufts University Diet & Nutrition Letter*, February 1992, 9(12):1.

Vegetarian diet for rheumatoid arthritis (tips from other journals). *American Family Physician*, February 1992, 45:880.

CHAPTER EIGHT—GALLBLADDER

Allen, M.J., Borody, T.J., Bugliosi, T.G., et al. Rapid dissolution of gallstones by methyl tert-butyl ether. *New England Journal of Medicine*, 1985, 312:217.

Eating fatty foods not only increases risk of heart disease, it can also give you gallstones. *The Lancet*, 1990, 336:1235–1237.

Ell, C.H., Kerzel, W., Schneider, H.T., et al. Piezoelectric lithotripsy: Stone disintegration and follow-up results in patients with symptomatic gallbladder stones. *Gastroenterology*, 1990, 99:1439–1444.

Gallbladder stones: Management. *The Lancet*, November 2, 1991, 338(8775):1121.

Laparoscopic or minilaparotomy cholecystectomy (education and debate). *British Medical Journal*, February 29, 1992, 304(6826):559.

New options for treating gallstone disease. *American Family Physician*, October 1991, 44(4):1295.

Prevention and treatment of kidney stones (consensus conference). *Journal of the American Medical Association*, August 19, 1988, 260(7):977.

Stone prone (gallbladder disease in women). *Ladies Home Journal*, May 1992, 109(5):140.

Urology (reviews of major advances and issues in medical specialties over the last 12 months). *Journal of the American Medical Association*, June 19, 1991, 265(23):3175.

CHAPTER NINE—CONSTIPATION

Bran-new ideas (adding high-fiber to the diet). *Saturday Evening Post*, March–April 1992, 264(2):16.

Carpenter, D. Beyond oat bran: From what we hear about psyllium, you'd be silly not to try it. *Men's Health*, June 1990, v(2):31.

Goldfinger, S. The hard facts (Part 1, constipation). *Harvard Health Letter*, February 1991, 16(4):1.

Lack of fluid, fiber may be cause of constipation (Special Report, constipation). *The Brown University Long-Term Care Letter*, July 23, 1991, 3(14):5.

Lipman, M. Relieving constipation—if you really have it. *Consumer Reports Health Letter*, November 1990, 2(11):84.

Spiller, R. Management of constipation: 2—When fiber fails. *British Medical Journal*, April 21, 1990, 300(6731):1064.

Taylor, R. Management of constipation: 1—High fiber diets work. *British Medical Journal*, April 21, 1990, 300(6731):1063.

CHAPTER TEN—CATARACTS

Anti-oxidizing vitamins prevent the "protein clumping" that leads to cataract formation. *Science News*, 1989, 135.

Guyton, D. L., et al. *Ophthalmology*, September 1991, 98:1469.

How vitamin E slows cataracts. *Health News & Review*, July–August 1989, 7(4):2.

Robertson, J. M. Vitamin E intake and risk of cataracts in humans, abstract of paper read at the vitamin E biochemistry and health implications seminar, New York, 1988.

Vitamins C & E reduce risk of cataracts. *Today's Living*, April 1, 1989, 20(4):16.

Vitamin C or E supplement may cut risk of cataracts. *Medical World News*, August 28, 1989, 30(16):20.

Vitamins may help prevent cataracts. *Nutrition Health Review*, Winter 1990, 53:12.

Winograd, A. Antioxidant vitamins may help prevent cataracts. *New York Academy of Sciences*, November 2, 1988.

CHAPTER ELEVEN—FERTILITY

Frisch, R. E. Fatness and fertility. *Scientific American*, March 1988, 258(3):88.

Frisch, R. E. Body fat, menarche, fitness and fertility. *Human Reproduction*, 1987, 2(6):521.

Gonzalez, E. R. Sperm swim singly after vitamin C therapy. *Journal of the American Medical Association,* 1983, 249(20):2747.

Kennedy, E. T., Gershoff, S., et al. Evaluation of the effect of WIC supplemental feeding on birth weight. *Journal of the American Diet Association*, 1982, 80:220–227.

Mahajan, A. K., Abbasi, A. A., et al. Effect of oral zinc therapy on gonadal function in hemodialysis patients. *Internal Medicine*, 1982, 97(2):257.

Stowers, S. L. Development of a culturally appropriate food guide for pregnant Caribbean immigrants in the United States. *Journal of the American Dietetic Association*, March, 1992, 92(3):331.

CHAPTER TWELVE—ANEMIA

Agarwal, K.N. Impact of anaemia prophylaxis in pregnancy on maternal haemoglobin. *Journal of the American Medical Association,* February 5, 1992, 267(5):642.

Beling, S. Anemia revisited (column). *Vegetarian Times*, December 1991, 172:16.

Dallman, P. R., Yip, R., and Johnson, C. Prevalence and causes of anemia in the United States. *American Journal of Clinical Nutrition*, 1984, 39(3):437–445.

From paralysis to fatigue (book review). *The Economist*, February 1, 1992, 322(7744):100.

Kummer, C. Lack of iron in vegetarian diet. *The Atlantic*, June 1991, 267:106.

Laliberte, R. Vital secrets. *Men's Health*, December 1991, 6(6):48.

The myths of science. *The Lancet*, May 26, 1990, 335(8700):1267.

Nickerson, H. J., Holubets, M. C., Weiler, B. R., et al. Causes of iron deficiency in adolescent athletes. *Journal Pediatry*, 1989, 114(4, pt. 1):657–663.

Old diet myths die hard. *Journal of Chiropractic*, September 1990, 27(9):28.

Parr, R. B., Bachman, L. A., and Moss, R. A. Iron deficiency in female athletes. *Physician Sportsmedicine*, 1984, 12(4):81–86.

Pilch, S. M., and Senti, F. R. Assessment of the iron status of the U.S. population based on data collection in the second National Health and Nutrition Survey 1976–1980. Center for Food Safety and Applied Nutrition, Food and Drug Administration, Department of Health and Human Services, 1984.

Risser, W. L., and Risser, J. H. Iron deficiency in adolescents and young adults. *The Physician and Sportsmedicine*, December 1990, 18(12):87.

CHAPTER THIRTEEN—IMMUNITY

Are your defenses down? Cycling's surprising effect on the immune system. *Bicycling*, March 1989, 30(2):170.

Boosting immunity in the elderly. *Agricultural Research*, November 1991, 39(11):27.

Cold & flu fighters (nutrients that strengthen the immune system). *Better Nutrition for Today's Living*, January 1992, 54(1):13.

Exercise and the immune system. *Executive Health's Good Health Report*, April 1992, 28(7):6.

Food safety crucial for people with lowered immunity. *FDA Consumer*, July–August 1990, 24(6):7.

Hinds, A. Nutrients as modulators of immune function. *Canadian Medical Association Journal*, July 1, 1991, 145(1):35.

Immunity starts in your kitchen. *Total Health*, February 1989, 11(1):52.

Mice developed could mimic human immune system. Massachusetts Institute of Technology *AIDS Weekly*, April 1992, 27(2):11.

Ozone loss hurts immune systems, scientists say (United States Congress). *AIDS Weekly*, December 1991, 2:4.

Peripheral stem cells made to work (editorial). *The Lancet*, March 14, 1992, 339(8794):648.

Study shows yogurt may improve immune defense. *Dairy Foods Newsletter*, April 6, 1992, 47(24):1.

Zinc/immune system link. *Arthritis Today*, March–April 1992, 6(2):15.

APPENDIX A

Primer on Proteins

Each recipe chart in *Magic Meals* provides the amino acid range for the essential amino acids (EAA). The range rather than specific percentages is used to avoid confusion. Anything over the basic requirement provides the same benefits.

Nutritional research has determined that proteins do not make the best fuel for our bodily system. Proteins also leave a number of different residues, which our bodies have to eliminate. For this reason, it would probably be best if we could limit our intake of proteins to only what is necessary. We could then vary our carbohydrate input to provide the needed calories. This makes sense because carbohydrates make the most efficient fuel.

Protein makes up practically all our living tissue, with the exception of our bones. Proteins are made up of chains of amino acids. When protein is digested, it's broken down into amino acids, which are later reassembled to meet the various needs of the body. If during reassembly, some of the necessary amino acids are not available, our body has the capacity to manufacture them. The body can manufacture only 11 of them. The 9 so-called essential amino acids must be obtained outside the body from food sources.

Foods that supply a sufficient amount of the nine essential amino acids provide complete proteins. Animal proteins fall into this category. Plant proteins which would include vegetables, grains, legumes, and fruits are not complete in one or more of the EAA. But plant-derived foods can be excellent sources of protein if eaten in complementary combinations that supply adequate amounts of all EAA. When any recipe in the book falls short of all EAA, you will always find a complementary food recommended to fulfill the EAA requirement. The amino acids lacking in a vegetable can be provided by a grain, another vegetable, or an animal-derived protein—at the same meal or later in the day.

Many of the recipes in *Magic Meals* depend on plant rather than animal protein to avoid heavy fat consumption. For example, lima beans are weak in the amino acid combination methionine/cysteine, so we need a food that is strong here. Your complementary food suggestions are designed to counterbalance any shortfalls.

Nutritionists say you should never accept a daily regimen whose analysis reveals that even one of the amino acids is not present to at least 100 percent. If you do not have sufficient protein intake, your body will forgo the least important rebuilding activities in favor of the most important. Among the least important are such rebuilding activities as hair growth and muscle maintenance.

This is not a problem for most of us and certainly not a problem for anyone cooking from the recipes in *Magic Meals*, as your chart keeps you informed of the EAA for each meal.

APPENDIX B

Primer on USRDAs and RDAs

RDA means Recommended *Dietary* Allowances, nutritional requirements that are set by the National Research Council's Food and Nutrition Board. A committee of scientists designated by the National Academy of Sciences' Food and Nutrition Board reviews the world's literature on the nutrient requirements of human beings.

The research they look at includes studies of individuals who are deficient in particular nutrients and those who are not. Summarizing these and other studies, the committee can estimate the average daily requirements for each nutrient. Because there are variations in individual requirements, before coming up with a final figure, scientists increase the average to cover the upper limits of people's needs.

It is this kind of precaution that makes it highly unlikely that any healthy person will need more than the RDA for a nutrient. The RDAs are guidelines for average amounts of nutrients that are to be consumed over a period of time.

The RDA varies based on age and sex, and the figures may differ for children, friends, males, and females.

The difference between the RDA and USRDA (U.S. Recommended *Daily* Allowances) is that the USRDA is a single number that does not vary with age and sex. It is set by the Food and Drug Administration. At the beginning of each chapter in *Magic Meals* you will see an RDA chart for the mineral or vitamin featured in that chapter. The figures listed in this chart are the RDAs organized by group/age and sex. The charts that follow the recipe within the chapter use the USRDA figures, the single number that does not vary with age or sex.

The FDA developed the USRDAs in 1973 by condensing the 17 separate RDAs that exist for each of the various age and sex groups; they tend to be higher than the RDAs because the FDA generally chose the largest RDA for each nutrient as the standard by which to measure a product's nutrient content. If, for example, a product supplies 100 percent of the USRDA for zinc, that means it supplies the 15 milligrams recommended for men and women, not the 10 milligrams suggested for children 1–6 years of age or the 20 recommended for pregnant women.

The USRDA is an easy method used by food manufacturers when giving nutrition information on their labels. It would take up too much space to include the RDA percentage for each age and sex group, so they use the one USRDA standard to measure nutrient percentages in their products. You get both figures in this book.

The RDAs are not quotas that you must meet every day to be healthy. Nutritionists generally become concerned when there is a consistent consuming of less than 70 percent of the RDA for a vitamin mineral or protein. Of course, the longer and farther you deviate from the RDA for a nutrient (such as going on a long fast), the greater the possibility that you will develop symptoms of a deficiency.

In this country, it is reported that it is next to impossible to go over the RDA limits or overdose with foods alone.

The RDAs are under revision from time to time, and certain numbers may be lowered or raised. Vitamins and minerals not currently listed may some day be included.

Recent changes include those for the calcium figures, which have been raised from 800 milligrams a day to 1,200 milligrams for men and women 19 through 24 years old. Researchers have found that too little calcium in the body can eventually lead to osteoporosis.

It is estimated that women take in way under these figures. Women are advised to increase their calcium intake by drinking more skim and/or low-fat milk and eating more low-fat yogurt as well as green vegetables.

The new RDA also lowered the level of iron in women's diets: 15 milligrams, rather than 18, is now considered sufficient to meet the requirements of nearly all healthy, nonpregnant women. The call to increase the milligrams of vitamin C to 100 as opposed to 60 is suggested only for smokers who seem to deplete this vitamin more than nonsmokers.

No doubt changes and revisions will be announced in the future; there is even some suggestion that the RDAs be modified all together. For now, however, the advice on dietary patterns is the same as in the past.

APPENDIX C

Primer on Meat

Although meat, especially red meat, is not utilized as the main ingredient in most of the recipes in *Magic Meals*, it does not mean that you have to forgo eating meat.

We know that meat is a major source of saturated fat, although dairy products can contain more saturated fat per ounce than red meat. It is also known that for many of us, it is unrealistic to give up eating meat. We can, however, minimize the percentage of saturated fats when we do eat meat.

The "good" and "select" cuts have less fat, fewer calories, and less cholesterol. Meat grading is determined by the fat content of the entire carcass. It is voluntary, so not all pieces are graded. If "select" is not available, choose "choice" cuts.

The USRDA suggests that the worst cuts of meat, from a health standpoint, are beef short ribs and well-marbled steaks. "Prime" and "choice" cuts are the highest in cholesterol. What makes them so tender and juicy is the fat. Top round, flank, and sirloin are better choices.

People are advised to limit portion sizes—3 to 4 ounces after cooking; a 3-ounce serving is about the size of a deck of cards. You will probably notice that all recipes in *Magic Meals* that do use meat recommend conservative amounts. The 3-ounce serving in the recipes refers to cooked meat that is trimmed of all visible fat and all bones. Meat generally shrinks during cooking by about one fourth, so a 3-ounce portion of cooked meat will have started as 4-ounces of raw meat. If you trim away all the visible fat on your steak, you can remove almost half its fat. Remove the fat before cooking.

Make a note that if the name includes loin or round, you will be getting a lean beef cut.

COMPARING MEATS (3.5 OUNCES, COOKED AND WELL TRIMMED)

TYPE	CALORIES	FAT (GRAMS)	% CALORIES FROM FAT
Beef			
Eye of round, select (e.g., minute steak)	178	6	30
Top round, choice (e.g., London broil)	194	6	28
Chuck, select (e.g., pot roast)	222	9	36
Top loin, select (e.g., New York or strip steak)	190	9	38
Sirloin, choice (e.g., top sirloin)	211	9	38
Tenderloin, select (e.g., filet mignon)	208	10	43
Chicken			
Breast, no skin	165	4	21
Breast, with skin	197	4	36
Drumstick, no skin	172	6	31
Thigh, no skin	209	11	47
Wing, with skin	290	19	59
Lamb			
Leg	191	8	38
Loin chop	202	10	45
Shoulder	204	11	48
Tenderloin	166	5	27
Center loin	190	8	38
Turkey			
Breast, no skin	135	1	7
Breast, with skin	153	3	18
Leg, no skin	108	2	17
Wing, no skin	207	10	43
Veal			
Leg	150	3	18
Sirloin	168	6	32
Loin chop	175	7	36
Shoulder roast	170	7	37

INDEX

A

Acne, 152
Age spots, 242
Aging people, 126
Airplane cabin air, 208
Alcohol, effects of, 114, 236
Almonds, 44
   with avocados and beansprouts, 178
   with spaghetti, asparagus and beetgreens, 54
American Diabetes Association (ADA), 137, 166
Anemia, 24, 106, 352, 379, 408
Animal fats, 74
Antibodies, reduction of, 416
Antioxidants, 309, 322
"Antisterility vitamin," 343
Aphrodisiacs, 358
Apple juice, 288
Apples, 158
   juicing the seeds, 334
   and peanuts, 212
   and pork, 294
   with turnips, 356
Arsenic poisoning, 334
Arthritis
   broccoli soup for, 210
   cause of, 224
   foods that aggravate, 207, 214
   heat rubs for, 24
   nutrients to help, 212
   olive oil, treatment with, 234
   protein gluten and, 222
   remedies that are health frauds, 226
   saturated fats and, 220
Asparagus
   with broccoli, corn and almonds, 368
   with carrots and celery, 20
   with cheese, 324
   with lentils, 144
   with peppers, 18

Asparagus *(cont'd.)*
   with red peppers, 42
   with shiitake mushrooms, 76
   with spaghetti and beetgreens, 54
   with tofu, 116
Aspirin, effects of, 40, 236
Avocados, 34, 178, 190

B

Back fractures, 182
Back pain, 330, 364
Bacteria, 186, 198
Baking soda, 156
Baldness, 366
Bananas, 68, 138, 282
Barley
   and the cardiovascular system, 118
   fiber and lowering cholesterol, 99
   with greens and rice bran, 346
   with kidney beans and groat, 48
   with okra, zucchini, and tomatoes, 118
   salad with okra and mushrooms, 138
   with shiitake mushrooms, 84
   soup with lentils and shiitake mushrooms, 298
   soup with tofu and mushrooms, 358
Beans, 84
   baked navy, pinto, and kidney, 46
   fava and ham, 70
   fava with chicken, 400
   green and chick peas, 256
   green and shiitake mushrooms, 162
   green with parsnips and potatoes, 248
   iron and, 66
   kidney, mango and chicken livers, 330
   kidney and cracked wheat (groats), 48
   kidney with brussels sprouts, 142
   kidney with chicken, 290

Beans (cont'd.)
    lima with okra, 260
    navy, 130
    navy with spinach, 278
    soup with, 266
    with tofu, 58, 140
    See also blackeye peas
Beansprouts, 178
Beef, 244
    with chicken and bok choy, 380
    chopped with lentils, 402
    fillet with chick peas and carrots, 250
    ground with cabbage, 398
    labeling of, 244
    with pork meatballs, 394
    raw ground, 356
Beetgreens, 54, 160
Beets, 10, 332
Beta-carotene, 3-4
    in asparagus, 20
    in broccoli, 12
    in greens, 6
    and heart attacks, 112
    and strokes, 112
    in sweet potatoes, 174
Bile, 239, 244
Birth control pills, 244
Birth defects, preventing, 94, 372
Birth defects and mother's age, 344
Blackeye peas, 66
Black fungus mushrooms
    with corn and peas, 216
    and lima bean soup, 40
    with scallops, 312
    with squash, brussels sprouts and walnuts, 226
    with tuna, 370
Blood coagulation, 24
Blood pressure, 68, 76, 92, 246
    diet for, 24
    garlic as therapeutic for, 88
    high, causes of, 86, 314
    how to reduce, 80, 82, 84
    low, 246
    sodium restriction and, 78
Bluefish, 234, 416
Body growth, 24, 198
Bok choy, 110, 148, 172, 188, 380
Bones, building, 171
Bowel movements, 304

Bran, 275, 288, 292, 294
Breast cancer, 3, 46, 254
"Breast disease," 26, 56
Breast-feeding, 38, 388
Broccoli, 68, 210
    with asparagus, corn and almonds, 368
    and blood pressure, 68
    with carrots, 166
    with chicken and sprouts, 352
    with chicken breast, 258
    with pepper and onion, 12
    with salmon, 174
    and sauteed vegetables, 198
    soup for arthritis pain, 210
Brussels sprouts
    with black fungus mushrooms, squash and walnuts, 226
    with cheese, 186, 196
    with grains, 344
    with kidney beans, 142
    with onions and spices, 26
Buckwheat, roasted (Groats), 182
Burns, 300
Butter, 94, 300, 434
B vitamins, 72

C

Cabbage
    baked with potatoes, 422
    in beet soup, 10
    with carrots, 276
    with fruit and seeds, 362
    with ground beef, 398
    and pork, 34
    and potatoes, 4, 6
    with rice, shiitake mushrooms and corn, 228
    and sauteed vegetables, 198
    soup, 4
    steamed, 22
Calcium
    canned fish and, 102
    in cheese, 130, 196
    extra in the diet, 178
    in frozen desserts, 252
    intake to prevent osteoporosis, 180
    levels consumed, 190
    menopause and, 396

Calcium *(cont'd.)*
  osteoporosis and, 192
  in salmon, 210, 230
  sources of, 188, 194, 228
  for teens, 198, 200
  women and, 171, 176, 456
Calories
  and digestion, 344
  and fertility, 374
  and vitamins, 4
Cancer
  coffee and, 56
  low levels of Vitamin C and, 126
  protection against, 3
Canned foods, shelf life, 262
Canola oil, 222
Cantaloupe , 190
Carbohydrates, 137, 142, 156, 158
  complex, 280
  dietary guidelines for, 266
Cardiac risk, lowering, 110
Cardioartery disease (CAD), 348
Carotenoid, 12
Carrots
  with asparagus and celery, 20
  with beef fillet, 250
  with broccoli, 166
  with cabbage, 276
  with ham and onions, 436
  with turnips and squash, 126
  with zucchini and leeks, 122
Cataracts
  antioxidants and, 326, 328, 330
  diet for, 336
  formation of, 318
  lens inhibitors, 324
  prevention of, 312, 332, 334
  vitamin deficiency and, 314, 316
  Vitamin E and, 310
Cauliflower, 184
  with curry and spices, 24
  with haddock, 406
  with macaroni and okra, 150
  and sauteed vegetables, 198
  with sprouts, zucchini, and mushrooms, 222
Cavities, 172
Cayenne pepper, 22
Cereals, bran, 290
Cervical cancer, 3-4, 94
Chard, 152

Cheese, 172, 180, 290
  with brussels sprouts, 186, 196
  cottage, 130
  part-skim, 180
Chicken
  baked with greens, fruits and nuts, 426
  with bean curd, 100
  with beef and bok choy, 380
  breasts with broccoli, 258
  breasts with broccoli and sprouts, 352
  breasts with fruit, 384
  breasts with lemon, 112
  breasts with onions, 404
  breasts with shiitake mushrooms, 314
  with fava beans, 400
  with kidney beans, 290
  with lemon and lettuce, 112
  livers, 94, 160
  livers and kale, 390
  livers and mango, 330
  livers with shiitake mushrooms, 374
  preparation of, 128
  with pumpkin, 428
  yellow-skinned, 196
Chick peas, 80, 110, 158
  and beans, 256
  with beans and spinach, 278
  with beef fillet, 250
  with steak, 382
  with tuna, 208
Chocolate, 124, 152, 192
Cholesterol
  children and, 164
  in the diet, 31, 48, 94, 144
  exercise and, 38
  gallstones and, 239, 256
  high, causes of, 100
  in lean meat, 260
  level and almonds, 44
  level and beans, 66, 70, 130
  level and garlic, 88, 99
  level and mushrooms, 76
  level in shellfish, 270
  levels and zinc, 250
  nuts and, 92
  poultry vs. beef, 188
  reading specific measurements, 239
  saturated fat and, 104
Circumcision, 350
Clams, 320

Codfish stew, 438
Coffee and breast disease, 56
Coffees, flavored, 108
Colds, 256, 418
Collagen, 402
Collard greens, 152, 200, 426
Colon cancer, 12, 102
Communication and blood pressure, 86
Conception, 350
Constipation, 275, 278, 304, 328
Cooking methods to preserve vitamins and
        minerals, 400
Copper, 34
Corn
    with broccoli, asparagus and almonds, 368
    with mushrooms and peas, 216
Cottage cheese, 130, 290
Couscous, 282, 300
Crab, 252
Cravings, 16, 258

D

Deficiency disease, 122
Defrosted food, 284
Depression, 386
Diabetes, 137, 154
    adult-onset (type II), 137, 154
    bran for, 292
    controlling with spices, 152
    diet for, 137, 156, 158
    exercise and, 154
    fish oil supplements and, 146
    intake of proteins, 162
    smoking and, 158
    sugar and, 142
Diarrhea, 418
Diet
    cancer prevention, 3
    children's, 276
    fasting and, 10
    guidelines for a healthy heart, 65
    iron in women's, 456
    iron poor, effects of, 404
    risks for gallstones, 254
"disability zone," 126
Disease prevention, xxiv
    cancer, 3
    cataracts and, 312, 332, 334

Disease prevention (cont'd.)
    heart disease, 108
    and the immune system, 411
    osteoporosis, 171, 202
    strokes, 36
DNA (Deoxyribonucleic Acid), 26

E

Eating patterns, 78, 260
Eggs, 162, 214, 322, 416
Elderly, 126, 192
Elimination, 300
Energy, 4, 122, 360
Eskimos and heart disease, study of, 102
Esophagus, cancers of, 3
Essential amino acids (EAA), 453-54
Estrogen, 176, 244
Exercise, 66, 82, 108, 275, 278, 292, 390
Exhaustion, 386
Eye infections, 426

F

Fasting, 10, 200, 216
Fat, 100
    beans and, 84
    in butter,
    daily consumption of, 104, 164, 412
    in dark and white meat, 44
    grapefruit burning, 404
    percentage of calories from, 40, 74, 434
    polyunsaturated, 232
    role in the diet, 3, 31, 34
    saturated, 100
    in starchy foods, 408
    in tofu, 70
    types of, 48, 74, 124
Fatigue, 24, 394
Fatty accumulations, 146
Fatty acids and arthritis, 220
Fertility
    calories needed for, 374
    deficiency in vitamins and minerals and,
        343, 352, 354
    obstacles to, 348
    Vitamin E, study of, 370
Fever, 294

Fiber, 48, 70, 84, 140
   barley and cholesterol, 99
   constipation and, 275
   foods high in, 82, 124, 138
   insoluble, 282, 300
   intake of, 137, 160, 252, 258, 288
   nutritional value of, 284
   pills and powders, 148
   in rice, 90
   soluble, 138, 142
   sources of, 258, 298
Fibrocystic disease, 26, 56
Figs, 68
Fingernails, 116, 184, 402
Fish, 52, 92, 128
   baking, 236
   bluefish, 234
   blue with parsnips and juice, 416
   canned, 102
   cod stew, 438
   with curried rice, 192
   flounder, 348
   haddock and cauliflower, 406
   halibut, 176, 310
   halibut with blackeyed peas, 408
   halibut with greens and mushrooms,
     412
   with omega-3 fatty acids, 207
   salmon, 174, 210, 230
   sardines, 232
   sole, 264, 386
   trout with fruit, 440
   tuna, 180, 208
   tuna and cabbage, 444
   tuna and macaroni, 180
   tuna with mushrooms, 370
   See also shellfish
Fish oils, 207, 234
Fish oil supplements, 146, 230
Fitness, 194, 386
Flank steak with chick peas, 382
Flounder, 164, 348
Fluid intake, 232, 286, 346
Flu shots, 228
Folic acid, 20, 94, 198, 228, 234, 400
Foodborne illness, 8
Food chart ranking, xxv
Foods, addictive, 172
Free radicals, 26, 320, 322, 434
Frozen desserts, 252

Frozen vegetables, methods for cooking,
   226
Fruit juices, 436
Fruit juice to sweeten foods, 230
Fruit salad, 432

G

Gallbladder disease, 244, 246, 264
Gallbladder operations, 268
Gallstones, 239
   prevention of, 260
   reasons for, 250, 254, 256, 266
   symptoms of, 262, 264
Garlic, 65, 88
   with broccoli, 68
   and the cardiovascular system, 65, 72
   and cholesterol, 99
   with fish, 92
   with lentils, 86
   with onion, 60
   with pork, 72
   with potatoes and onions, 420
   with rice, carrots and curry, 74
   soup, 202
   with spinach and tomatoes, 106
Germs in airplanes, 208
Ghee, 94
Glasses, non-prescription, 320
Gout, 207, 214
Grain, 36, 242, 266, 344
Greens, 6, 110, 152, 254
   and beta-carotene, 6
   with chicken, fruit and nuts, 426
   with ground beef, 200
   with rice, 90
   with rice bran and barley, 346
   and stroke, 31
Guidelines for selecting recipes, xxiv
Gums, aching, 40

H

Haddock
   with cauliflower, 406
Hair, 58
Hair growth, 438, 454
Halibut, 160, 310

Halibut *(cont'd.)*
    with blackeyed peas, 408
    with greens and mushrooms, 412
    stir-fry, 160
    with swiss chard, 176
Ham with spinach, 338
Hay fever, 32, 418
Headaches, 42
Headstands, 104
Healing foods, xxiii
Heartbeat, regulating, 99
Heart disease
    causes of, 390
    diet for, 99, 128
    reducing the risk of, 108
    and women, 150
Heat rubs for muscle soreness or
    arthritis, 24
Heme iron, 379-80
Hemoglobin, 408
High blood pressure, 31
High Density Lipoproteins (HDL), 18, 38, 50,
    120, 240, 250
Honey, 424
Honey vs. sugar, 220
Hot drinks to keep warm, 232
Hot flashes, 420
Hypertension, 65, 92, 314

I

Immune system, 411, 422, 436
Impotence, 343
Inactivity, 66, 278
Intelligence, 20
Iron, 72, 148
    anemia and, 379
    in beans, 48, 66, 142
    deficiency of, 414
    and the immune system, 414
    largest source of, 36
    and the risk of a heart attack, 110
    sources of, 140, 242, 379, 380, 396
    types of, 379-80
    ways to increase, 22
Iron-deficiency anemia, 72
Iron pots and skillets, 22, 140
Irritable bowel syndrome, 282, 300

J

Jam, 286

K

Kale, 16, 254
    with chicken livers, 390
    with turkey, 334
    and turnips, 214
Kidney beans, 46, 48, 142
Kidney stones, 160

L

Labels on food, 310, 324, 426, 428, 432, 456
Larynx, cancers of, 3
Laxatives, 302
LDL cholesterol, 66, 118
Lead ink in bread wrappers, 22, 224
"Lean meat," 178
Leeks, 122
Lentils, 82, 280
    with asparagus, 144
    with chopped beef, 402
    with garlic, 86
    with potatoes, celery and peppers, 50
    with turkey, 354
Lettuce, 239
Light scanning, 254
Linguine with kale and mushrooms, 156
Liver, calf's with mushrooms, 392
Liver spots, 242
Lobster, 270
Lung cancer, 12
    and sweet potatoes, 14

M

Macaroni
    with okra and cauliflower, 150
    with tuna, cheese and peppers, 180
Mackerel, 102, 236
Magnesium
    and heart disease, 116
    and kidney stones, 160
    sources of, 99

Mammography, 254
Mango, 330
Margarine, 246
Mayonnaise, 88, 354
Meats, 457
    comparing calories and fat (chart), 458
    iron rich, 380
    ranked for cholesterol, 272-73
    red, 100, 264, 398
    See also specific meat
Melanoma, 418
Memory, 20
Men, rate of bone loss for, 202
Menopause, 114, 171, 176, 388, 390, 396, 422
Menstruation, 336, 379, 382, 398
Milk, 34, 80, 90, 186
Millet, 242
Mineral deficiency, 184
Mineral oil, 328
Miscarriage, chance of, 346, 366
Misting of produce, 12
Moles, 382, 418
Monounsaturated fat, 44
Mouth, cancers of, 3, 54
MSG (monosodium glutamate), 42
Muscle growth, 384
Muscle maintenance, 454
Mushrooms
    poisonous, 268
    See also Shiitake; Black fungus
Mustard greens, 200, 426

N

Navy beans, 46, 130
Newborns sensitivity to pain, 370
Nightshade family foods, 208
Nonheme iron, 379-80
Nutritional charts, how to read,
    xxvi
Nutritional deficiency, 184
Nutritional requirements, how to maintain, xxiv
Nuts, 92, 110, 188, 194, 226

O

Oat bran, 292, 294
Oats, 284

Obesity, 266, 332
Okra, 70
    with barley, zucchini and tomatoes, 118
    with lima beans, 260
    with macaroni and cauliflower, 150
Olive oil, 120
Omega-3 fatty acids, 102, 128, 146, 438
    arthritis and, 207
    best fish for, 230
    cancer and, 3
    reduction in death rate and, 99
Omega-6 fatty acids, 232
Onions
    with broccoli and onion, 12
    with brussels sprouts and spices, 26
    with chicken breasts, 404
    with garlic, 60
    with ham and carrots, 436
    with potatoes and garlic, 420
    with potatoes and peppers, 104
    with spaghetti and potato, 32
    with sweet potatoes, 154
Organic food, 114, 296
Osteoporosis, 102, 171, 456
    definition of, 186
    intake of calcium, 180
    men and, 202
    smoking and, 182
Overeating, 74
Overweight, 137, 250
Oysters, 148, 246, 350, 424
    with shiitake mushrooms and turkey, 430

P

Pancreas, cancers of, 3
Parsnips, 262
    with fish and juice, 416
    with green beans and potatoes, 248
Pasta, 8
    with asparagus and beetgreens, 54
    with kale and shiitake mushrooms, 156
    with okra and cauliflower, 150
    with potato and onion, 32
    sauce with red peppers, 8
    and shiitake mushrooms, 224
    with tuna, cheese and peppers, 180
Pasteurization, 186
Peak bone mass, 174

Peanuts, 212
Pearl barley, 138
Peas, 138
    blackeyed with halibut, 408
    with black fungus mushrooms and corn, 216
    with potatoes and tomatoes, 56, 124
Peppers, 8, 372
    with asparagus, 18, 42
    with beans, 256
    with broccoli and onion, 12
    with potatoes and onions, 104
    with prunes, 302
    with shiitake mushrooms, 434
    with sprouts, 364
    with tuna, cheese and macaroni, 180
Perch, 322
Physical exam, 298
Pimples, 152
Pinto beans, 46
Pork
    with apples, 294
    with beef meatballs, 394
    and cabbage, 34
    with garlic, 72
    and prunes, 36, 296
Potassium
    blood pressure and, 84
    stroke-associated deaths and, 60
    strokes and, 31-32, 36, 42, 50
Potatoes, 174
    baked with cabbage, 422
    baked with wheat germ, 366
    and cabbage, 6
    with lentils, celery and peppers, 50
    with onions and garlic, 420
    with parsnips and green beans, 248
    with peas and tomatoes, 56
    with peppers and onions, 104
    and sauteed vegetables, 198
    with spaghetti and onion, 32
    with tomatoes and peas, 124
    See also sweet potatoes
Poultry, 44, 196
Prenatal nutrition, 234
Pretzels, 444
Processed food, 296
Protein, 72, 106, 142, 453-54
Proteins, complementary, 86
Prunes, 158

Prunes *(cont'd.)*
    with peppers, 302
    with pork, 36, 296
Psyllium, 296
Puberty, 420
Purines, 207, 214

R

Ragweed, 32
Recommended dietary allowance (RDA), xxiv–xxv, 455-56
    for calcium, 171
    for iron, 379
    for magnesium, 99
    for potassium, 31, 65
    for proteins, 384
    for sodium, 65
    for vitamin C, 3
    for vitamin E, 309
    for zinc, 343
Rectum, cancers of, 3
Refrigerating foods, 8, 12, 34, 262, 356, 414
Regularity, 292
Research information tips, xxv
Rest, 126
Rheumatoid arthritis (RA), 207, 222
    diet for, 218
    fasting and, 216
    and the immune system, 438
Rice, 74, 78, 304
    with almonds and mushrooms, 194
    with greens, 90
    with salmon, 192
    wild, 118, 228, 316
Roaches, 316

S

Salad, 138, 190
Salmon, 102, 128, 210, 230
    with broccoli, 174
    with curried rice, 192
Salmonella, 162, 198
Salt, 440
Salt preference, 14
Sardines, 232
Sauce, pasta with peppers, 8

Scallops
   with black fungus mushrooms, 312
Seafood. *See* Fish; Shellfish
Sea salt, 18
Selenium, 32, 270, 430
Shampoos, 58
Shelf life of food, 262
Shellfish, 52
   clams, 320
   crab, 252
   lobster, 270
   oysters, 148, 246, 350, 424
   oysters and mushrooms, 430
   scallops, 312
   shrimp, 172, 244
   shrimp stew, 360
Shiitake mushrooms
   with asparagus, 76
   baked with peppers, 434
   with barley, 84
   with bean sprouts, cauliflower and
      zucchini, 222
   with chicken breasts, 314
   with chicken livers, 374
   with fish and greens, 412
   and green beans, 162
   with lentils, 82
   with linguine and kale, 156
   with mackerel, 236
   and pasta, 224
   with rice, cabbage and corn, 228
   with rice and almonds, 194
   salad with barley and okra, 138
   soup with barley, 298
   soup with tofu and barley, 358
   with sweet potatoes, 108
   with tofu, greens and beans, 140
   with zucchini and carrots, 268
Shrimp, 244
   stew, 360
   with sunflower seeds and bok choy, 172
"Silent killer," 65
Skin, healthy, 218
Sleep, 379, 392, 394
Smoking, 31, 54, 456
   diabetes and, 158
   and estrogen levels, 182
   menopause and, 348
Sneezing, 190
Snuff, 54

Sodium, 90, 440, 444
   in tofu, 58
Sole, 264
   with cucumber, 386
Sorbitol, 406
Soup
   barley, tofu and shiitake mushroom,
      358
   barley with shiitake mushrooms, 298
   with beans, 266
   beet, 10
   broccoli for arthritis, 210
   cabbage, 4
   lima bean, 40
Soybeans, 146
Spaghetti
   with asparagus and beetgreens, 54
   with potato and onion, 32
Spices helping to control diabetes, 152
Spinach, 66, 80, 152
   with beans and chick peas, 278
   with chick peas and beans, 278
   with fruit, 418
   with ham, 338
   and iron, 36
   with tomatoes, 106
Sports injuries, 248, 292
Squash, 218
   baked acorn, 239
   with brussels sprouts, black fungus
      mushrooms and walnuts, 226
   with turnips and carrots, 126
Squid, 318
Steam cooking, 10
Stearic acid, 124
Stomach, cancers of, 3
Stomach cramps, 442
Strawberries, 72
Strength training, 150
Stress, 106, 166, 314, 330
Strokes
   causes of, 54
   diet for, 24, 31-32, 42
   estrogen and, 52
   potassium and (study), 60
   prevention of, 36, 56
   reduction in mortality rate of, 58
Sugar, 210, 428
Sugar and diabetes, 142
"Sugar free," 430

Sugar free foods, 154
Sugar metabolism, 150
Sugar vs. honey, 220
Surimi, 368
Sweet potatoes, 14, 132, 326, 328
    with apricots, 442
    calories in, 174
    with juice, 414
    with onions, 154
    with peach nectar, 220
    with shiitake mushrooms, 108
Swordfish, 52

T

Talking and blood pressure, 86
Taste perceptions, 148
Tea and iron deficiencies, 72
Thymus, 416
Tofu, 70
    with asparagus, 116
    with beans, 58
    with greens, beans, and shiitake
        mushrooms, 140
    soup, 202
    soup with barley and mushrooms, 358
Tomatoes
    with barley, okra and zucchini, 118
    with peas and potatoes, 56
    with potatoes and peas, 124
    with spinach, 106
    stuffed with tuna, 120
Tongue, taste perception of, 140
Toothpaste, 156
Trans fatty acids, 246
Trout, 92
    with fruit, 440
Tuna
    baked with cabbage, 444
    with chick peas, 208
    with macaroni, cheese and peppers,
        180
    steaks with black fungus mushrooms,
        370
    with tomatoes, 120
Turkey
    breast and lentils, 354
    breast with oats and seeds, 44
    ground with kidney beans, 396

Turkey (cont'd.)
    with kale, 334
    with oysters and mushrooms, 430
    with wheat germ and mushrooms, 38
    with zucchini and cauliflower, 388
Turnips, 114, 336
    with carrots and squash, 126
    with fruit, 356
    and kale, 214

U

Ulcers, 90
U.S. Recommended Daily Allowances
    (USRDA), 184, 455-56
Uterine cervix, cancers of, 3

V

Varicose veins, 60
Vegetable fats, 74
Vegetables
    moldy, 338
    ranked for calcium, 204
    ranked for dietary fiber, 168, 306
    ranked for magnesium, 134
    ranked for potassium, 62
    ranked for sodium, 96
    ranked for vitamin C, 28
    storage of, 270
    See also specific vegetables
Vegetarians, 86, 106, 380
Vitamin A
    breast cancer and, 46
    cancer and, 3, 6
    heart disease and, 122
    sources of, 132
Vitamin B6, 160, 440
Vitamin C
    cancer and, 3-4, 6
    care of food with, 16
    and cataracts, 309
    fertility and, 343, 360
    illness and, 432
    iron absorption and, 402
    low levels of, 126
    men and, 372
    and nitrosamine, 26

Vitamin C *(cont'd.)*
   smokers and , 456
   vegetables ranked in (chart), 28
   women and, 18
Vitamin D, 176
Vitamin deficiencies, 184, 416
Vitamin E, 362
   as an antioxidant, 326
   cancer and, 3-4
   cataracts and, 309-10
   fertility and, 343
   foods ranked in order for, 340
   male sperm and, 364
   sources of, 428
Vitamin loss, 6
Vitamins, 4, 112, 122, 132
   determined by growing soil, 6
   shots for, 352
   See also specific name of

W

Waffles, 144
Walking, 38, 390
Weight control, 10, 142, 343, 362
Weight-lifting, 82, 150, 312
Wheat, bulgar, 286
Wheat bran, 288
Wheat germ, 174, 366

Women
   and age of menopause, 422
   anemia and, 379
   diet deficiencies of, 406
   fertility and, 343
   gallbladder disease and, 244, 250
   and menstruation, 336, 382, 398
   and osteoporosis, 180, 192
   pregnancy and, 234, 258

Y

Yams, 326
Yeast infections, 212
Yogurt, 130, 418, 444

Z

Zinc, 72, 148
   fertility and, 343, 356, 358
   foods ranked in order for, 376
   and the immune system, 412, 424, 430
   males and, 368
Zucchini
   with barley, okra and tomatoes, 118
   with carrots and leeks, 122
   with carrots and mushrooms, 268
   with mushrooms, sprouts and cauliflower, 222